Cornelia Heisterkamp

Cornelia Heisterkamp

130.—

Decision Making in Small Animal Orthopaedic Surgery

Veterinary Titles

Allen/Kruth:
: Consultation in Small Animal Cardiopulmonary Medicine

Auer/Morris:
: Orthopaedic Radiology of the Foal

Binnington/Cockshutt:
: Decision Making in Small Animal Soft Tissue Surgery

Farrow:
: Decision Making in Small Animal Radiology

Farrow:
: Emergency Small Animal Radiology

Horney:
: Decision Making in Large Animal Alimentary Tract Surgery

Latshaw:
: Veterinary Developmental Anatomy: A Clinically Oriented Approach

Sumner-Smith:
: Decision Making in Small Animal Orthopaedic Surgery

Thomson:
: Special Veterinary Pathology

Decision Making in Small Animal Orthopaedic Surgery

G. Sumner-Smith, B.V.Sc., M.Sc., F.R.C.V.S.

Professor, Ontario Veterinary College, University
of Guelph, Guelph, Ontario, Canada; Veterinary
Consultant, Labor für Experimentelle Chirurgie
Forschungsinstitut, Davos, Switzerland

1988

B.C. DECKER INC • Toronto • Philadelphia

Publisher

B.C. Decker Inc.
3228 South Service Road
Burlington, Ontario L7N 3H8

B.C. Decker Inc.
P.O. Box 30246
Philadelphia, Pennsylvania 19103

Sales and Distribution

United States and Possessions	**The C.V. Mosby Company** 11830 Westline Industrial Drive Saint Louis, Missouri 63146
Canada	**The C.V. Mosby Company, Ltd.** 5240 Finch Avenue East, Unit No. 1 Scarborough, Ontario M1S 4P2
United Kingdom, Europe and the Middle East	**Blackwell Scientific Publications, Ltd.** Osney Mead, Oxford OX2 OEL, England
Australia	**CBS Publishing Australia Pty. Limited** 9 Waltham Street Artarmon, N.S.W. 2064 Australia
Japan	**Igaku-Shoin Ltd.** Tokyo International P.O. Box 5063 1-28-36 Hongo, Bunkyo-ku, Tokyo 113, Japan
Asia	**CBS Publishing Asia Limited** 10/F, Inter-Continental Plaza Tsim Sha Tsui East Kowloon, Hong Kong

Decision Making in Small Animal Orthopaedic Surgery   ISBN 0–941158–80–2

© 1988 by B.C. Decker Incorporated under the International Copyright Union. All rights reserved. No part of this publication may be reused or republished in any form without written permission of the publisher.

Library of Congress catalog card number: 87–71769

10 9 8 7 6 5 4 3 2 1

for Jack and Candy

CONTRIBUTORS

ALLEN G. BINNINGTON, D.V.M., M.Sc.

Diplomate A.C.V.S., Associate Professor, Ontario Veterinary College, University of Guelph, Guelph, Ontario, Canada

JOANNE R. COCKSHUTT, D.V.M., M.Sc.

Assistant Professor, Ontario Veterinary College, University of Guelph, Guelph, Ontario, Canada

JON F. DEE, D.V.M., M.S.

Diplomate A.C.V.S., Hollywood Animal Hospital, Hollywood, Florida, U.S.A.

LARRY G. DEE, A.B., D.V.M., Dip. A.B.V.P.

Diplomate A.C.V.S., Hollywood Animal Hospital, Hollywood, Florida, U.S.A.

CRAIG W. MILLER, D.V.M., M.V.Sc.

Diplomate A.C.V.S., Assistant Professor, Ontario Veterinary College, University of Guelph, Guelph, Ontario, Canada

W. DIETER PRIEUR, Dr. med. vet.

Director, A.O. Vet Zentrum, Institute Straumann Waldenburg, Switzerland; Adjunct Professor, School of Veterinary Medicine, Michigan State University, East Lansing, Michigan, U.S.A.

GEOFF SUMNER-SMITH, B.V.Sc., M.Sc., F.R.C.V.S.

Professor, Ontario Veterinary College, University of Guelph, Guelph, Ontario, Canada; Veterinary Consultant, Labor für Experimentelle Chirurgie Forschungsinstitut, Davos, Switzerland

PREFACE

In the area of small animal orthopaedics, the neophyte is often overwhelmed by the recent explosion in the literature. As a result, it is often difficult for the uninitiated to find a "critical path" through the textual material, and, thus, difficult for him or her to make treatment decisions based on their reading.

Recently trained veterinary surgeons, however, have been exposed to the Problem Oriented Medical (POM) approach in their handling of case records, and consequently, rather than employing the somewhat hit-and-miss technique of previous generations of surgeons, tend to apply this approach in their everyday practice. In addition, the advent of computers, which now are used in all aspects of learning, has reinforced the critical pathway approach because they solve problems in much the same manner. Thus, in a busy clinical environment, the use of decision making texts has much to advocate it because their use can lead the surgeon to perform the required task and ensure that no signs, relevant to the diagnosis and treatment, are missed. To quote Dryden:

> Errors, like straws, upon the surface flow;
> He who would search for pearls must dive below.
> John Dryden
> 1631 – 1700

However, even with its leads and clean pathways of thought, there is a danger, inherent in this type of text, in that their use encourages the reader to remain an empiricist, and I warn that such texts add to the application of knowledge, but not to the art of orthopaedic surgery. This latter element, which is essential to the development of good judgment, comes with diligent study and even more with time and experience.

ACKNOWLEDGEMENTS

To the publisher, Mr. Brian Decker and his staff, I wish to extend my thanks for their invitation to edit this book. My initial reaction was that the task would be simple , one taking only a few weeks. How wrong I was! The style of the Decision Making series requires an entirely different approach from the one used in preparing a normal manuscript. My Associate Medical Editor at B.C. Decker was Mrs. Agnes McIvor who, with tolerance and good humor, suffered my peccadillos and kept me on the proper path. To this lady my special thanks are due.

Lloy Osburn and Dr. Clive Eger produced the figures nearly all of which are original. Their contributions have added much to the text. Finally, it will become obvious to the reader that, without the labors of the contributors, the book would never have seen the light of day. To these colleagues my heartfelt thanks.

Geoff Sumner-Smith
Everton, August 1987

CONTENTS

LOCOMOTION

Normal Locomotion 2
Geoff Sumner-Smith

Forelimb Action 4
Geoff Sumner-Smith

Hind Limb Action 6
Geoff Sumner-Smith

Lameness Work-Up 8
Allen G. Binnington

Lameness 10
Geoff Sumner-Smith

Foreleg Lameness in the Young Animal 12
Craig W. Miller

Hind Limb Lameness in the Young Animal 14
Craig W. Miller

ARTHROSES

Degenerative Joint Disease 16
W. Dieter Prieur
Geoff Sumner-Smith

Arthritis 18
Geoff Sumner-Smith

Septic Arthritis 20
Geoff Sumner-Smith

Immune-Mediated Arthritis 22
Craig W. Miller

Osteochondritis Dissecans 24
Craig W. Miller

FRACTURE MANAGEMENT

Principles of Fracture Management 26
Geoff Sumner-Smith

Fracture Suspected in Immature Animals 28
Geoff Sumner-Smith

Fracture in the Young Animal Involving
a Growth Plate 30
Geoff Sumner-Smith

Limb Deviation Caused by Growth Plate
Injury and Premature Closure 32
Geoff Sumner-Smith

Pathologic Fracture 34
Geoff Sumner-Smith

Hematogenous Osteomyelitis 36
Craig W. Miller

Traumatic Osteomyelitis 38
Craig W. Miller

FORELIMB DISORDERS

Shoulder Pain 40
Craig W. Miller

Scapular Fracture 42
Craig W. Miller

Proximal Humeral Fracture 44
Craig W. Miller

Humerus Shaft Fracture 46
Craig W. Miller

Distal Humeral Fracture 48
Craig W. Miller

Elbow Pain 50
Geoff Sumner-Smith

Arthritis of the Elbow 52
Geoff Sumner-Smith

Elbow Dislocation 54
Geoff Sumner-Smith

Antebrachial Fractures 56
Geoff Sumner-Smith

Acute Antebrachiocarpal Luxation–
Subluxation 58
Jon F. Dee

Styloid Fracture 60
Jon F. Dee

Accessory Carpal Bone Fracture 62
Jon F. Dee

Radial Carpal Bone Fracture and
Luxation 64
Jon F. Dee

Carpal Arthrodesis 66
Jon F. Dee

Metacarpal (Metatarsal) Fracture 68
Jon F. Dee

Metacarpal or Metatarsal-Phalangeal
Subluxation, Luxation 70
Larry G. Dee

Phalangeal Luxation 72
Larry G. Dee

Phalangeal Fracture 74
Jon F. Dee

Hind Limb Disorders

Hip Pain 76
Geoff Sumner-Smith

Pelvic Trauma 78
Allen G. Binnington

Pelvic Fracture 80
Joanne R. Cockshutt

Acetabular Fracture 82
Joanne R. Cockshutt

Fractures Involving the Hip Joint 84
W. Dieter Prieur

Pelvic Fracture Complications 86
Allen G. Binnington

Coxofemoral Luxation 88
Allen G. Binnington

Traumatic Hip Luxation 92
W. Dieter Prieur

Hip Dysplasia 94
Joanne R. Cockshutt

Canine Hip Dysplasia 96
W. Dieter Prieur

Slipped Capital Epiphysis 100
W. Dieter Prieur

Avascular Necrosis of the Femoral Head
(Legg-Calvé-Perthes Disease) 102
W. Dieter Prieur
Geoff Sumner-Smith

Sepsis in Total Hip Replacement 104
Geoff Sumner-Smith

Femoral Head and Neck Fracture 106
W. Dieter Prieur

Femoral Neck Fractures 108
W. Dieter Prieur

Proximal Femur Fracture 110
W. Dieter Prieur

Femoral Shaft Fracture 112
W. Dieter Prieur

Distal Femur Fracture 114
W. Dieter Prieur

Fracture of the Patella and Rupture of the
Patella Ligament 116
Geoff Sumner-Smith

Chronic Swelling of the Stifle Joint 118
Geoff Sumner-Smith

Stifle Ligament Injury 120
Geoff Sumner-Smith

Meniscal Injury 122
Geoff Sumner-Smith

Patella Luxation 124
Geoff Sumner-Smith

Tibial Plateau Fracture 128
Geoff Sumner-Smith

Proximal Tibial Growth Plate Fracture in
Young Animals 130
Geoff Sumner-Smith

Tibial Shaft Fracture 132
Geoff Sumner-Smith

Nomenclature of the Tarsal Joints 134
Jon F. Dee

Malleolar Shearing Injury 136
Jon F. Dee

Malleolar Fracture 138
Jon F. Dee

Proximal Intertarsal Subluxation 140
Jon F. Dee

Talus Fracture 142
Jon F. Dee

Calcaneus Fracture 144
Jon F. Dee

Intertarsal Subluxation 148
Jon F. Dee

Tarsocrural Arthrodesis 152
Jon F. Dee

Central Tarsal Bone Fracture 154
Jon F. Dee

Second Tarsal Bone Fracture 156
Jon F. Dee

Third Tarsal Bone Fracture 158
Jon F. Dee

Fourth Tarsal Fracture 160
Jon F. Dee

Tarsometatarsal Joint Subluxation 162
Jon F. Dee

DISORDERS OF THE SPINE

Atlantoaxial–Complex Congenital Lesions 164
Geoff Sumner-Smith

Atlantoaxial Fracture 166
Geoff Sumner-Smith

Cervical Spine Fracture 168
Geoff Sumner-Smith

Thoracolumbar Spine Fracture 170
Geoff Sumner-Smith

Sacral Injuries 172
Joanne R. Cockshutt

INJURY OF THE CRANIUM

Cranial Fracture 174
Craig W. Miller

Mandibular Fracture 176
Geoff Sumner-Smith

Conditions of the Mandible 178
Geoff Sumner-Smith

Temporomandibular Joint Pain 180
Geoff Sumner-Smith

Teeth

Conditions of Growing Teeth 182
Geoff Sumner-Smith

Periodontal Tissue Disease 184
Geoff Sumner-Smith

Malocclusion 186
Geoff Sumner-Smith

Diseases of the Teeth 188
Geoff Sumner-Smith

Trauma to Musculoskeletal Tissue

Bite Wounds 190
Geoff Sumner-Smith

Gunshot Wound to the Limb 192
Geoff Sumner-Smith

Tendon Injury 194
Geoff Sumner-Smith

The Severely Injured Patient: Part I 196
Geoff Sumner-Smith

The Severely Injured Patient: Part II 198
Geoff Sumner-Smith

Appendices

Appendix I 200

Appendix II 201

Appendix III 202

INTRODUCTION

The production of a multiauthored book is not without its tribulations. One of these is the possible overlap of information. In this text there are a few areas of overlapping, but I have left them in place, believing that the reader might enjoy and benefit from slightly different views on the same topic.

The text may be employed in two ways. The first is in the emergency situation when a clinician may feel the need for a guiding hand to pilot a route through a maze of problems; in such situations the text must be used in conjunction with its soft-tissue counterpart. Secondly, in chronic conditions the text should serve a useful role in providing a check list and hence permit the clinician to ensure that nothing has been overlooked.

If time is taken to study the system presented in this book, it may well reward the reader when time is not of the essence. In normal circumstances, its place is close to the emergency room.

NORMAL LOCOMOTION

Geoff Sumner-Smith

A. A stride is considered to be a whole cycle from one point of that cycle back to the same point. We speak of the Stance Phase (retraction) and the Swing Phase (protraction); the Contact Point, when the foot touches the ground and the Lift Point, when it leaves the ground (Fig. 1). The forelimbs support and arrest the body; the hind limbs propel the body, but they also initiate deceleration, particularly of the faster gaits. The gait patterns are shown in Figure 2.

B. The walk is a slow symmetrical rotatory gait with either two, three, or four legs supporting the body. Short-coupled, long-legged dogs sometimes walk with the ipsilateral limbs nearly together in the Swing Phase.

C. The trot is a two-beat gait in which the diagonally opposite limbs alternately support the body. This is an extremely useful gait with which to examine an animal for lameness. Toy dogs tend to use the trot as their "normal" gait unless they are walking extremely slowly.

D. The pace is a gait adopted by some large and giant breed animals, although a slow pace may be seen in some smaller animals. Although some dogs pace preferentially, they will also trot. The pace is said to be less tiring, but it probably permits less overall speed than does the trot.

References

Adrian MJ, Roy WE, Karpovich PV. Normal gait of the dog: an electrogoniometric study. Am J Vet Res 1966; 27:90–95.

Alexander RM. Animal mechanics. London: Sidgwick & Jackson, 1968.

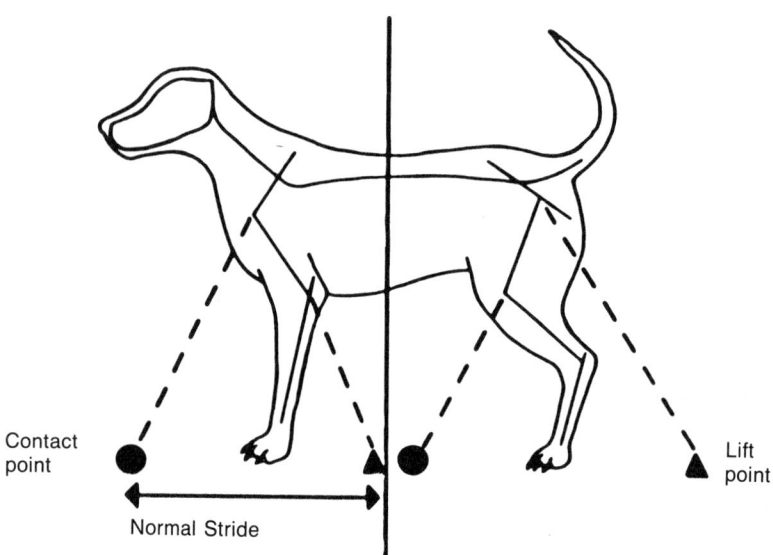

Figure 1 Contact Point and Lift Point in a normal stride.

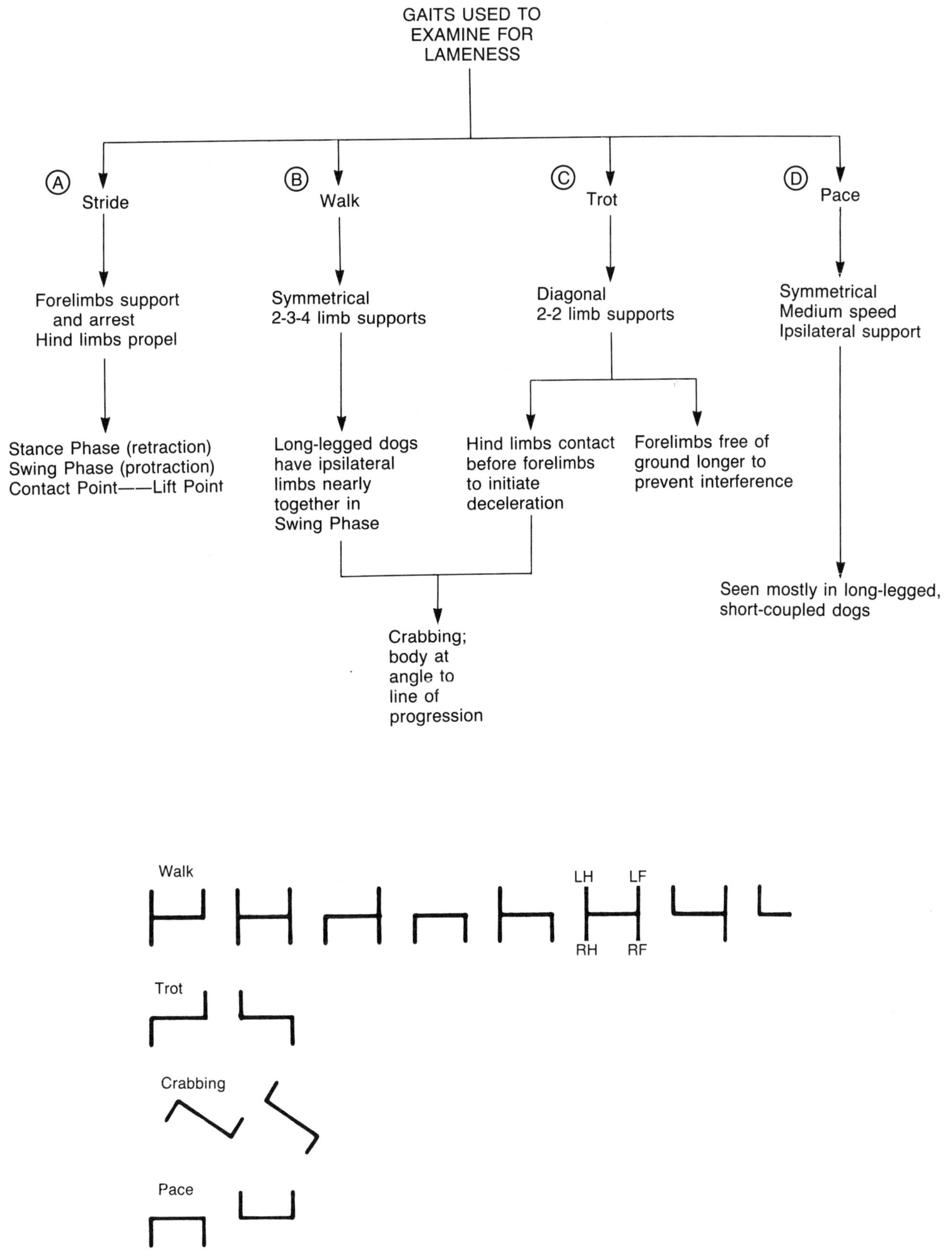

GAITS USED TO EXAMINE FOR LAMENESS

Ⓐ Stride
- Forelimbs support and arrest
- Hind limbs propel
  - Stance Phase (retraction)
  - Swing Phase (protraction)
  - Contact Point——Lift Point

Ⓑ Walk
- Symmetrical 2-3-4 limb supports
  - Long-legged dogs have ipsilateral limbs nearly together in Swing Phase
    - Crabbing; body at angle to line of progression

Ⓒ Trot
- Diagonal 2-2 limb supports
  - Hind limbs contact before forelimbs to initiate deceleration
  - Forelimbs free of ground longer to prevent interference
  - Crabbing; body at angle to line of progression

Ⓓ Pace
- Symmetrical Medium speed Ipsilateral support
  - Seen mostly in long-legged, short-coupled dogs

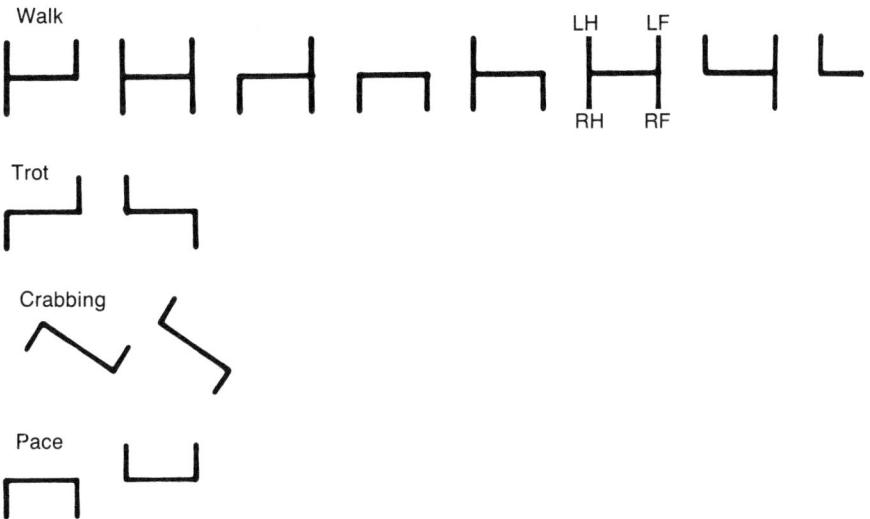

Figure 2 Gait patterns.

FORELIMB ACTION

Geoff Sumner-Smith

A. The forelimb is attached to the body by the muscles of the thorax, and is literally slung between the scapulae. Such a joint is known as a synsarcosis. A cat's clavicle does not form a true arthrodeal joint with other bones. It is vestigeal and is embedded within the pectoral group of muscles. The synsarcosis is an ideal joint to absorb the concussion produced when the forelimbs hit the ground, and it allows the forelimb to move nearly 180 degrees on the thoracic wall. The normal angles of the joints of the forelimb are shown in Figure 1. The scapulo-humeral joint angle changes very little during the stride of the forelimb in either the walk or trot, although it also absorbs some of the concussion at the Contact Point through the first half of the Stance Phase (Fig. 2).

B. The elbow joint is a complex mechanical component of the forelimb; three bones are involved, each articulating with the other two. The radius and ulna form a hinge with the humerus and are also capable of a small amount of supination and pronation with one another. The hinge joint shows little change of joint angle until the end of the Stance Phase.

C. The carpus functions for the most part as a hinge joint, although all of the components do move among themselves. For the purposes of locomotion the radial, carpal, and intercarpal joints are considered as one. The "combined joint" is flexed at the beginning of the Swing Phase and is somewhat hyperextended at the end of that phase (Fig. 3).

D. The foot consists of many joints between the various components of the phalanges, but for the purposes of locomotion and assessing lameness, they are considered as an integral unit, each element of the unit having an effect on the whole. Surprisingly the metacarpal pad is the first to contact the ground and the first to leave it; the final traction is applied by the toe nails.

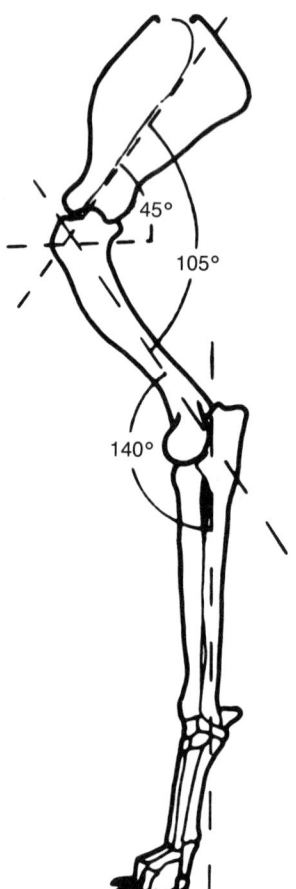

Figure 1 The normal angles of the joints of the forelimb taken from spark pen analyses of forelimb action.

TABLE 1 Locomotion: Action of Forelimb Joints

Location of Joint	Type of Joint	Joint Action During Locomotion
(A) Shoulder	Synsarcosis	Absorbs concussion. Allows 180° range of movement. Little change in joint angle throughout a stride
(B) Elbow	Ginglymus/plane	Little change in joint angle until the end of the Stance Phase
(C) Carpus	Ginglymus/plane	Flexed at the beginning of the Swing Phase. Hyperextended at the end of the Swing Phase
(D) Foot	Gliding/plane	Metacarpal pad contacts ground first and leaves ground first in every phase

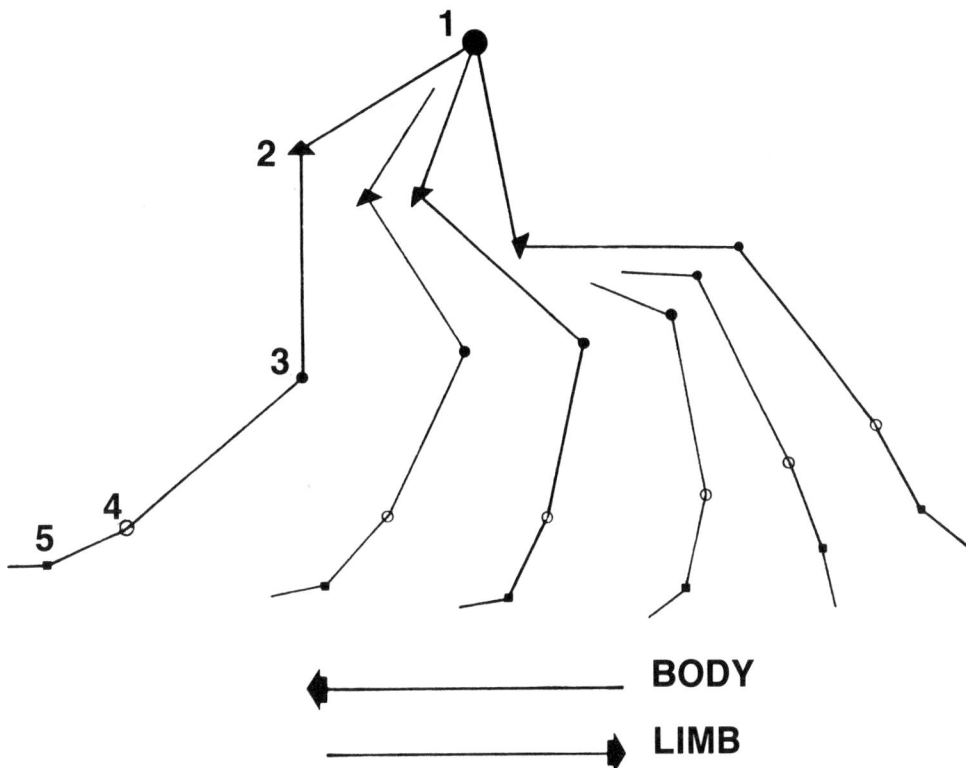

Figure 2 Normal goniometric angles of the dog's forelimb during the Stance Phase (Retraction). Pivoting takes place through the synsarcosis of the scapula on the thorax. 1. Pivot center of scapula on the thorax. 2. Shoulder joint. 3. Elbow Joint. 4. Carpal. 5. Metacarpal-phalangeal joint.

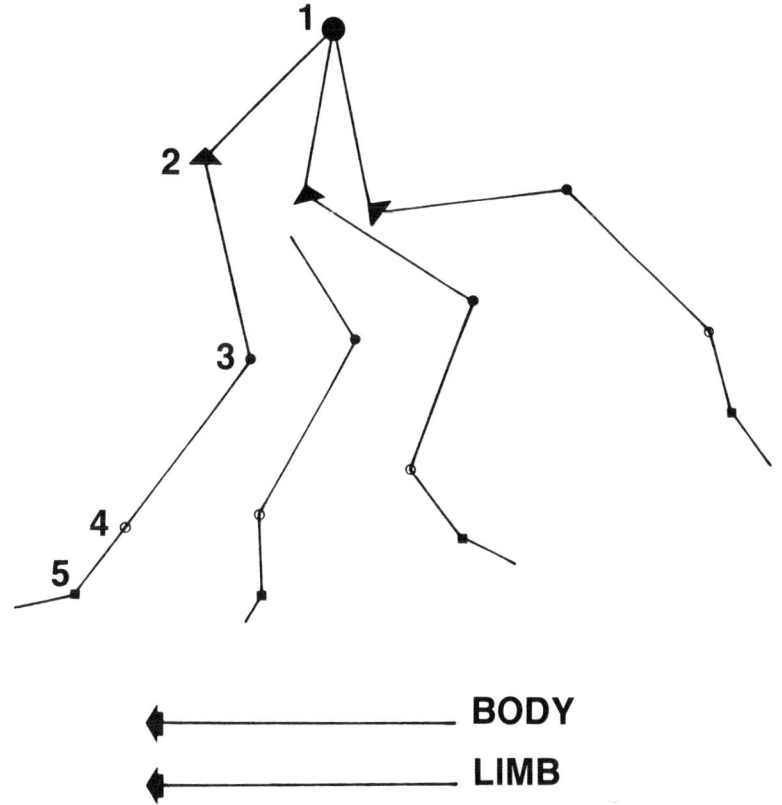

Figure 3 The same forelimb during the Swing Phase (Protraction).(Points are the same as for Figure 2.)

HIND LIMB ACTION

Geoff Sumner-Smith

A. The hip joint is categorically the most important joint in the body of an animal. Although orthopaedic surgeons will consider arthrodesing other joints, the fused hip joint renders the relevant hind limb totally functionless. The hip joint produces nearly all of the excursion of the Swing and Stance Phases and the concussion of the hind limb is absorbed through the craniodorsal aspect of the acetabulum. The normal goniometric angles and the normal joint angles are shown in Figures 1 and 2.

B. The stifle joint consists of the hinge joint between the femur and the head of the tibia and fibula, and the gliding pulley joint of the patella on the trochleal groove, as it guides the action of the quadriceps muscles. In the walk and trot there is little change in the joint angle until the end of the Stance Phase and the beginning of the Swing Phase. Much more use is made of the joint at the faster gaits.

C. The metatarsal joint is complex, but it too acts as a hinge. During the walk and trot there is little change in the joint angle. However, at the faster gaits the joint is used considerably to finalize the propulsion exerted by the hind limbs.

D. The remarks made for the forefoot are, in the main, applicable to the hind foot (p 4).

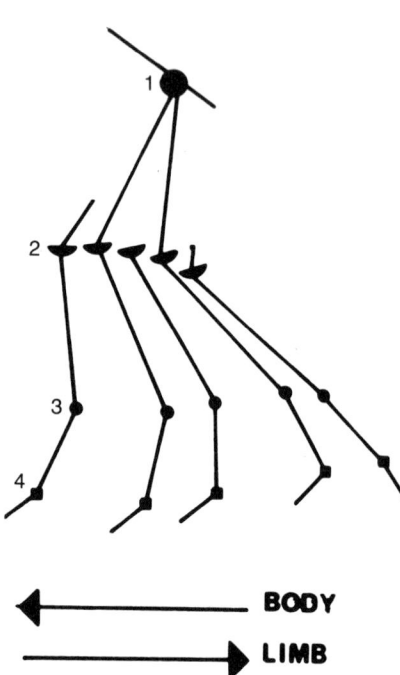

Figure 1 Normal goniometric angles of the hind limb during the Stance Phase. 1. Hip. 2. Stifle. 3. Hock. 4. Metatarsal joint.

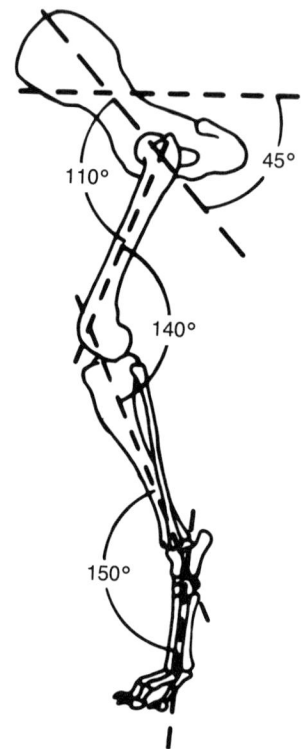

Figure 2 Normal joint angles of the hind limb taken from a spark pen analysis.

TABLE 1 Locomotion: Action of Hind Limb Joints

Location of Joint	Type of Joint	Joint Action During Locomotion
Ⓐ Hip	Ball and socket	Produces nearly all of the excursion of the limb in both Swing and Stance Phases Absorbs concussion via the acetabulum
Ⓑ Stifle	Ginglymus/plane	Little change in joint angle until the end of the Stance Phase
Ⓒ Hock	Ginglymus/plane	Little change in joint angle until the end of the Stance Phase
Ⓓ Foot	Gliding/plane	Metacarpal pad contacts ground first and leaves ground first in every phase

LAMENESS WORK-UP

Allen G. Binnington

A. Age, weight, breed, and sex are essential to the signalment of a lameness work-up.

B. The owner should be questioned regarding the rate of lameness onset and as to whether the animal is acutely or chronically lame, weight-bearing or nonweight-bearing. If there is a history of trauma, the following indications should be considered: (1) Is the lameness continuous or intermittent? (2) Does the animal "warm out" of it or does the lameness worsen with exercise? (3) Is the lameness limited to one limb, multiple limbs, or is it a shifting lameness? (4) Does it change with temperature or weather changes? (5) Does the animal have trouble rising, climbing stairs, or jumping?

C. To examine the gait, the animal is required to walk, trot, run, and circle to the left and right. Signs to be watched for are: an altered gait, a favored limb, shortened stride, hyperextension of joints, abduction or adduction of a limb, the presence of head bob and its relation to limb replacement, shifting of weight from forelimbs to hind limbs or vice versa, and the width of the stance base—wide or narrow. The gait examination should pinpoint the limb involved and possibly identify the specific bone or joint.

D. After a complete physical examination, the normal and involved limbs should be palpated from distal to proximal in order to examine the nails, pads, skin, ligamentous, tendinous, muscular, and bony structures. Evidence of muscular atrophy, areas of swelling, pain, crepitus, heat, and decreased limits of joint motion on joint laxity should be noted. A neurologic examination may be indicated by the findings of this examination.

E. Lameness can be caused by a variety of nonorthopaedically related causes. Metabolic problems such as myasthenia gravis, hypoglycemia, myopathies caused by chronic hyperadrenocorticoidism, and chronic hyperthyroidism may be involved. Either upper or lower motor neuron deficits can cause lameness. Specific organ problems, such as prostatitis and nephritis, can lead to gait abnormalities that are presented as lameness by the animal's owner.

F. Radiography is used to confirm lesion location and to tentatively rule out specific etiologies of lameness that include developmental abnormalities, fractures, dislocation, and infectious, metabolic, degenerative, and neoplastic processes.

G. Muscle and tendon problems are usually the result of trauma. Lameness may be attributed to rupture of muscle bundles, avulsion of tendinous origins or insertions, muscle contusions with hematoma formation, or loss of function caused by contracture and fibrosis of specific muscle groups. Exploratory surgery of the involved muscles confirms the diagnosis and allows repairs, if possible. A muscle biopsy may be needed to establish a diagnosis in certain neuromuscular diseases.

H. A bone biopsy may be necessary to differentiate between a neoplastic, infectious, or metabolic bone process. Skeletal radiography may be required to rule out metastasis or to confirm a systemic bone problem.

I. Use of special manipulative procedures, such as anterior drawer movement, stress radiography (especially for carpal problems), and image intensification of joint movement may pinpoint ligamentous injuries. Joint taps with synovial fluid analysis and culture and sensitivity should be considered, as should exploratory arthrotomies with biopsies if necessary. Autoimmune diseases may be confirmed with antinuclear antibody and rheumatoid factor tests.

Reference

Leach D, Sumner-Smith G, Dagg AI. Diagnosis of lameness in dogs: a preliminary study. Can Vet J 1977; 18(3):58.

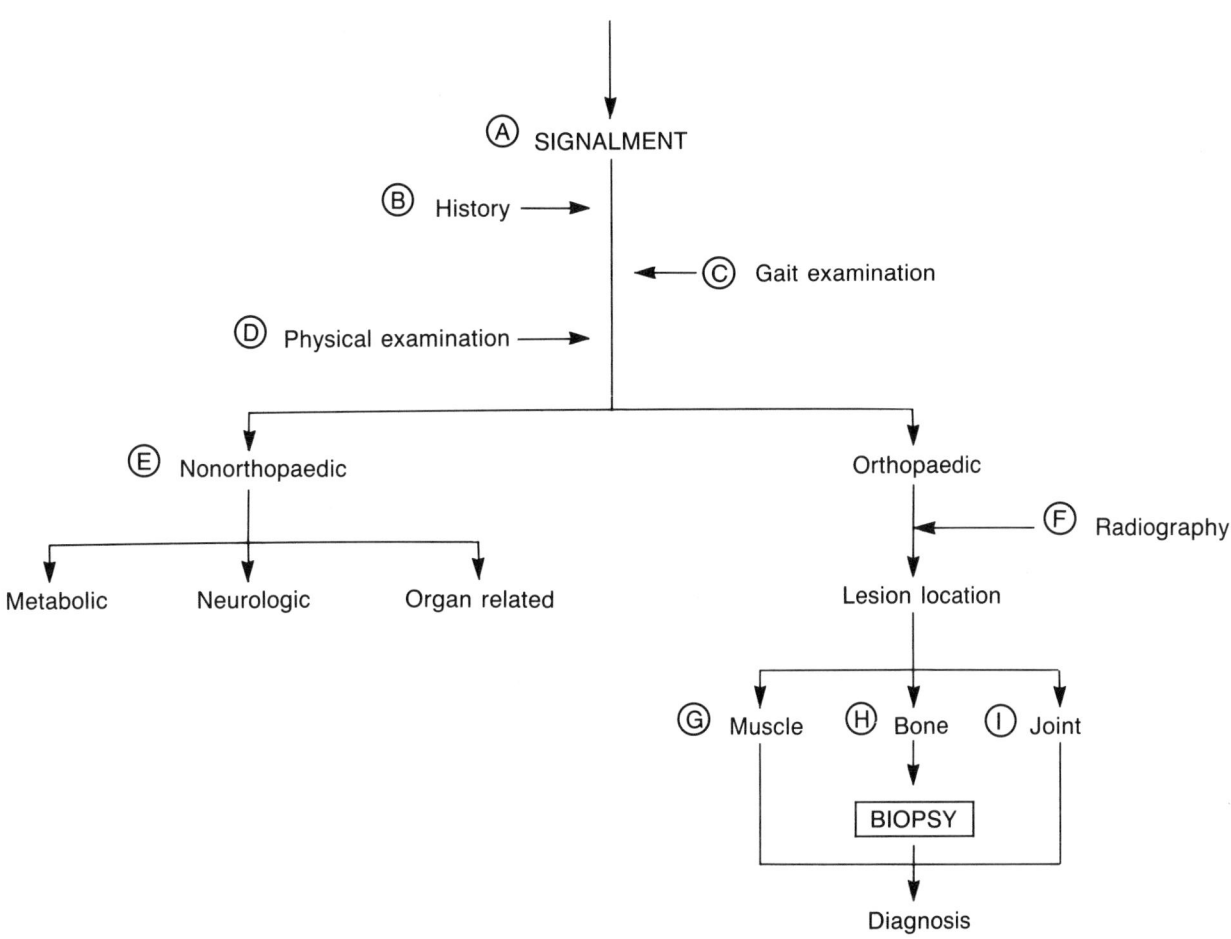

LAMENESS

Geoff Sumner-Smith

A. In order to assess the cause of lameness, patients should be observed going away from the observer, from both sides, and with the animal approaching. A lame animal shifts weight to the side of the sound limb and hence increases the oscillation of its center of gravity. The observer should learn to "play back" an animal's action in slow motion in his mind and then watch the animal move again. This technique requires practice but can be very useful to analyze the site of lameness. Some forms of lameness, which are not visible when the animal walks, often show when it trots.

B. In lifting the head on the unsound limb the animal appears to "lurch over" that forelimb (Fig. 1).

C. The observer should watch the animal over a sufficient number of steps to ensure that the presence or absence of all of these signs is checked. "Freezing" of the shoulder joint is a term employed to indicate that motion of the joint is stilled, with all motion taking place elsewhere in the limb (Fig. 2A).

D. Elbow lameness due to pain in the elbow results in a marked decrease of even the minimal movement normally present in the joint. The humerus, radius, and ulna appear almost to move as if they were one bone, with a bend in the middle and the whole limb moving as one bone against the thorax. Some relative increase in movement of both the shoulder joint and the carpus may take place as a compensatory mechanism.

E. Usually lameness originating from the foot joints is easier to diagnose than elsewhere in the limb. The action of the limb is normal until the foot is required to contact the ground. The toe is used if the pain is present in the palmar or plantar aspect of the foot. If toes are involved the reaction is immediate as soon as the foot touches the ground; in all but the mild cases, the patient prefers to walk on three legs, carrying the affected forelimb.

F. Hind limb lameness is characterized by the shifting of weight mentioned under A. In order to accomplish this, the animal carries its head much lower than normal to initiate a cantilever effect through the shoulder and the thoracic and lumbar portions of the spine.

G. When the lameness originates in a hip, the animal attempts to decrease the excursion of the femoral head in the acetabulum. Hence it adopts an oscillating gait, bending the spine laterally on the affected side in order to assist in the forward placement of the foot. Bilateral hip lameness elicits lateral bending in both directions (Fig. 2B and Fig. 3).

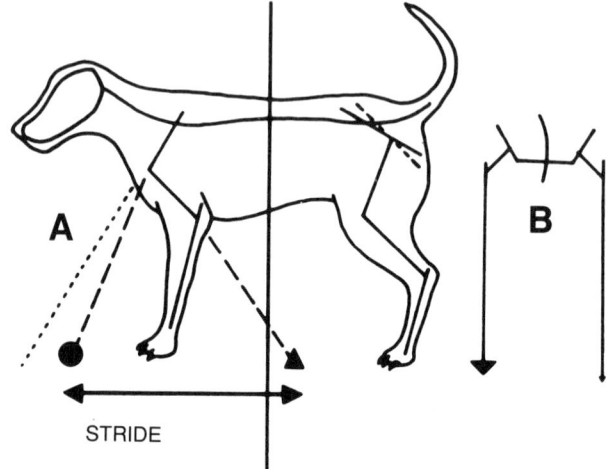

Figure 2 *A,* Shortening of the stride in the Swing Phase of a dog with shoulder lameness. Tilting of the pelvis in lameness is due to hip problems. *B,* There is lateral oscillation of the pelvis in all hind limb lameness. (From Leach D, Sumner-Smith G, Dagg AI. Diagnosis of lameness in dogs: a preliminary study. Can Vet J 1977; 18(3):58.)

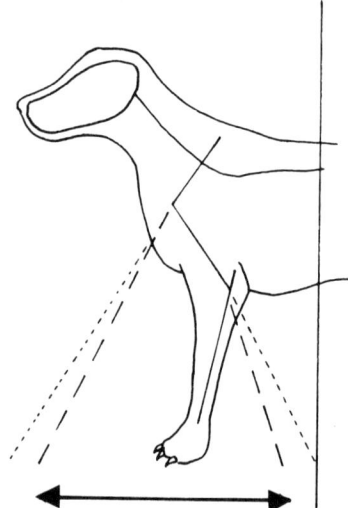

Figure 1 Diagram of lameness in the left forelimb. The normal length of the Stance Phase is reduced in length and extension. (From Leach D, Sumner-Smith G, Dagg AI. Diagnosis of lameness in dogs: a preliminary study. Can Vet J 1977; 18(3):58.)

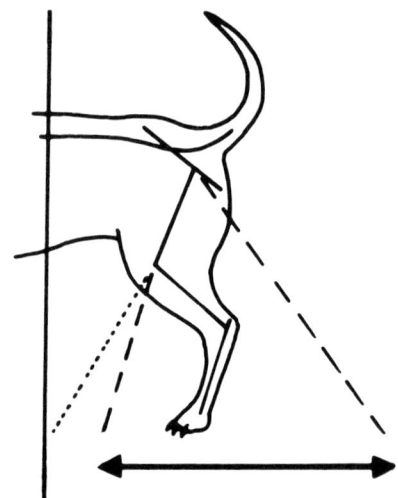

Figure 3 Shortening of the Swing Phase in hind limb lameness. (From Leach D, Sumner-Smith G, Dagg AI. Diagnosis of lameness in dogs: a preliminary study. Can Vet J 1977; 18(3):58.)

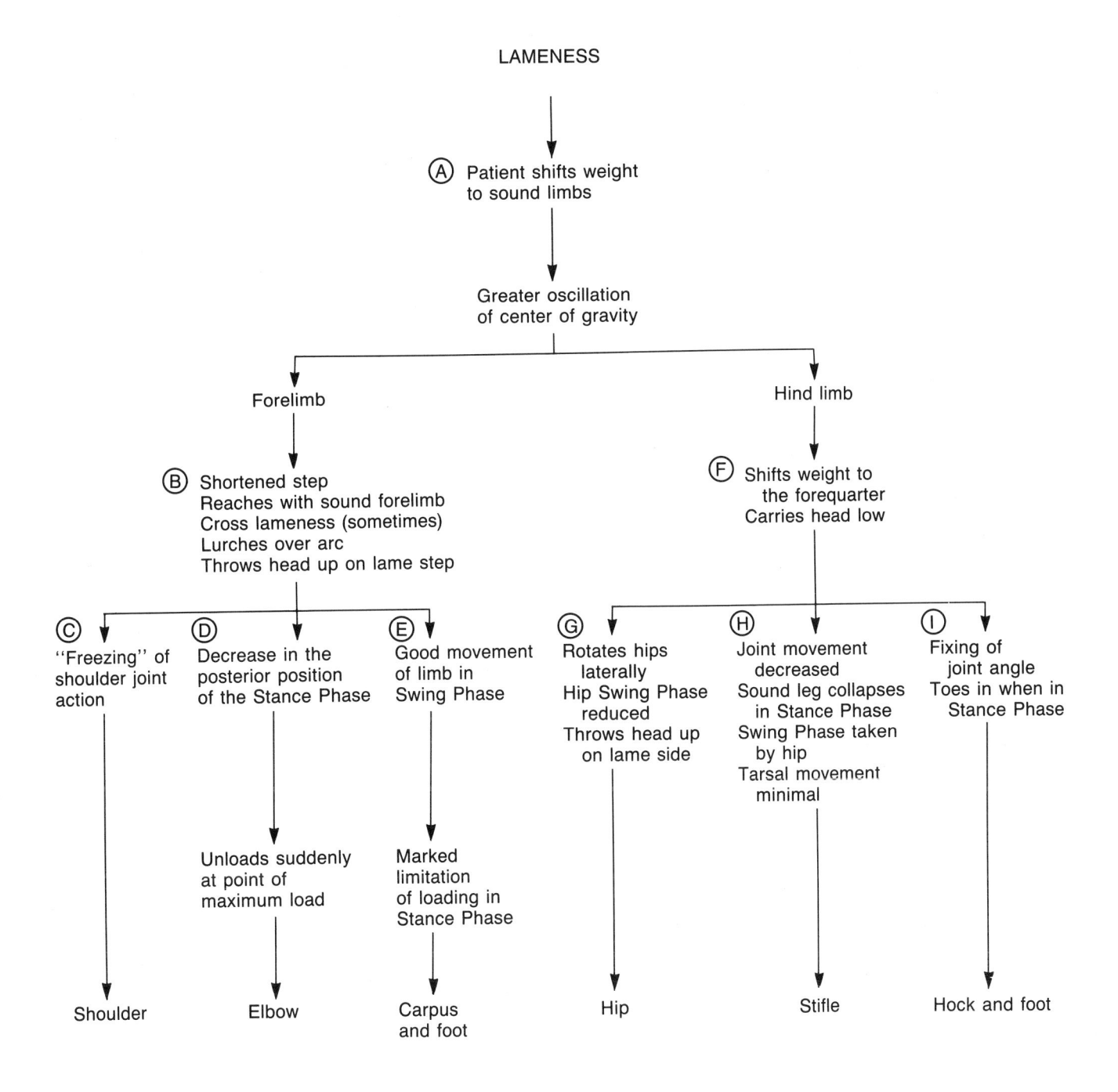

LAMENESS

- **A** Patient shifts weight to sound limbs
  - Greater oscillation of center of gravity
    - **Forelimb**
      - **B** Shortened step
        Reaches with sound forelimb
        Cross lameness (sometimes)
        Lurches over arc
        Throws head up on lame step
        - **C** "Freezing" of shoulder joint action → **Shoulder**
        - **D** Decrease in the posterior position of the Stance Phase → Unloads suddenly at point of maximum load → **Elbow**
        - **E** Good movement of limb in Swing Phase → Marked limitation of loading in Stance Phase → **Carpus and foot**
    - **Hind limb**
      - **F** Shifts weight to the forequarter
        Carries head low
        - **G** Rotates hips laterally
          Hip Swing Phase reduced
          Throws head up on lame side → **Hip**
        - **H** Joint movement decreased
          Sound leg collapses in Stance Phase
          Swing Phase taken by hip
          Tarsal movement minimal → **Stifle**
        - **I** Fixing of joint angle
          Toes in when in Stance Phase → **Hock and foot**

H. The stifle joint carries its maximum load at the midpoint of the Stance Phase when the foot is under the hip. It is at this point that the limb appears to collapse, throwing weight on the opposite sound limb. Bilateral stifle lameness is particularly crippling; the patient adopts a shuffling gait, which is often mistakenly diagnosed as resulting from lumbar disc disease.

I. Hock joint lameness shows up quite readily if the pain is severe, but in mild cases it may be necessary to see the animal move at quite a fast pace, even a lope, in order to extend fully the joint and hence to demonstrate the lameness.

Reference

Leach D, Sumner-Smith G, Dagg AI. Diagnosis of lameness in dogs: a preliminary study. Can Vet J 1977; 18(3):58.

FORELEG LAMENESS IN THE YOUNG ANIMAL

Craig W. Miller

A. Skeletal abnormalities can be induced by deficiencies or excesses of many nutrients. The most common nutrients implicated in skeletal disease are calcium, phosphorus, and vitamin D. However, a myriad of other dietary components, which include copper, zinc, manganese, fluorine, vitamin A, vitamin C, protein, and carbohydrates, have been implicated also. In most cases, dietary correction of nutritional skeletal disease consists of placing the animal on a well-balanced, commercial diet.

B. Treatment of pathologic fractures secondary to nutritional imbalance is best done, if possible, by coaptation. In these cases, the poor quality of bone cortices makes application of internal or external fixation devices difficult.

C. Asynchronous growth of the radius and ulna has been reported to cause humeroradial subluxation in large, rapidly growing dogs. This has been attributed to an osteochondrosis-like lesion in the radial growth plates, which slows radial growth. Correction of severe cases is similar to that for traumatic retardation of the radial growth plates.

D. Retained cartilaginous cores in the distal ulnar growth plate are postulated to be manifestations of osteochondrosis in the rapidly growing dog. This defect in endochondral ossification is capable of slowing ulnar growth and producing angular and rotational limb deformities. Correction of clinically significant deformities is similar to those of traumatic origin.

E. Carpal hyperextension in young animals is often caused by inadequate exercise and poor flooring. The problem usually resolves if these conditions are corrected. Padded bandages can be used if pressure sores develop on the palmar aspect of the carpus. As rigid immobilization can cause increased ligamentous laxity, it should be avoided.

F. Panosteitis is a self-limiting disease that affects the long bones of young, rapidly growing dogs. The etiology is unknown, but the disease appears to originate in the adipose bone marrow. The disease can effect more than one limb and more than one bone in a single limb. Shifting lameness, from one leg to another, is a common manifestation of this disease. A presumptive diagnosis of panosteitis can be made when pain is elicited upon deep palpation of one or more long bones. The diagnosis can be confirmed radiographically. The disease is self-limiting; however, some dogs are severely affected. Nonsteroidal anti-inflammatory drugs are recommended in such cases.

G. Bone cysts (monostotic or polyostotic) are rare in dogs. The reported cases occurred in young, large dogs and had a predisposition for the metaphyses of the forelimb. Large lesions are best treated by curettage and cancellous bone grafting.

H. Hypertrophic osteopathy is a disease that involves the metaphyses of large, growing dogs. Many etiologies have been postulated for this disease, but none have been proved. The disease is self-limiting, but severe cases can be treated with nonsteroidal anti-inflammatory agents. Correct any dietary imbalances.

References

Newton CD, Nunamaker DM. Normal and abnormal gait. In: Newton CD, Nunamaker DM, eds. Textbook of small animal orthopaedics. Philadelphia: JB Lippincott, 1985:1083.

Olsson S-E. Osteochondrosis in the dog. In: Current veterinary therapy VI. Philadelphia: WB Saunders, 1980:807.

Shires PK, Hulse DA, Kearney MT. Carpal hyperextension in the two-month-old pup. JAVMA Jan 1985; 186(1):49.

FORELEG LAMENESS IN THE YOUNG ANIMAL

History →
Physical examination →

(A) Abnormal diet

- **No fractures** → Correct Diet
- **Fractures** → (B) **REPAIR FRACTURES** → Correct Diet

Normal diet

Shoulder → Radiography
- Congenital luxation → Shoulder Pain (p 40)
- Osteochondritis dissecans → Osteochondrosis (p 24)

Elbow → Radiography
- Fragmented coronoid process (p 50, 52)
- Ununited anconeal process (p 50, 52)
- (C) Elbow subluxation → Growth plate injury (p 54)

Carpus
- Valgus deformity → Radiography → (D) Retained cartilage cores
- Hyperextension → Ligamentus laxity → (E) Conservative Management
  - Successful → Continue Conservative Management
  - Unsuccessful → Bandage

Long bone → Radiography
- (F) Panosteitis → Medical Therapy
- (G) Bone cyst
  - Small defect → Observe → Resolution / No resolution
  - Large defect → CURETTAGE AND BONE GRAFT
- Osteomyelitis (p 36)
- (H) Hypertrophic osteodystrophy → Medical Management

13

HIND LIMB LAMENESS IN THE YOUNG ANIMAL

Craig W. Miller

A. Genu valgum is a developmental abnormality seen in young, rapidly growing, large breeds of dogs. The etiology is unclear, but a failure in endochondral ossification at the distal femoral and proximal tibial growth plates has been postulated. The condition is seen in conjunction with coxofemoral abnormalities such as coxa valga and increased anteversion of the femoral neck.

B. A lateral patellar luxation is caused by an abnormally aligned quadriceps mechanism. In cases with minor angular deformity, realignment of the quadriceps pull by means of transposition of the tibial tuberosity, accompanied by deepening of the trochlear groove by means of wedge recession, may be sufficient correction to allow good function.

C. Animals with significant angular or rotational deformity may require correctional femoral osteotomy in order to gain adequate rear limb function.

References

Newton CD. Genu valgum. In: Newton CD, Nunamaker DM, eds. Textbook of small animal orthopaedics. New York: JB Lippincott, 1985:633.

Slocum B. Trochlear recession for patellar stabilization. Proceedings of the 15th Annual Meeting of the American College of Veterinary Surgeons 1980.

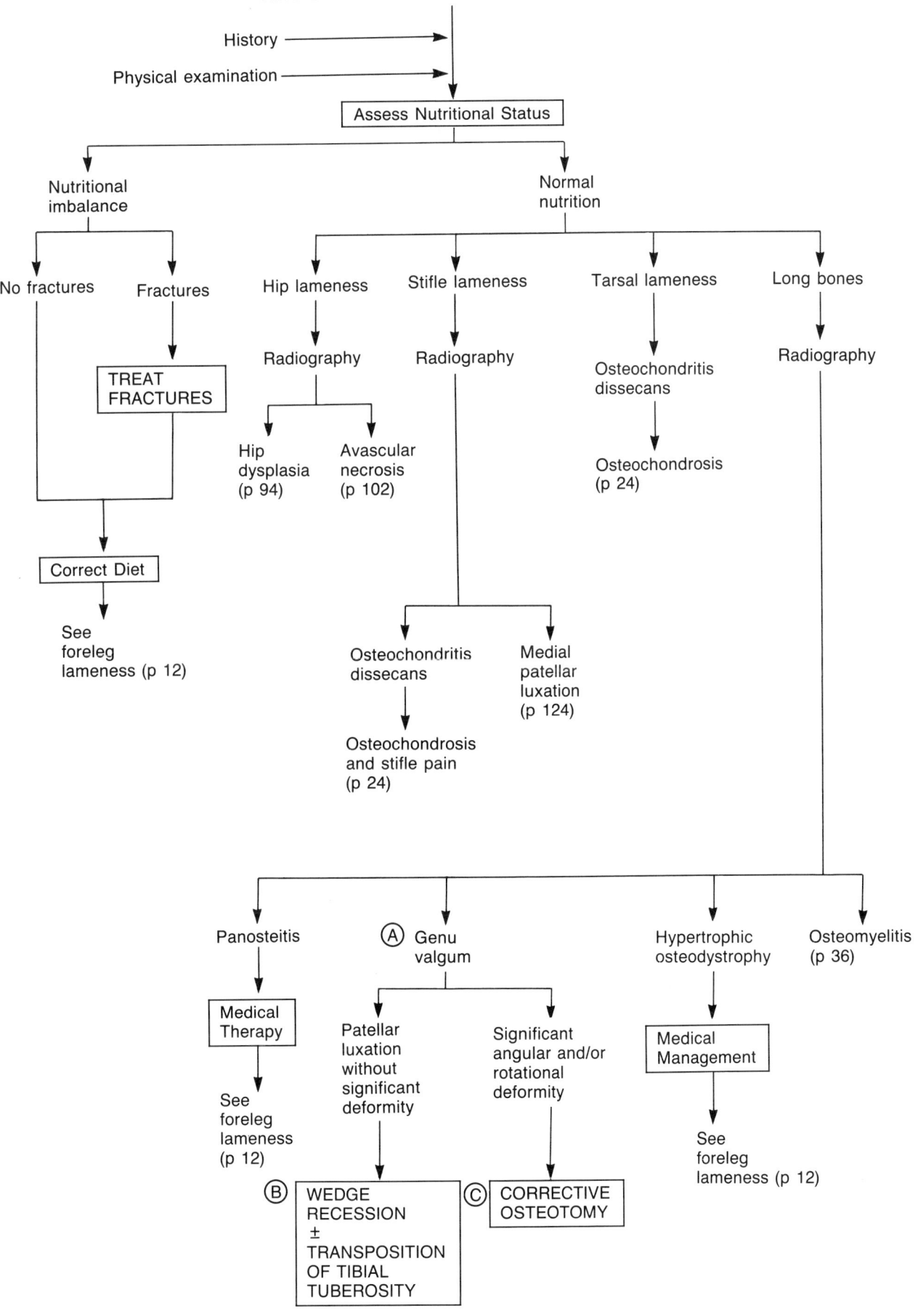

DEGENERATIVE JOINT DISEASE

W. Dieter Prieur
Geoff Sumner-Smith

Although a treatment protocol is not given in the text of this chapter, it is included to give the reader a primer of the development of the condition of degenerative joint disease. The algorithm has been written in linear form, but it is possible to take any point on the algorithm and to move in either direction. The term "a vicious cycle" is very appropriate to the condition of degenerative joint disease (DJD).

A. The cartilage of a joint may be damaged as the result of direct trauma, which can be extrinsic, such as in fractures and ruptured ligaments. Alternatively the damage may be the result of metabolic changes within the joint, that is, intrinsic trauma. Both types of trauma result in changes in joint metabolism.

B. Significant changes occur in the synovial membrane, which initially becomes inflamed and thickened. These changes result in further damage to the cartilage by metabolic waste products. Later, as a result of the synovitis, toxins and enzymes are excreted and accumulate within the synovial fluid. Subsequent retinacular fibrosis occludes and decreases the blood flow to the synovial membrane, further exacerbating the thickening.

C. The reciprocal damage of chondrocytes and matrix by overstressing causes loss of proteoglycans by enzymatic degradation damage to the matrix, attributably to loss of water, which hence damages the chondrocytes. Damage also occurs as the result of the toxic metabolites and enzymes that develop within the synovial fluid themselves and which stems from the general condition and inflammatory products of the synovial membrane (glycopenia).

D. All of the above result in evinced pain, which is a major sign of degenerative joint disease—the result of numerous changes in and around the joint as follows: from muscle contracture of the periarticular muscles as well as other muscles of the appendicular skeleton, from the synovitis, from capsular fibrosis and arising from joint instability that causes intermittent stretching of the retinaculum. Additionally, the pain causes a decrease in normal joint motion.

E. The changes in the components of the tissues result in joint stress, which further disturbs joint mechanics and joint instability with the result of further decreasing the nutrition of the cartilage, increasing damage to the matrix, and changing congruity in the joint surfaces.

F. Subsequent to the above changes, there is a further increase in retinacular fibrosis.

G. Further muscle contracture occurs at this point.

H. Further joint deformation occurs, with osteophyte formation due to the instability and tearing of the Sharpe's fibers.

References

Olsson SE. Degenerative joint disease: a review with special reference to the dog. J small Anim Pract 1971; 12:333.

Pedersen NC, Paul R. Canine joint disease. Vet Clin North Am 1978; 8:465.

Pond MJ. Normal joint tissues and their reaction to injury. Vet Clin North Am 1971; 1:523.

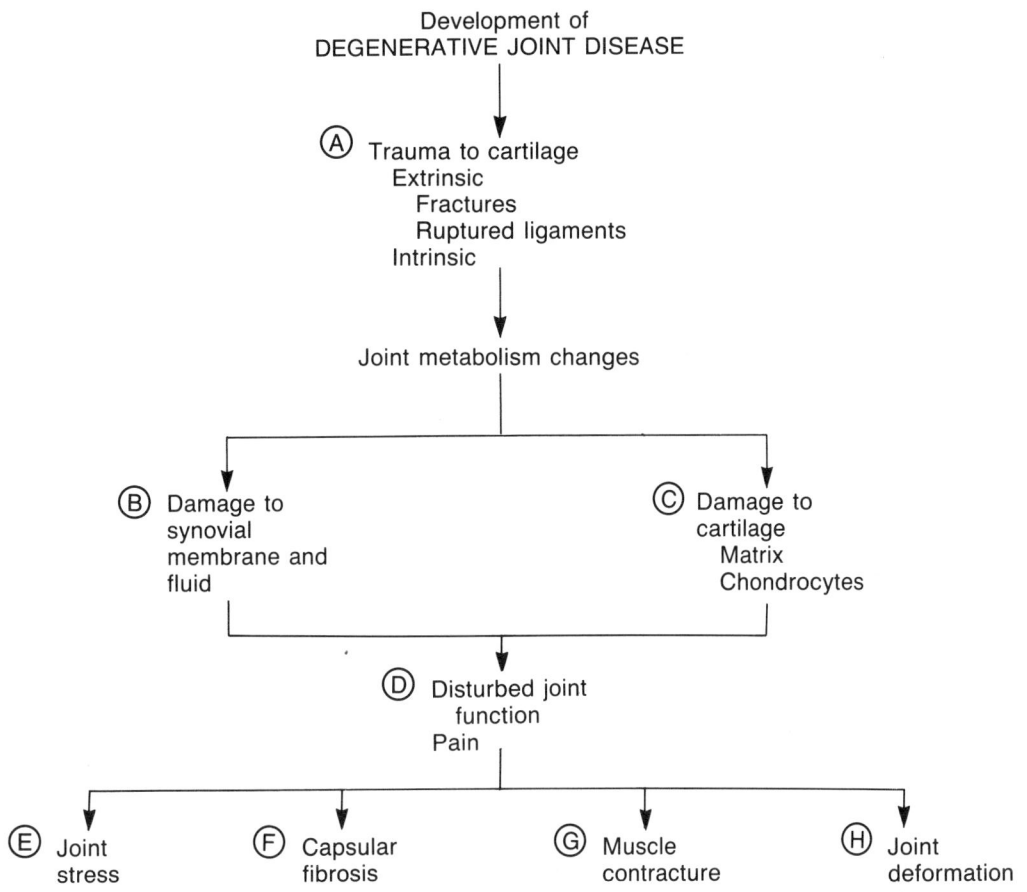

ARTHRITIS

Geoff Sumner-Smith

The term arthritis may be defined as inflammation of a joint that is accompanied by pain. The finite diagnosis depends upon the particular type.

A. Degenerative joint disease results from prolonged stresses over a long period. These may be exacerbated by congenital malformation, e.g., hip dysplasia, ununited coronoid process, and ununited anconeal process. In severe cases that do not respond to palliative therapy, surgical excision, joint replacement, or fusion may be necessary.

B. Rheumatoid arthritis causes proliferative synovitis that gradually destroys the joint. Medical treatment may be palliative (p 22). In severe cases, more radical joint surgery may be required. In animals, this usually takes the form of arthrodesis except in the hip, wherein excision or total joint replacement may be suitable.

C. Osteochondritis dissecans is the inflammatory response to osteochondrosis. It has been diagnosed in most joints of the appendicular skeleton, as well as in the cervical vertebrae of dogs. In young animals, excision of loose bodies and the removal of attached cartilage flaps are recommended. In older animals, surgery may not be necessary provided the joint does not lock. In such cases exercise can promote healing (p 16).

References

Alexander JW, Begg S, Dueland R, et al. Rheumatoid arthritis in the dog: clinical diagnosis and management. JAAHA 1976; 12:727.

Mankin HJ. The reaction of articular cartilage to injury and osteochondritis. N Engl J Med 1974; 291:1335.

Pedersen WC, Weisner K, Castles JJ, et al. Noninfectious canine arthritis: the inflammatory non-erosive arthritides. JAVMA 1976; 109:304.

ARTHRITIS Suspected

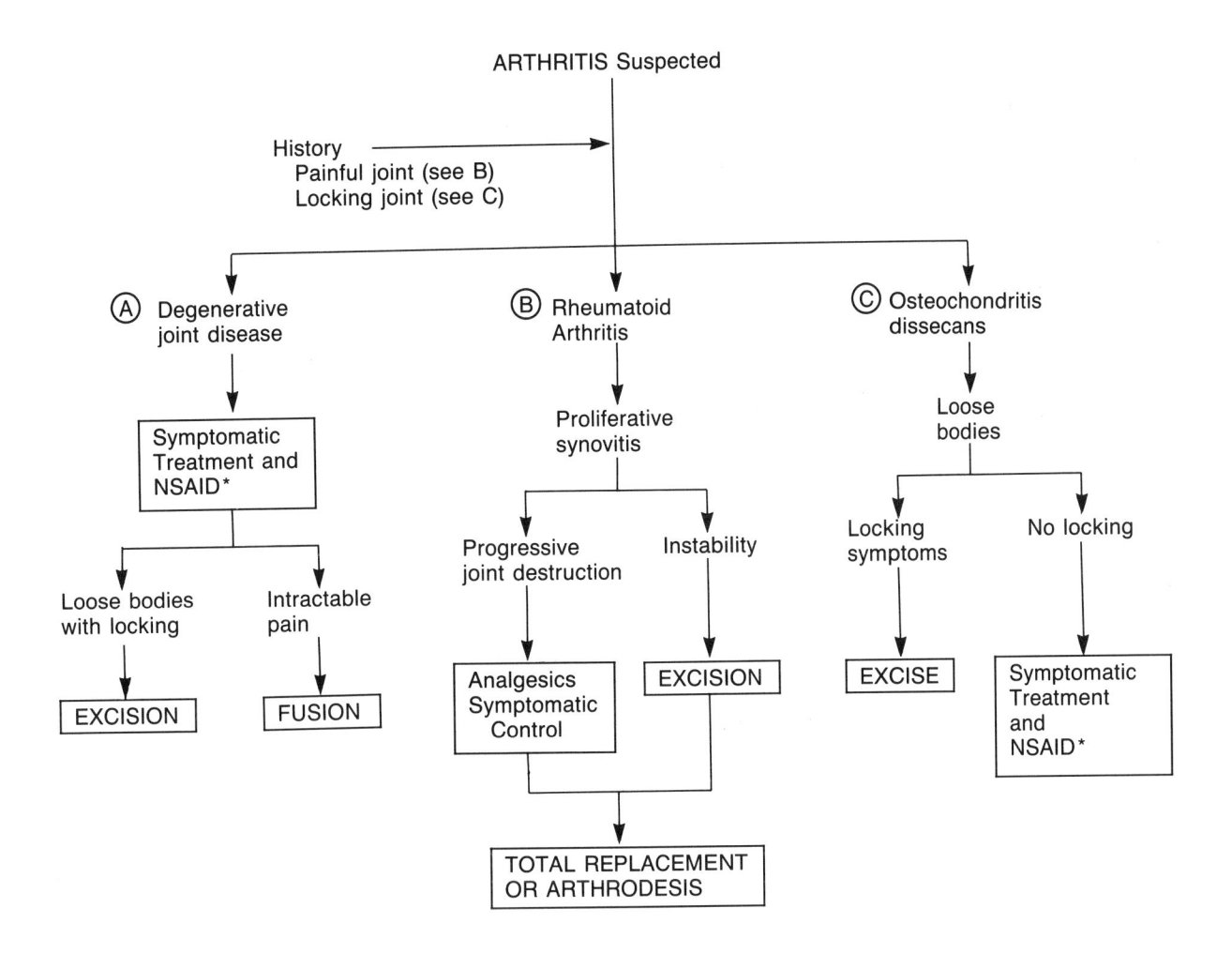

History
- Painful joint (see B)
- Locking joint (see C)

A. Degenerative joint disease
→ Symptomatic Treatment and NSAID*
- Loose bodies with locking → **EXCISION**
- Intractable pain → **FUSION**

B. Rheumatoid Arthritis
→ Proliferative synovitis
- Progressive joint destruction → Analgesics Symptomatic Control
- Instability → **EXCISION**
→ **TOTAL REPLACEMENT OR ARTHRODESIS**

C. Osteochondritis dissecans
→ Loose bodies
- Locking symptoms → **EXCISE**
- No locking → Symptomatic Treatment and NSAID*

*NSAID = Nonsteroidal anti-inflammatory drugs

SEPTIC ARTHRITIS

Geoff Sumner-Smith

Although in small animals the condition is not seen commonly, when it does occur septic arthritis has a devastating effect on the joint. Knowledge of the root of contamination, hematogenous or exogenous, is important.

A. A joint aspirate should be drawn for both physical and bacteriologic examination, including sensitivity tests. Infected synovial fluid is cloudy, thin, and has an increased protein and a decreased glucose content. The leucocyte count is usually >50,000.

B. Usually hematogenous infection occurs in young animals. The bacteremia may originate from pneumonia, diarrhea, umbilical infection, or endocarditis. Occasionally hematogenous spread may take place from a neighbouring septic epiphysitis or from a contiguous osseous surface with subsequent penetration of the cartilage.

C. Exogenous septic arthritis results from wounds that penetrate the synovial capsule. Bite wounds are particularly serious since invariably there is little or no drainage from the area. The carpal and tarsal joints of the areas are common sites for bites. Direct contamination of the joint may also occur as the result of automobile accidents, gunshot wounds, contaminated surgery, and iatrogenic intraarticular injection. The injection of corticosteroids intraarticularly predisposes to infection; particularly by extension from a contiguous source, such as metaphyseal or soft tissue infection.

D. A broad-spectrum antibiotic should be employed intravenously at the start of treatment; definitive therapy must await the results of cultures of the synovial fluid and blood. Subculturing is sometimes necessary following exogenous infection because of the multiplicity of contaminating bacteria. Intravenous antibiotic administration should be continued until the crisis has been controlled, followed by oral antibiotic therapy until the leucocyte picture and the sedimentation rate have returned to normal or near normal.

E. The two most important tasks in the treatment of septic arthritis are the resolution of infection and the removal of all enzymes and breakdown products that, if left in place, will continue to injure the cartilage. Early mild cases may be treated by distention irrigation, but it is usually necessary to perform surgical drainage of the joint. Severe cases also require surgical debridement. A drain should be left in position for only 24 to 48 hours; longer is not advisable as movement of the joint may result in tracking of further contamination from the skin's surface.

F. A sequel to chronic infection, or resistant organisms, may be that poor mobility of the joint remains, although the infection eventually resolves. Provided that there is no evidence of remaining infection, a joint that remains very stiff and painful because of the local laying down of fibrous tissue may be arthrodesed in an attempt to ease the discomfort.

G. Despite persistent treatment, some joints remain chronically infected with concomitant fistula formation. Although the persistence of infection may be caused by the local walling off of the bacteria during treatment, it is more likely because of financial constraints that prevent expensive long-term therapy; euthanasia may be considered for an animal that continues to suffer.

References

Alexander JW. Septic arthritis: diagnosis and treatment. JAAHA 1978; 14:499.

Carb A. Suppurative arthritis. In: Bojrab MJ, ed. Pathophysiology in small animal surgery. Philadelphia: Lea & Febiger, 1981.

Curtiss PH. The pathophysiology of joint infections. Clin Orthop 1973; 96:129.

Pedersen NC. Synovial fluid collection and analysis. Vet Clin North Am 1978; 8:495.

SEPTIC ARTHRITIS Suspected

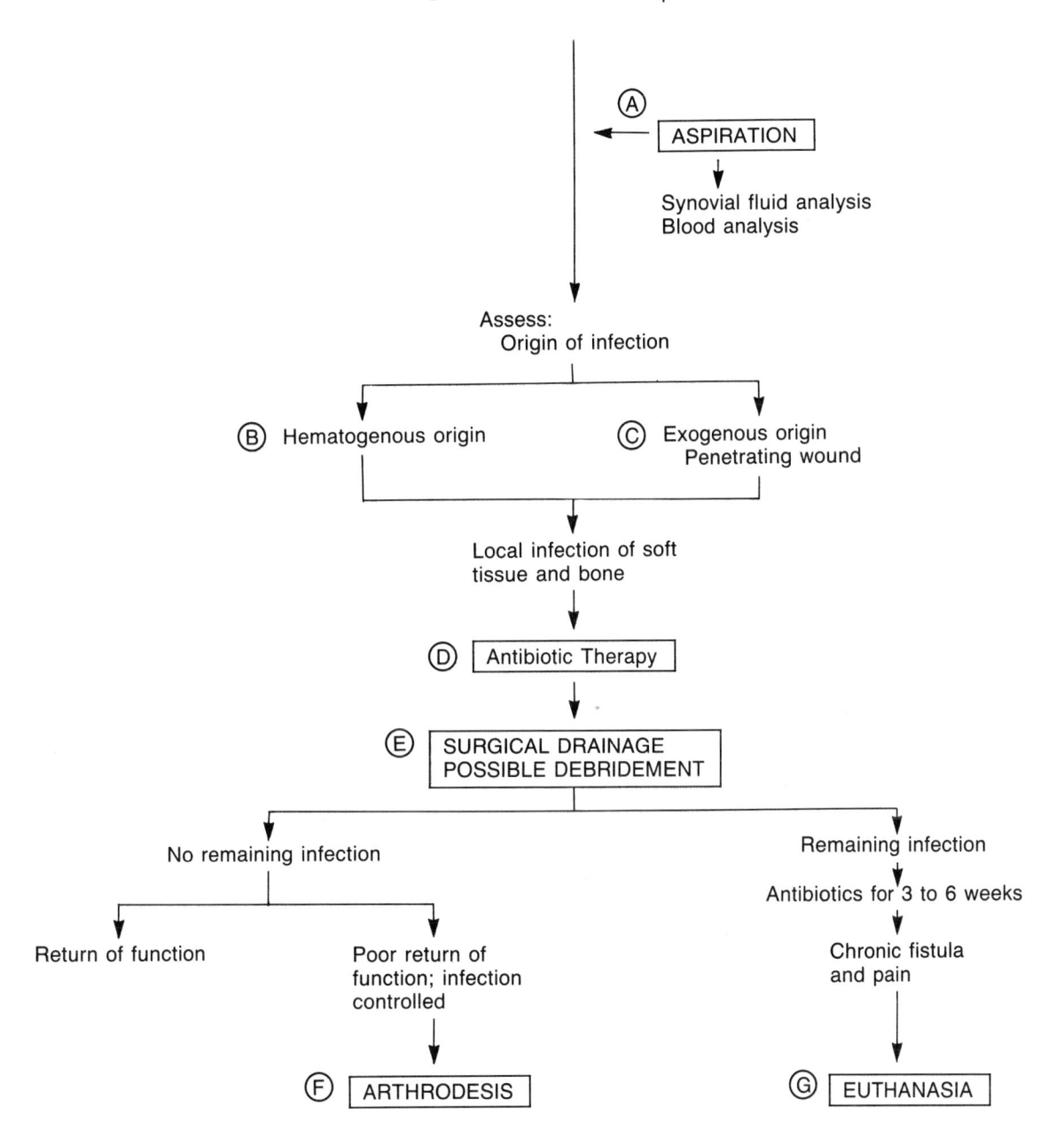

- Ⓐ **ASPIRATION**
  - Synovial fluid analysis
  - Blood analysis
- Assess: Origin of infection
  - Ⓑ Hematogenous origin
  - Ⓒ Exogenous origin / Penetrating wound
- Local infection of soft tissue and bone
- Ⓓ **Antibiotic Therapy**
- Ⓔ **SURGICAL DRAINAGE POSSIBLE DEBRIDEMENT**
  - No remaining infection
    - Return of function
    - Poor return of function; infection controlled
      - Ⓕ **ARTHRODESIS**
  - Remaining infection
    - Antibiotics for 3 to 6 weeks
    - Chronic fistula and pain
      - Ⓖ **EUTHANASIA**

IMMUNE-MEDIATED ARTHRITIS

Craig W. Miller

A. A thorough history should be recorded in all cases of suspected joint disorder. Cyclical episodes of fever that are unresponsive to antibiotic therapy, and which are accompanied by malaise, lameness, or stiffness should alert the clinician to the possibility of immune-mediated arthritis.

B. A complete physical examination is essential in order to recognize immune-mediated joint disease. Multiple joints are often involved, especially distal ones such as the tarsus or carpus. However, immune-mediated arthridites can involve single joints. The identification of involved joints on physical examination is essential before performing diagnostic radiography and arthrocentesis. Some immune-mediated arthridites, such as systemic lupus erythematosus or chronic infections, are manifestations of systemic disease. A thorough physical examination is necessary in order to detect such abnormalities. Include a complete blood count (CBC) and biochemical profile in the initial examination.

C. Synovial fluid analysis of affected joints is necessary in order to identify immune-mediated arthridites. These arthridites are classified as noninfectious inflammatory diseases. The characteristic changes in synovial fluid include an increased number of inflammatory cells, especially nondegenerative neutrophils. It is often not possible to distinguish between the various immune-mediated joint diseases based on routine synovial fluid analysis. Lupus erythematosus (LE) cells are an inconsistent finding in the synovial fluid of dogs that are affected with systemic lupus erythematosus (SLE). Ragocytes, as described in human patients with rheumatoid arthritis, are not definitively described in dogs.

D. Employ radiographs, synovial biopsy, and immune serologic tests in order to distinguish between erosive and nonerosive arthritis. Radiographic changes associated with erosive arthritis include soft tissue swelling and progressive destruction of subchondral bone, both centrally and peripherally, in the affected joint. Nonerosive diseases usually exhibit little to no radiographic changes in the articular cartilage. Synovial biopsy can be performed by arthrotomy or under arthroscopic control. The characteristic pathologic lesions of erosive arthritis consist of villous hyperplasia of the synovial membrane, dense lymphocytic and plasmacytic infiltrates of the synovial membrane, and marginal articular erosion. The nonerosive forms of arthritis usually demonstrate a mild mononuclear cell infiltrate with a more pronounced superficial polymorphonuclear cell infiltrate. Villous hyperplasia and marginal articular erosions are not prominent features. Immune serologic tests include rheumatoid factor, antinuclear antibody, and LE cell preparations. Rheumatoid factor is present in only about 25 percent of cases of canine erosive arthritis; thus, in contrast to human patients, it is not considered a contributory test. The presence of antinuclear antibody is suggestive of systemic lupus erythematosus, and other body organs such as the kidneys and skin should be carefully evaluated for concurrent disease. The presence of LE cells in synovial fluid or peripheral blood is also suggestive of systemic lupus, but it is much less consistent than ANA.

E. Aspirin seems to have little therapeutic impact on cases of canine rheumatoid-like arthritis. Steroids often result in a short-term improvement. The most consistent results are seen after treatment with a combination of prednisolone, cyclophosphamide, and azothioprine.

F. Occasionally severe deformity may necessitate arthrodesis of one or possibly two joints. Arthrodesis is not advised if there is a generally poor response to therapy or if more than two joints require fusion.

G. The arthritis associated with systemic lupus erythematosus is usually steroid responsive. Systemic lupus erythematosus is a polysystemic immunologic disease with many possible manifestations. Besides causing a nonerosive arthritis, SLE can be expressed as hematologic disorders, glomerulonephritis, dermal lesions, or other less common findings. Routine hematologic and biochemical tests are variable in cases of SLE, depending upon organ involvement. The presence of antinuclear antibody is the immunologic test most widely used at present. As some cases may test ANA negative, the presence of characteristic multisystem involvement even with a negative ANA is strongly suggestive of SLE. Corticosteroids are used to treat the arthritis caused by SLE. Refractory cases are treated with a combination of steroids, cytotoxic, and immunosuppressive drugs such as cyclophosphamide and azothioprine.

H. Nonerosive immune-mediated arthritis may be associated with chronic systemic diseases. Though the diseases may differ, the pathogeneses are probably similar. Chronic mycoplasmic, bacterial, or fungal infections have been associated with joint disorders in dogs. The management of these diseases entails treating the underlying disease. Steroids may improve the inflammatory joint manifestations, but they should be avoided if there is an underlying infectious etiology.

I. Idiopathic immune-mediated arthritis is the most common of the nonerosive arthridites. The disease is termed idiopathic after underlying systemic diseases such as chronic infections or systemic lupus erythematosus have been ruled out. This disease is classically manifested as cyclical fever, malaise, anorexia, and lameness or stiffness. The disease most commonly involves several joints. The distal joints (carpus, tarsus) are most frequently involved, but if the disease is monoarticular, the elbow is most often affected. The treatment of choice is cor-

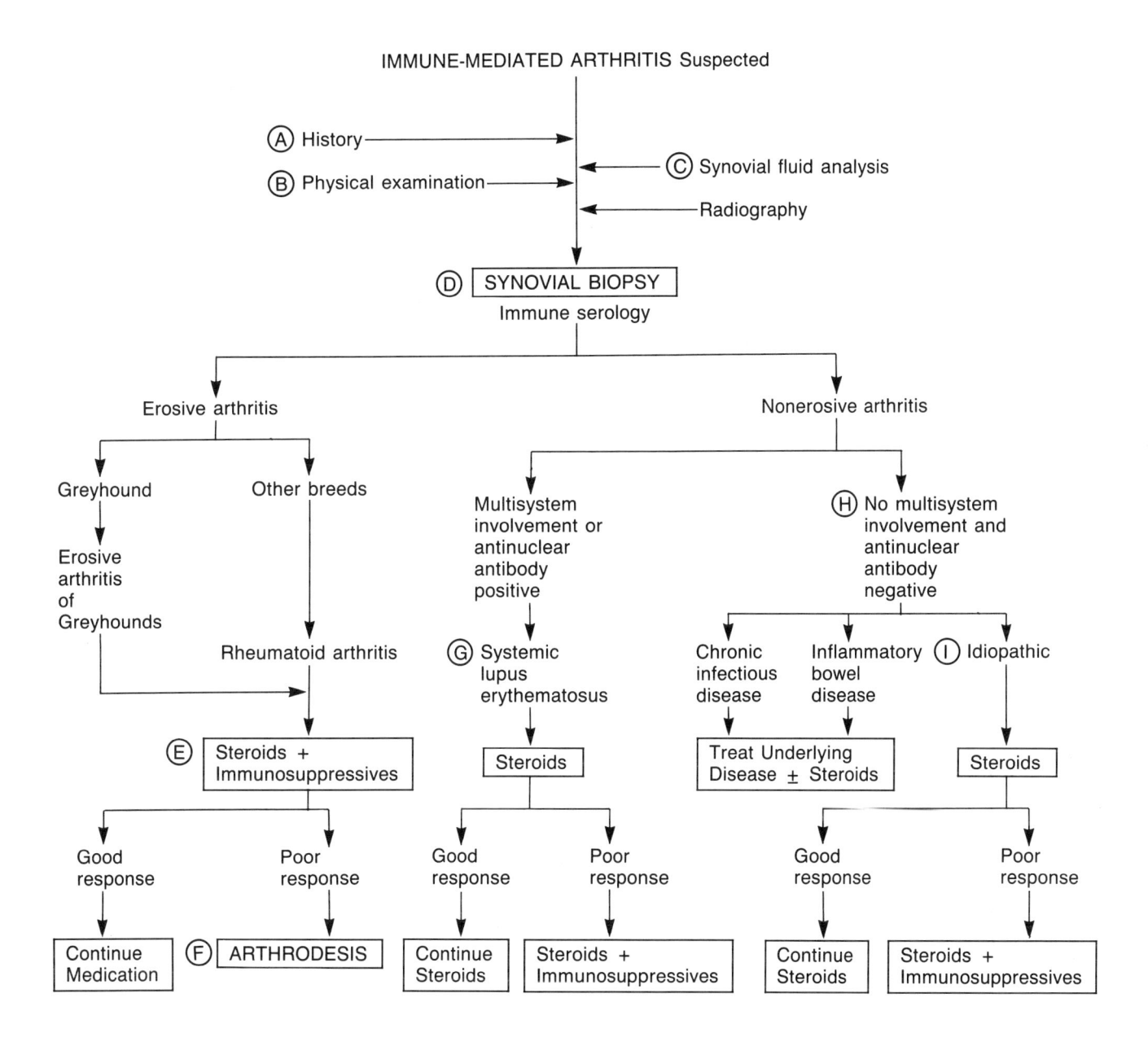

IMMUNE-MEDIATED ARTHRITIS Suspected

- (A) History
- (B) Physical examination
- (C) Synovial fluid analysis
- Radiography

(D) **SYNOVIAL BIOPSY**
Immune serology

Erosive arthritis

- **Greyhound** → Erosive arthritis of Greyhounds
- **Other breeds** → Rheumatoid arthritis

(E) **Steroids + Immunosuppressives**
- Good response → Continue Medication
- Poor response → (F) **ARTHRODESIS**

Nonerosive arthritis

Multisystem involvement or antinuclear antibody positive
- (G) Systemic lupus erythematosus → **Steroids**
  - Good response → Continue Steroids
  - Poor response → Steroids + Immunosuppressives

(H) **No multisystem involvement and antinuclear antibody negative**
- Chronic infectious disease
- Inflammatory bowel disease
  → Treat Underlying Disease ± Steroids
- (I) Idiopathic → **Steroids**
  - Good response → Continue Steroids
  - Poor response → Steroids + Immunosuppressives

---

ticosteroids, which often give dramatic clinical relief. If the response to treatment is poor, more powerful immunosuppressive drugs such as azothioprine can be added. Approximately 30 to 50 percent of dogs have clinical recurrence after medication is discontinued.

References

Pedersen NC, Pool RR, O'Brien TR. Naturally occurring arthropathies of animals. In: Resnick D, Niwayama G, eds. Diagnosis of joint disorders, Vol I. Philadelphia: WB Saunders, 1981.

Perman V. Synovial fluid analysis. In: Kaneko JJ, ed. Clinical biochemistry of domestic animals. 3rd ed. New York: Academic Press, 1980:232.

OSTEOCHONDRITIS DISSECANS

Craig W. Miller

A. A thorough history should be a part of every orthopaedic evaluation. Particular points of enquiry should include diet, onset of lameness, and affected litter mates.

B. The physical examination is important in order to isolate the painful joint. Panosteitis, or other orthopaedic problems of young, rapidly growing dogs, can often be differentiated by physical examination. Pain, joint effusion, decreased range of motion, and crepitation are important findings in suspected cases of osteochondritis dissecans (OCD).

C. The diagnosis of OCD is most commonly confirmed by radiographs, although some lesions may be difficult to visualize by means of standard projections. These cases may require multiple oblique views in order to clearly delineate the defect. Contrast arthrography has been reported to demonstrate subchondral defects not visible on plain films. Radiographs of the contralateral joint are useful as osteochondritis dissecans often occurs bilaterally.

D. If clinical lameness is apparent, but radiographs do not reveal a lesion, repeat the physical examination. If the original findings are validated, then several different radiographic views may be used to delineate a lesion. If the further radiographs still do not reveal a lesion, perform an arthroscopic examination of the relevant joint in an attempt to detect osteochondritis dissecans or other joint pathology.

E. Conservative therapy is reserved for cases with small radiographic lesions and minimal clinical signs or for animals that are nearing skeletal maturity and have only mild signs. Lesions in the shoulder that are of less than 1 cm in diameter and less than 3 mm deep have reportedly been managed conservatively with good success. Such animals should also be free of visible "joint mice."

F. Reevaluation at 4 to 6 weeks should demonstrate an improvement in clinical signs and a static or decreased radiographic lesion. If these criteria are not met, surgical intervention is indicated.

G. Most cases of osteochondritis dissecans seen by the veterinarian can be placed in this category. Surgical intervention is indicated in the majority of clinically lame dogs presented with osteochondritis.

H. Surgery in most cases of OCD involves arthrotomy, excision of the undermined cartilage flap, and removal of any cartilage fragments within the joint. The edges of the defect should be made perpendicular to the articular surface. Leave healthy granulating surfaces intact. Curettage or drilling (forage) of the defect should be limited to areas of subchondral eburnation. The prognosis for surgical intervention is best in the shoulder joint. The outcome is less predictable in the elbow and stifle joints. A recent report indicates that surgical intervention in the tibiotarsal joint for osteochondritis dissecans may be contraindicated. The author recommends arthrotomy and flap excision using a caudomedial approach.

I. Young dogs with obvious degenerative joint disease secondary to osteochondritis dissecans may still be helped by arthrotomy and flap excision. The prognosis in such cases must be more guarded than in animals that show minimal degenerative changes.

J. Occasionally a dog may be presented late in the course of the disease with severe degenerative joint disease. It is often impossible to ascertain the etiology, but osteochondritis dissecans may be suspected. Medical management that combines low impact exercise (e.g., swimming) with nonsteroidal anti-inflammatory medication (e.g., aspirin) may benefit the animal.

K. Cases of severe degenerative joint disease that do not respond to medical management may require arthrodesis of the affected joint. This procedure results in loss of function of the joint, but in most cases, the animal is able to use the limb without pain.

References

Lenahan TM, Van Sickle DC. Canine osteochondrosis. In: Newton CD, Nunamaker DM, eds. Textbook of small animal orthopaedics. Philadelphia: JB Lippincott, 1985:981.

Smith MM, Vaseur PB, Morgan JP. Clinical evaluation of dogs after surgical and nonsurgical management of osteochondritis dissecans of the talus. JAVMA 1985; 187:1,31.

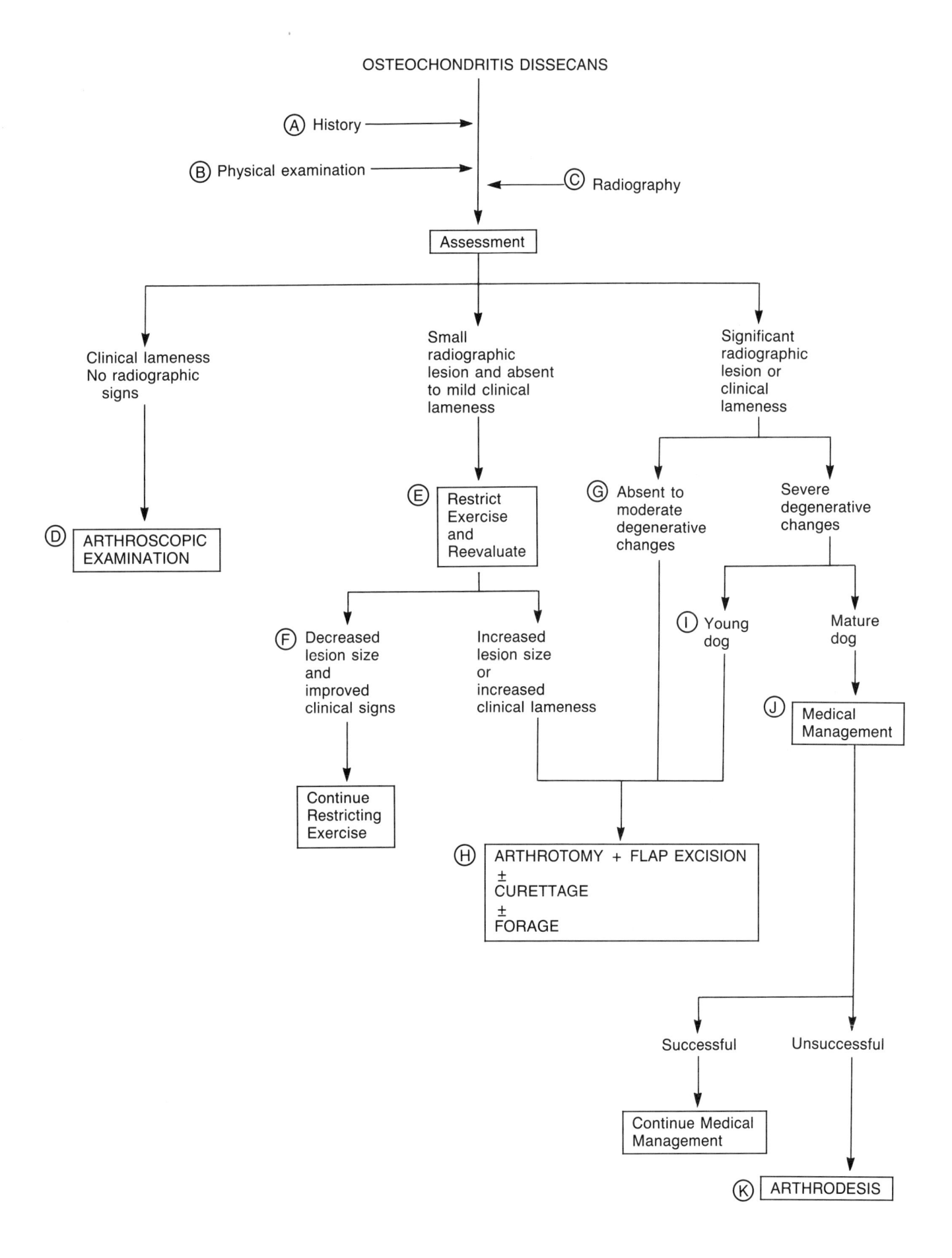

OSTEOCHONDRITIS DISSECANS

- (A) History
- (B) Physical examination
- (C) Radiography

↓

Assessment

- **Clinical lameness, No radiographic signs**
  - (D) ARTHROSCOPIC EXAMINATION

- **Small radiographic lesion and absent to mild clinical lameness**
  - (E) Restrict Exercise and Reevaluate
    - (F) Decreased lesion size and improved clinical signs → Continue Restricting Exercise
    - Increased lesion size or increased clinical lameness → (H) ARTHROTOMY + FLAP EXCISION ± CURETTAGE ± FORAGE

- **Significant radiographic lesion or clinical lameness**
  - (G) Absent to moderate degenerative changes → (H) ARTHROTOMY + FLAP EXCISION ± CURETTAGE ± FORAGE
  - Severe degenerative changes
    - (I) Young dog → (H) ARTHROTOMY + FLAP EXCISION ± CURETTAGE ± FORAGE
    - Mature dog → (J) Medical Management
      - Successful → Continue Medical Management
      - Unsuccessful → (K) ARTHRODESIS

25

PRINCIPLES OF FRACTURE MANAGEMENT

Geoff Sumner-Smith

A. Most fractures and luxations are not in themselves life-threatening. The establishment of a patent airway, control of hemorrhage, and preservation of tissue perfusion take precedence over the stabilization of fractures and luxations. The blood loss into areas of large muscular mass may constitute up to 40 percent of an animal's normal circulatory volume; fractures of the pelvis or mandible may sever major vessels with consequent exsanguination of the patient if hemorrhage is not controlled. The amount of blood lost through an open fracture before presentation cannot be directly assessed but may be estimated during a general examination by monitoring blood pressure and capillary refill time.

B. The degree and severity of damage to soft tissue has a marked bearing on the treatment regimen implemented. It is often difficult to establish whether or not a fracture is compound without a very detailed examination; even very small puncture wounds should alert the veterinarian to a diagnosis of compound (open) fracture. When evaluating soft tissue, pay specific attention to the blood supply to more distal segments. An assessment of the neurologic competence of the body distal to the fracture significantly affects the choice of treatment. An initial negative neurologic evaluation of a distal segment should not be taken as unequivocal. Reassessment at 12-hour intervals sometimes shows return of nerve integrity to an area that previously showed a negative response.

C. Proper splinting of an animal is only possible below the elbow and below the stifle; however, the upper limb may be splinted against the trunk. Some immobilization of the neck and trunk, by splinting, prevents further damage to soft tissues. Displacement fractures should not be manipulated before radiographic examination, unless there are muscular or neuromuscular complications that require immediate correction.

D. When the patient is suitably stabilized, definitive radiography, in a minimum of two planes, enables a full assessment of the fracture. Before taking nonstandard radiographs in various positions, the dangers inherent in such situations should be assessed and the risk appreciated. Further damage to surrounding tissue increases the risk to the patient.

E. In an open fracture following the removal of gross contamination (preferably by irrigation), debridement of the whole area is essential. Judgement may require that this procedure be delayed for 24 hours. This will include an assessment of the animal's catabolic state and ability to withstand the onslaught of surgery. Nevertheless, when it is indicated, it should be meticulous and ensure that only viable tissue remains. Meanwhile, high doses of broad-spectrum antibiotics should be administered parenterally.

F. The "proper" regimen of treatment for a fracture depends on many factors. In veterinary orthopaedics, these include: the competence of the surgeon, the availability of instrumentation, and the owner's ability to fund the procedure. It is preferable that a case be referred to a competent specialist rather than have the animal receive less than ideal treatment.

References

Brinker WO, Hohn RB, Prieur WD. Manual of internal fixation in small animals. New York: Springer-Verlag, 1984:85.

Brinker WO, Piermattei DL, Flo GL. Handbook of small animal orthopedics and fracture treatment. Philadelphia: WB Saunders, 1983:2.

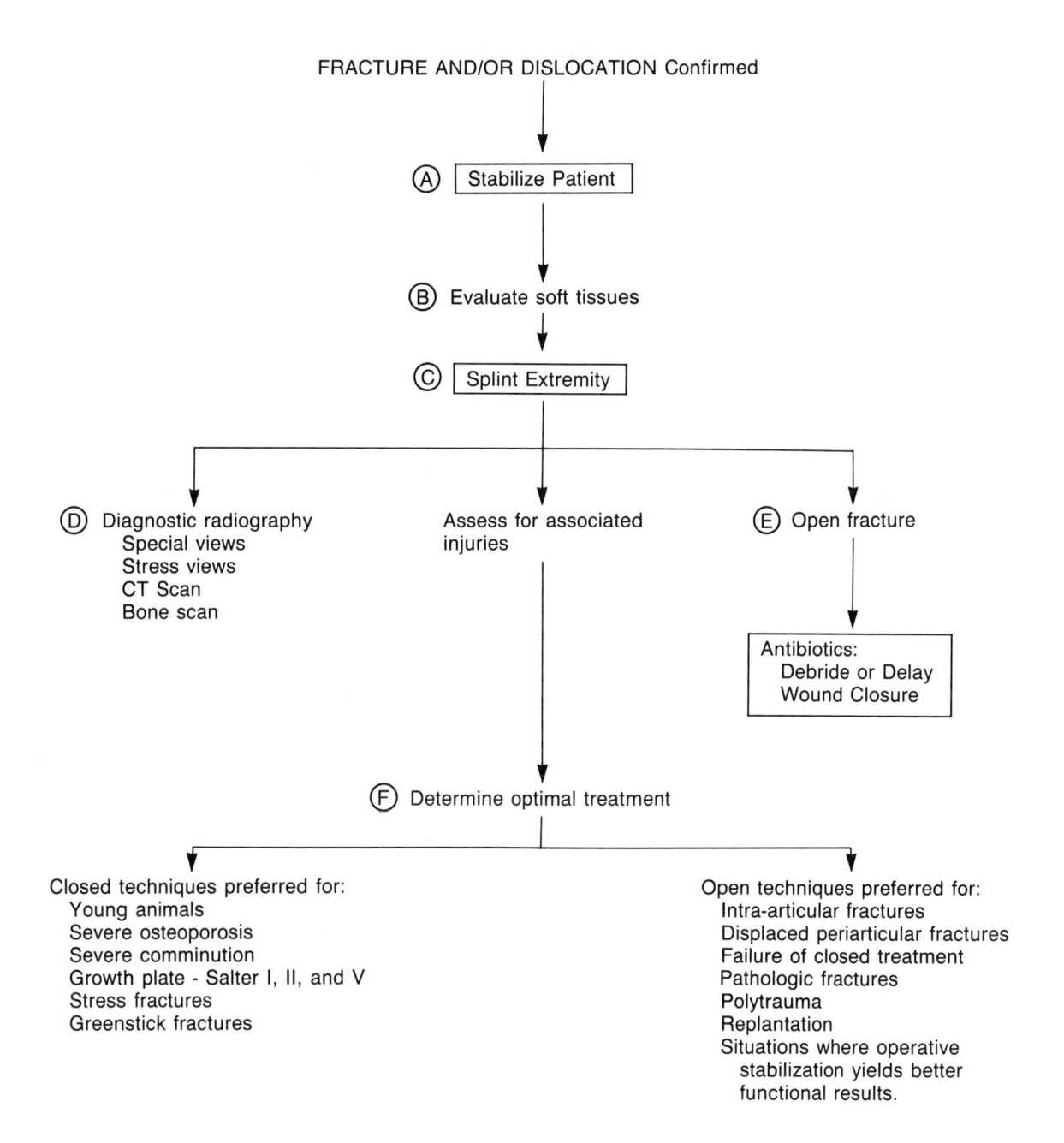

FRACTURE AND/OR DISLOCATION Confirmed
↓
(A) Stabilize Patient
↓
(B) Evaluate soft tissues
↓
(C) Splint Extremity
↓

- (D) Diagnostic radiography
  - Special views
  - Stress views
  - CT Scan
  - Bone scan
- Assess for associated injuries
- (E) Open fracture
  ↓
  Antibiotics:
  Debride or Delay
  Wound Closure

↓
(F) Determine optimal treatment

Closed techniques preferred for:
- Young animals
- Severe osteoporosis
- Severe comminution
- Growth plate - Salter I, II, and V
- Stress fractures
- Greenstick fractures

Open techniques preferred for:
- Intra-articular fractures
- Displaced periarticular fractures
- Failure of closed treatment
- Pathologic fractures
- Polytrauma
- Replantation
- Situations where operative stabilization yields better functional results.

FRACTURE SUSPECTED IN IMMATURE ANIMALS

Geoff Sumner-Smith

Fractures in the immature animal present the following problems not seen in the adult: (1) presence of a growth plate; (2) presence of growth plate "scar-line", dense growth line, secondary centers of ossification, and large nutrient foramina; any of which may confuse the radiographic diagnosis of a fracture; (3) incomplete fractures ("greenstick") which may occur because of the elasticity and plasticity of juvenile bone; (4) the very rapid healing that occurs following fracture and the ability of the bone to remodel so much while it is still young; (5) the frequency of occurrence, which is possibly more common than appreciated; (6) stronger and more active periosteum; (7) special problems in diagnosis, e.g., possible disappearance of lameness after a few days and less tolerance of major blood loss; (8) reaction of bone to compromised blood supply, e.g., decreased bone formation. Although immobilization of the fracture is normally necessary, one must also take into account that the bone is literally changing shape daily. Growth occurs at the growth plate, longitudinally, circumferentially, appositionally, in the epiphysis, and within the articular surface. In treating these fractures it is therefore necessary to bear in mind that these growth areas should not be compromised by the methods employed to stabilize the fracture while it heals.

A. In young animals a fracture may well stimulate local appositional growth and this must be borne in mind. If the fracture is "complete" the stimulation is usually circumferential and results in lengthening of the bone. If the fracture is "incomplete" resulting stimulation may result in malalignment of the limb. Because of the very rapid growth that occurs in young animals it is advisable to take frequent radiographs to monitor the healing pattern of the fracture.

B. Greenstick fractures are incomplete fractures where only one side of the cortex is fractured, the opposing cortex bending. Alternatively, just the outer surface of the cortex is affected and the endosteal surface bends. The conversion of a greenstick fracture to a "complete" fracture is a matter of judgment. A torus fracture is an incomplete fracture with buckling of the cortex, the result of impaction of the bone.

C. If there is minimal or no displacement, the animal is able to bear weight and has no deformity; rest and restriction of movement by cage confinement are usually adequate treatments.

D. Diaphyseal fractures, below the elbow or stifle may be treated by splinting, special bandages, or casts of various materials. Above those two joints conservative treatment may suffice. Occasionally internal fixation is required.

E. Internal fixation of incomplete fractures is rarely necessary, although subsequent treatment of growth plate injuries may require surgery (p 30).

F. Complete fracture of any bone in the immature skeleton may occur. Although the diagnosis and signs of the fracture in the immature skeleton differ little from those in the mature skeleton, the treatment may be different due to associated effects on further growth (p 32).

G. Knowledge of the normal commencement and conclusion periods of growth plate closure is mandatory in dealing with fractures through the growth plate (see Table 1). Although treatment of such fractures or dislocations is dealt with on p 30, reference here is made to the classification of such fractures according to the Salter-Harris terminology: Type I - displacement of the epiphysis, Type II - displacement of the epiphysis plus fracture of the metaphysis, Type III - fractures through the epiphysis to the growth plate, Type IV - fractures through the epiphysis and metaphysis, Type V - compression of the growth plate (see p 30, Fig. 1). Fracture stabilization devices must not restrict normal growth at the plate. Even if a growth plate is closed, appositional growth continues in the epiphysis. Consequently, any restricting device may bring about an alteration in the configuration in the epiphysis with a consequent malalignment of the articular surface that is reflected in the apposing articular surface.

H. Diaphyseal fractures may be quite simple to treat or may present the orthopaedist with many unexpected complications because of the continuing growth of the bone. Before embarking on a treatment regimen, the clinician should be cognizant of the following factors: (1) Longitudinal growth must not be impaired by the devices that are employed. Although very rapid remodeling occurs around devices that are fixed internally, there is slowing of growth on the side that is restricted. Very rapidly growing individuals may have the growth altered by external devices, such as plaster of Paris, with consequent distortion of the limb both at the growth plate and along the diaphysis. (2) Usually circumferential growth is not restricted by the devices used for fixation unless the healing time is particularly prolonged. (3) Appositional growth occurs in both longitudinal and lateral planes as the bone grows in size. Consequently, the comments given under B and C apply here. In young animals the subsequent effect on the joint can be disasterous if meticulous treatment is not followed (see p 32).

I. Multiple fractures, as well as those involving the metaphyses or epiphyses, require internal fixation as do displaced diaphyseal fractures that do not lend themselves to external immobilization, e.g., humerus and femur.

References

Brinker WO, Pierrmattei DL, Flo GL, eds. Handbook of small animal orthopedics and fracture treatment. Philadelphia: WB Saunders, 1983:195.

Sumner-Smith G. Management of fractures in growing animals. In: Skeletal diseases of growing animals. Perth: Murdoch University Foundation for Continuing Education, 1980:75.

Sumner-Smith G. Observations on epiphyseal fusion of the canine appendicular skeleton. J small Anim Pract 1966; 7:303.

LIMB FRACTURE IN IMMATURE ANIMALS

- Ⓐ History
- Radiography
- Physical examination
  - Lame on a particular limb
    - Partial weight-bearing
    - Unable to bear weight

- Ⓑ Incomplete fracture
  - Greenstick fracture
  - Torus fracture
  - Ⓒ Conservative Measures
  - Ⓓ External Immobilization
  - Ⓔ INTERNAL FIXATION

- Ⓕ Complete fracture
  - Ⓖ Fractures involving a growth plate (p 30)
    - Ⓓ External Immobilization
  - Ⓗ Intra-articular fracture (p 32)
  - Ⓘ INTERNAL FIXATION

TABLE 1 Summary of the Handling of Fractures in Young Animals

Goals	External Devices	Pin Splints	Internal Devices
To maintain apposition during healing	Plaster of Paris cast	External fixators (various models)	IM Pin
To allow joint movement during or after healing	Plastersplints		Multiple pinning
To avoid compromise of soft tissue	Splints (wooden and metal)		Rush pins
Toleration of treatment	Moldable plastics		Cross pins
Minimal aftercare	Aire-cast		Screws
Economical treatment	Thomas splint		Plates
	Robert Jones bandage		
	Lennox bandage		

FRACTURE IN THE YOUNG ANIMAL INVOLVING A GROWTH PLATE

Geoff Sumner-Smith

These fractures are usually divided into five types as described in the Salter-Harris classification (Fig. 1).

A. The Type I fracture shows separation through the growth plate with displacement of the epiphysis. Sites commonly involved are: the proximal humerus, proximal femur (caput), and the distal femur. Usually a form of cross-pinning is suitable for treatment of this displacement, provided that reduction has been achieved. If treated soon after the trauma, prognosis is good.

B. The Type II fracture is the same as Type I, but additionally incorporates a small portion of the metaphysis. Sites commonly involved are: the proximal humerus, distal femur, and proximal tibia. Provided they are treated early, these fractures also carry a good prognosis. Following reduction, cross-pinning of these fractures is usually satisfactory, but in very large animals, it is preferable and desirable to lag-screw the metaphyseal portion.

C. In the Type III fracture, the fracture extends into the joint, but does not involve the metaphysis. Part of the growth plate is also involved. Occasionally the epiphysis may separate into two fragments with both separated from the metaphysis through the growth plate. The distal humerus, distal femur, and distal tibia are sites where this type of fracture may occur. As the joint surface is involved, special attention to replacement of joint congruity is mandatory; otherwise, subsequent arthritis and malwear readily occur. Cross-pinning is usually a suitable method of treatment, but in order to obtain proper stability, it may be employed when the epiphysis is in two separate pieces. A lag screw, either above or preferably with an additional Kirschner wire, must be used to join the two together. It should be appreciated that a growth plate is positioned between the two condyles of the distal humerus, which will not be severely compromised if the animal is more than 18 weeks of age.

D. The Type IV fracture is virtually a combination of Types II and III. It is most commonly seen in the distal humerus and distal femur. Treatment, by the means described in paragraphs B and C, usually yields a good prognosis. If the fracture is not treated properly at an early age, the prognosis is decidedly poor; severe arthrosis is a direct outcome.

E. The Type V fracture is the most difficult to diagnose and treat in the early stages. It is virtually a compression of the growth plate with resultant damage to the activity of the osteoblasts in the formation of growing bone. Growth is irregular and, depending on the natural loading of the limb, growth plate closure occurs with subsequent deviation, which is usually of the valgus. Type V fracture is commonly seen in the distal femur or proximal tibia, but is even more common in the distal radius and/or ulna; severe deformities may result. For treatment see limb deformities (p 32). In young animals, if damage to the limbs is not diagnosed at the initial examination, it is essential to advise the owner that damage may have occurred and will show itself subsequently. The condition requires treatment as soon as it is observed. The golden rule in the treatment of these fractures is to avoid further compromise of the growth plate. Consequently, compression by restrictive devices of any sort (i.e., screws, plates) should not be used to span this area.

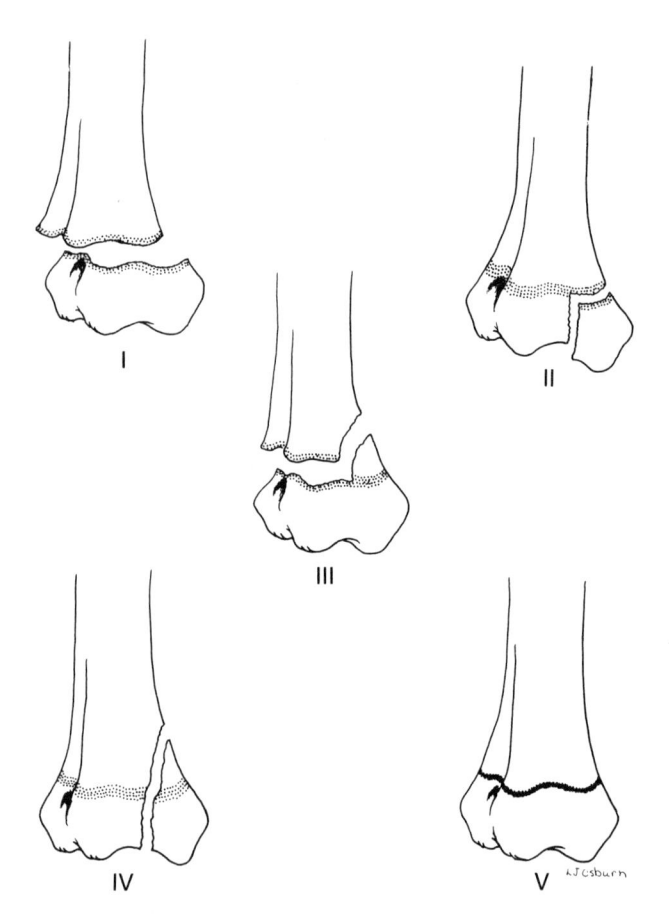

Figure 1 Salter-Harris classification of growth plate injuries.

References

Brinker WO, Piermattei DL, Flo GL. Handbook of small animal orthopedics and fracture treatment. Philadelphia: WB Saunders, 1983:195.

Sumner-Smith G. Management of fractures in growing animals. In: Skeletal diseases of growing animals. Perth: Murdoch University Foundation for Continuing Education, 1980:75.

Sumner-Smith G. Observations in epiphyseal fusion of the canine appendicular skeleton. J small Anim Pract, 1966; 7:303.

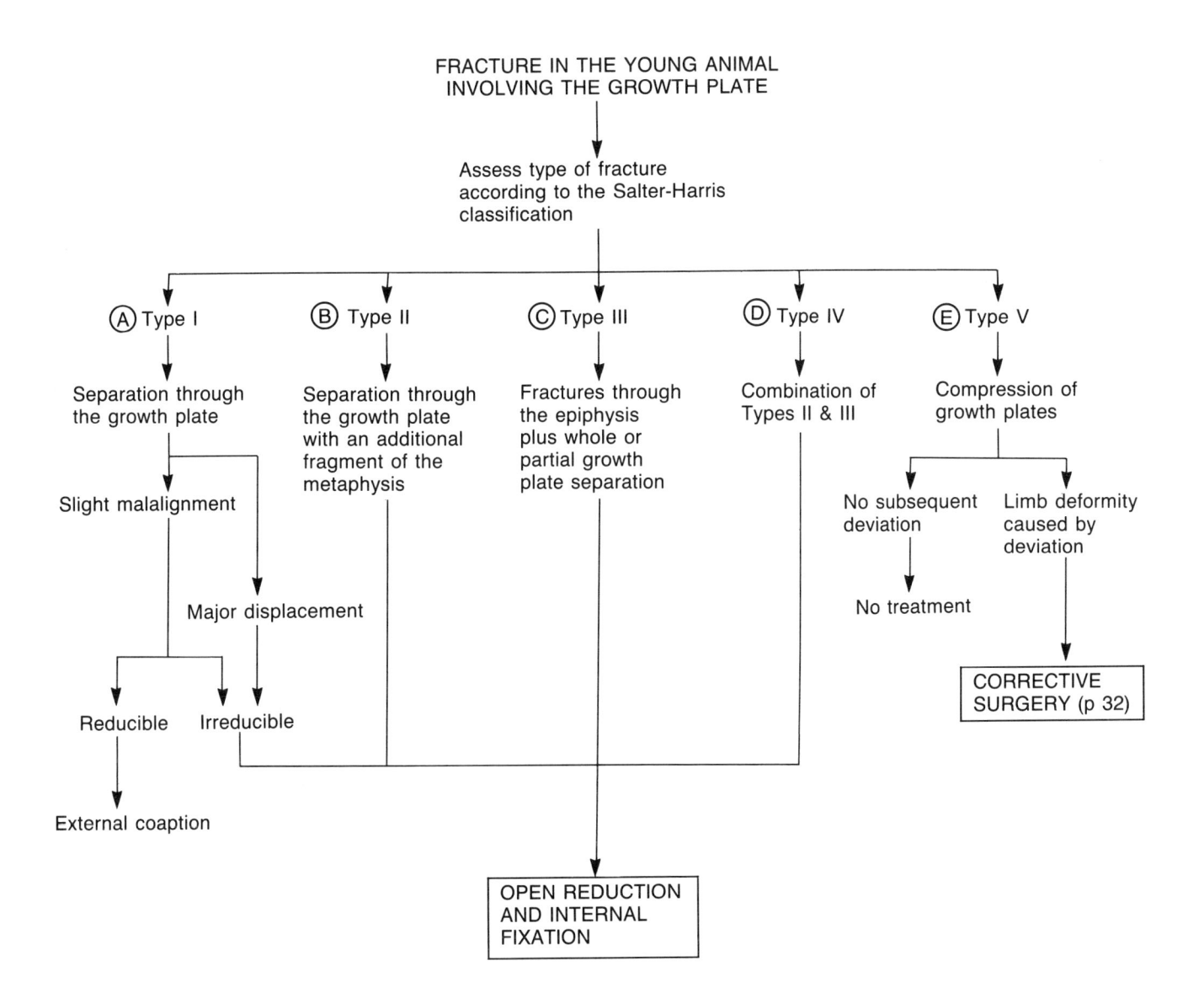

```
                    FRACTURE IN THE YOUNG ANIMAL
                    INVOLVING THE GROWTH PLATE
                                │
                                ▼
                    Assess type of fracture
                    according to the Salter-Harris
                    classification
                                │
    ┌───────────────┬───────────┼───────────┬───────────────┐
    ▼               ▼           ▼           ▼               ▼
 (A) Type I    (B) Type II  (C) Type III (D) Type IV   (E) Type V
```

(A) Type I — Separation through the growth plate
- Slight malalignment
  - Reducible → External coaption
  - Irreducible → OPEN REDUCTION AND INTERNAL FIXATION
- Major displacement → OPEN REDUCTION AND INTERNAL FIXATION

(B) Type II — Separation through the growth plate with an additional fragment of the metaphysis → OPEN REDUCTION AND INTERNAL FIXATION

(C) Type III — Fractures through the epiphysis plus whole or partial growth plate separation → OPEN REDUCTION AND INTERNAL FIXATION

(D) Type IV — Combination of Types II & III → OPEN REDUCTION AND INTERNAL FIXATION

(E) Type V — Compression of growth plates
- No subsequent deviation → No treatment
- Limb deformity caused by deviation → CORRECTIVE SURGERY (p 32)

LIMB DEVIATION CAUSED BY GROWTH PLATE INJURY AND PREMATURE CLOSURE

Geoff Sumner-Smith

A knowledge of the normal growth plate closure time is necessary before attempting to treat these conditions.

A. Premature closure of the proximal radius growth plate results in a shortening of the radius with a subsequent increase in the joint space between the condyles of the humerus and the radial head. A looseness develops, which can lead to degenerative arthrosis and a crippling lameness. An opening osteotomy of the radius is performed in order to bring the radial head into articulation with the humerus and is kept open by means of a suitable plate. In patients that are very young, the remaining growth in the distal radius may be such that a subsequent opening osteotomy is required.

B. In early cases of partial or total premature closure of the distal radius growth plate, spanning of the growth plate from the medial side by either one or two staples may suffice. In more advanced cases, or when little growth remains, a corrective osteotomy is required.

C. Premature closure of the distal ulna growth plate and/or
D. partial closure of the distal radius growth plate can result in lameness and severe deformities of both the radius and the ulna. In early cases, ulnar ostectomy that removes at least 1 cm from the proximal mid-third of the ulna frees the restrictive effect of the ulna and, if this is combined with stapling of the medial side of the radial growth plate, may suffice to realign the limb. In older cases when little growth remains, it is necessary to combine the ulnar ostectomy with corrective wedge osteotomy of the radius. Either plates or an external fixator may be employed for subsequent stabilization.

E. Partial premature closure of the distal femur growth plate is not common. Because of the small size of the distal femoral fragment that results from the osteotomy, a T-plate or reconstruction plate allows the insertion of sufficient screws to stabilize the area. Cancellous bone may be harvested from the proximal tibia to fill the gap, but if the latter is large, a wedge should be taken from the iliac crest.

F. In the case of partial premature closure of proximal tibial growth plate with valgus deviations, according to the amount of bone that remains in the proximal segment following the osteotomy, a "T-", "L-", or hook plate may be employed to acquire adequate stability. An external fixator is not recommended. A table of growth plate closure times appears in Appendix II.

References

Brinker WO, Piermattei DL, Flo GL. Handbook of small animal orthopedics and fracture treatment. Philadelphia: WB Saunders, 1983:202.

Leger L, Sumner-Smith G, Gofton N, Prieur WD. A.O. hook plate fixation for metaphyseal fractures and corrective wedge osteotomies. J small Anim Pract 1982; 23:209.

LIMB DEVIATIONS CAUSED BY GROWTH PLATE INJURY*

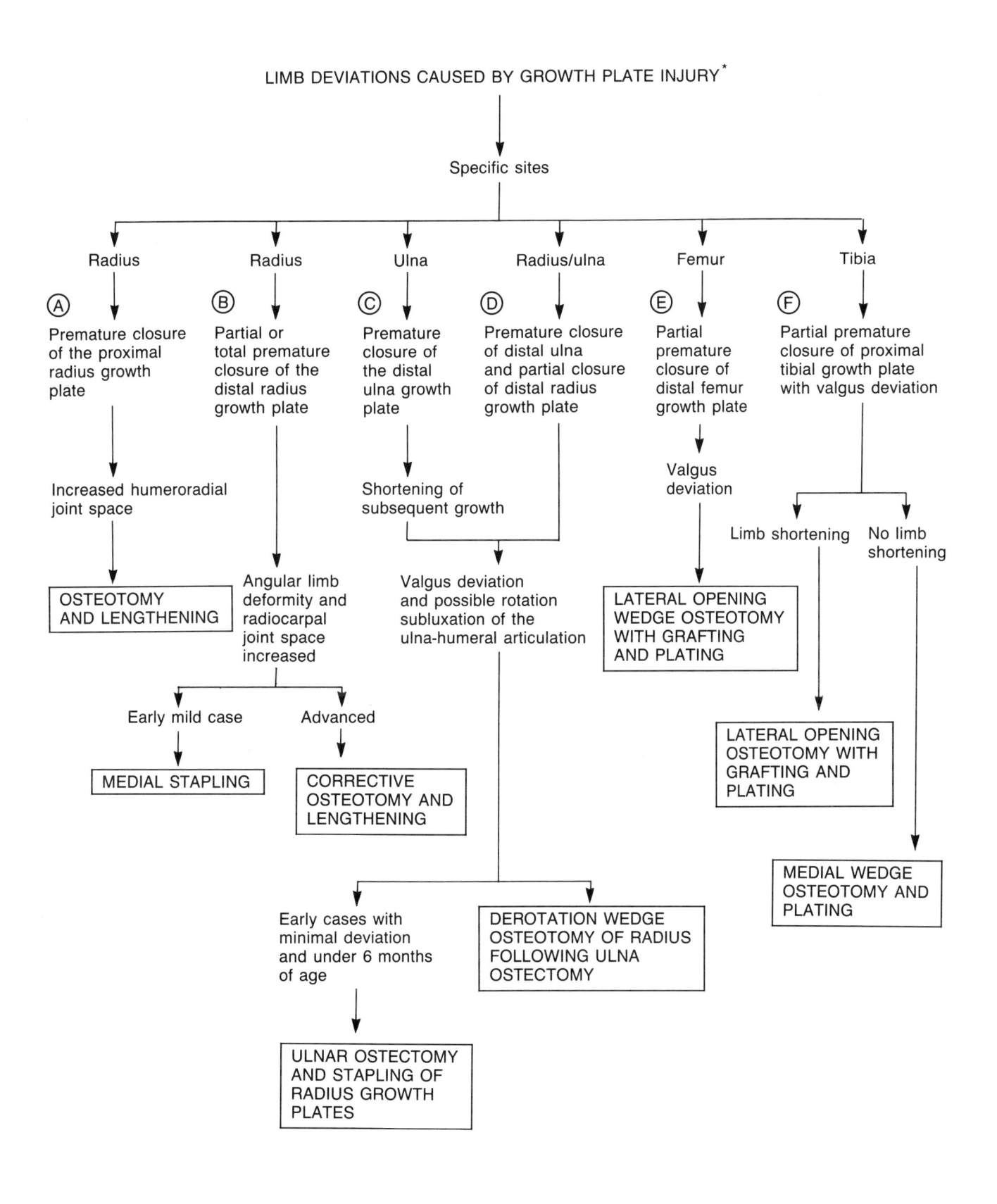

```
                                    Specific sites
                                          │
        ┌──────────┬──────────┬──────────┼──────────┬──────────┐
       Radius     Radius      Ulna    Radius/ulna   Femur      Tibia
        (A)        (B)        (C)       (D)         (E)        (F)
```

(A) Premature closure of the proximal radius growth plate → Increased humeroradial joint space → **OSTEOTOMY AND LENGTHENING**

(B) Partial or total premature closure of the distal radius growth plate → Angular limb deformity and radiocarpal joint space increased
- Early mild case → **MEDIAL STAPLING**
- Advanced → **CORRECTIVE OSTEOTOMY AND LENGTHENING**

(C) Premature closure of the distal ulna growth plate → Shortening of subsequent growth

(D) Premature closure of distal ulna and partial closure of distal radius growth plate → Valgus deviation and possible rotation subluxation of the ulna-humeral articulation
- Early cases with minimal deviation and under 6 months of age → **ULNAR OSTECTOMY AND STAPLING OF RADIUS GROWTH PLATES**
- **DEROTATION WEDGE OSTEOTOMY OF RADIUS FOLLOWING ULNA OSTECTOMY**

(E) Partial premature closure of distal femur growth plate → Valgus deviation → **LATERAL OPENING WEDGE OSTEOTOMY WITH GRAFTING AND PLATING**

(F) Partial premature closure of proximal tibial growth plate with valgus deviation
- Limb shortening → **LATERAL OPENING OSTEOTOMY WITH GRAFTING AND PLATING**
- No limb shortening → **MEDIAL WEDGE OSTEOTOMY AND PLATING**

*For additional description of types, see p 30.

PATHOLOGIC FRACTURE

Geoff Sumner-Smith

A. Preexisting conditions of the bone may bring about areas of local weakness. However, radiographs may demonstrate either generalized or isolated variations in bone density and structure. Except in educational institutes, the more sophisticated and sensitive techniques of bone scanning are rarely possible.

B. Biopsy of the area under suspicion is mandatory. The tissue removed should be subjected not only to histologic examination but also to culturing to confirm or refute the presence of osteomyelitis. The above techniques may be dispensed with in cases of certain conditions with appearances that are pathognomonic.

C. In young animals, pathologic fracture may be caused by benign osseous conditions such as juvenile osteomalacia. Treatment should be aimed at correcting the skeletal condition in order to allow the fracture to heal normally. Until proved otherwise, lesions in the mature animal should always be considered malignant. Benign dense lesions in mature bone, osteoma, may contribute to fracture at the periphery precipitated by sudden changes in the stiffness of the bone and the consequent production of a stress riser.

D. During histologic examination, the callous of a healing fracture may be mistaken for a primary osteosarcoma; particular care must be taken in obtaining the core sample. The casual orthopaedic oncologist should not attempt to do this, but should refer the case to a specialist who has not only the knowledge, but also the equipment available, for such examinations. Although amputation has long been the alternative to euthanasia, more recent progress has indicated that, in some circumstances, radical excision with attendant chemotherapy may also be attempted.

E. Radical excision in areas previously believed to be inoperable, i.e., the mandible and maxilla, is now quite frequent for both benign and malignant tumors, with most gratifying results. Nevertheless it should be borne in mind that malignant tumors in the canine skeleton are always more fulminating than similar pathologic conditions in the human skeleton. Long-term positive results are unfortunately not as frequent.

F. Apart from the normal osteoporosis of aging, elderly animals suffer from generalized osteoporosis because of sterilization in both males and females; there is no clear evidence that the incidence is more frequent in the female—as is the case in humans. Compression collapsed fracture of the spine or the long bone may occur in patients with osteoporosis or osteomalacia. Fulminating malignant bone neoplasms may be treated by radical excision and massive alografts or by amputation. Internal fixation of the associated fracture and defect is supplied by plates and screws. Defects in the metaphyseal area may be supported by subcortical bone cement.

G. Systemic bone disease in animals requires that the underlying condition be treated at the same time as the fracture receives attention. Delayed healing may be expected in such conditions as secondary nutritional hyperparathyroidism and osteoporosis.

References

Harrington K et al. The use of methylmethacrylate as an adjunct in the internal fixation of malignant neoplastic fractures. J Bone Joint Surg 1972; 54A:1665.

Sumner-Smith G, Waters EH. The adjunctive use of methylmethacrylate in the stabilization of multiple fractures. JAAHA 1976; 12:778.

Stevenson S et al. Fracture associated carcinoma in the dog. JAVMA 1982; 180:1189.

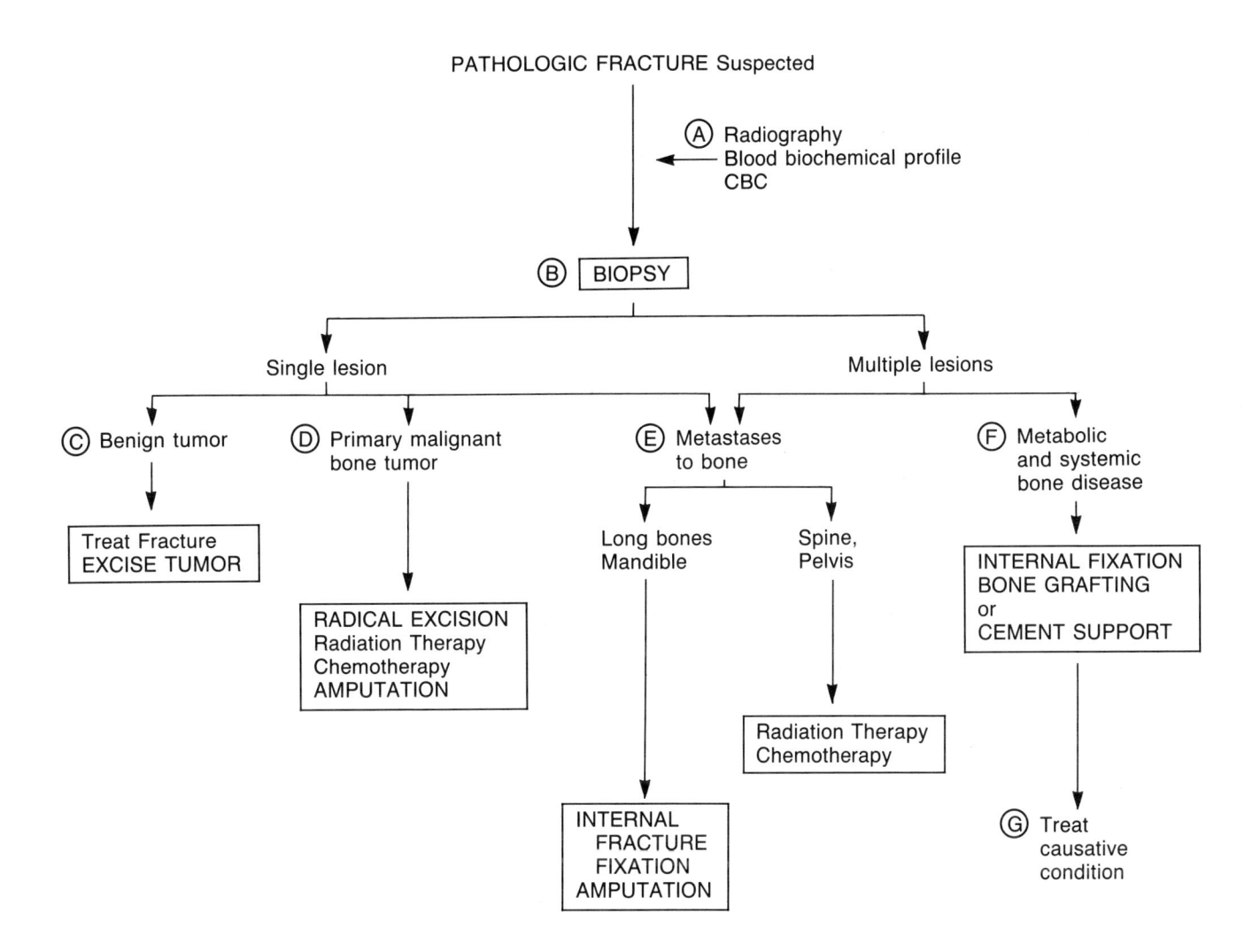

PATHOLOGIC FRACTURE Suspected

- **(A)** Radiography ← Blood biochemical profile, CBC
- **(B)** BIOPSY
  - Single lesion
    - **(C)** Benign tumor → Treat Fracture, EXCISE TUMOR
    - **(D)** Primary malignant bone tumor → RADICAL EXCISION, Radiation Therapy, Chemotherapy, AMPUTATION
    - **(E)** Metastases to bone
      - Long bones, Mandible → INTERNAL FRACTURE FIXATION, AMPUTATION
      - Spine, Pelvis → Radiation Therapy, Chemotherapy
  - Multiple lesions
    - **(E)** Metastases to bone (see above)
    - **(F)** Metabolic and systemic bone disease → INTERNAL FIXATION, BONE GRAFTING or CEMENT SUPPORT → **(G)** Treat causative condition

HEMATOGENOUS OSTEOMYELITIS

Craig W. Miller

A. Hematogenous osteomyelitis is less common in small animals than it is in large animals or man. It is most common in the young animal and originates from embolism of small metaphyseal vessels. Hematogenous osteomyelitis may extend to the nearby joint; this causes a septic arthritis that must be treated promptly and aggressively (Fig. 1). Elicit thorough history in all cases of suspected osteomyelitis. Information such as the type of trauma, time since the initial trauma, and initial treatment are important to the outcome of the case.

B. A thorough physical examination of the entire animal is essential. Rule out pathology of other body systems. The most common physical findings in cases of hematogenous osteomyelitis include fever, localized pain, lameness, and soft tissue swelling.

C. Radiographs are essential in identifying the focus and extent of the problem. Radiographic changes are not evident in the acute stages of osteomyelitis (10 to 14 days). As the disease progresses, one may see radiographic evidence of soft tissue swelling, periosteal elevation (Fig. 2), and bone lysis.

D. Bacterial culture and sensitivity are imperative in the treatment of osteomyelitis. A deep needle aspirate or tissue culture during debridement are often diagnostic. Blood cultures are indicated in cases of acute hematogenous osteomyelitis.

E. Initial treatment of osteomyelitis is ideally based on sensitivity results. Presumptive antibiotic therapy should be instituted if the suspicion of a bacterial etiology is high or if septic arthritis is suspected. Utilize a broad spectrum bacteriocidal antibiotic (e.g., cephalosporin).

F. A poor response to antibiotic therapy after 48 to 72 hours is an indication for surgical decompression and drainage of the medullary canal. This can be accomplished by drilling holes with a Steinman pin. Avoid the growth plate. A small portion of the cortex can be excised, if necessary, in order to establish drainage.

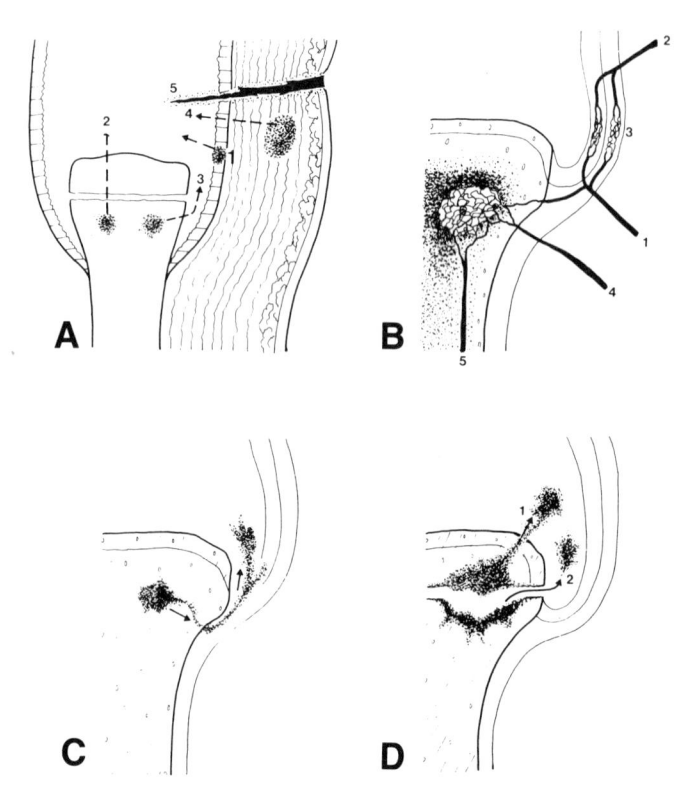

Figure 1 Septic arthritis: potential routes of contamination; A, hematogenous spread of infection to a joint can result from direct lodgement of organisma in the synovial membrane (1) or, as illustrated in B, direct vascular continuity between an infected epiphysis and the synovial membrane. Spread into the joint from a contiguous source can occur from a metaphyseal focus that extends into the epiphysis and from there into the joint (2); from the metaphyseal focus with extension into the joint when the growth plate is intra-articular (3); or from a contiguous soft tissue infection (4). Direct implantation following a penetrating wound (5) can also lead to septic arthritis; B, and C, hematogenous spread of infection to a joint can occur owing to vascular continuity between the epiphysis and the synovial membrane. In B, the vessels shown include arterioles (1), venules (2), and capillaries (3), of the capsule; periosteal vessels (4); the nutrient artery (5); and metaphyseal epiphyseal anastomoses (6). The synovial membrane may become infected from an osseous focus before the joint fluid is contaminated. This sequence of events is diagrammed in C; D, spread from a contiguous osseous surface can result from penetration of the cartilage (1) or pathologic fracture with articular contamination (2). In this situation, synovial fluid may become infected before the synovial membrane. (Redrawn with permission from Resnick D, Niwayama G. Diagnosis of bone and joint disorders. Philadelphia: WB Saunders, 1981.)

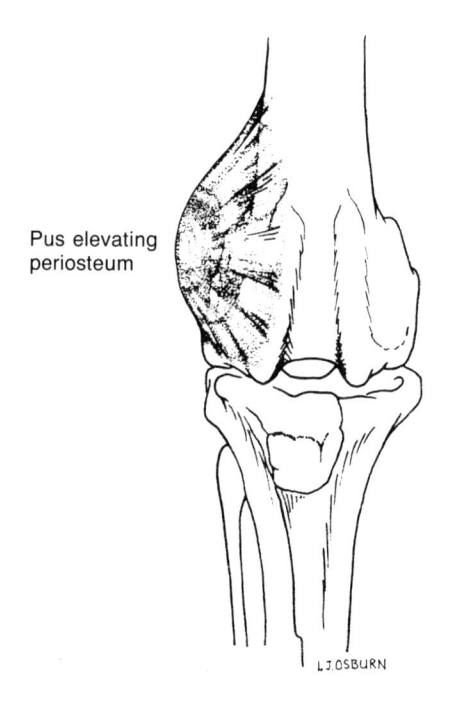

Figure 2 Appearance of a focus of osteomyelitis in a long bone; drawn from a radiograph.

```
                    HEMATOGENOUS
                 BACTERIAL OSTEOMYELITIS Suspected
                              │
         Ⓐ History ──────────→│
                              │
         Ⓑ Physical examination ──→│←── Ⓒ Radiography
                              │
                              │←── Ⓓ Culture and sensitivity
                              │
              ┌───────────────┴───────────────┐
              ↓                               ↓
       No radiographic changes         Radiographic changes
              ↓                               │
         Ⓔ [Antibiotics]                      │
              │                               │
        ┌─────┴─────┐                         │
        ↓           ↓                         │
   Good clinical  Poor clinical               │
   response       response                    │
        ↓           ↓                         │
  ┌──────────┐  ┌──────────────────────┐      │
  │Continue  │  │Ⓕ SURGICAL DECOMPRESSION│←────┘
  │Antibiotics│ │   and                 │
  │for 4 to 6 │ │   Reassess Antibiotics│
  │Weeks     │  └──────────────────────┘
  └──────────┘
```

References

Aron DN. Pathogenesis, diagnosis, and management of osteomyelitis in small animals. Comp Cont Ed 1979; 1:824.

Caywood DD, Wallace LJ, Braden TD. Osteomyelitis in the dog: a review of 67 cases. JAVMA 1978; 173:943.

Holmberg DL. The use of prophylactic penicillin in orthopaedic surgery: a clinical trial. Vet Surg 1985; 14:160.

TRAUMATIC OSTEOMYELITIS

Craig W. Miller

A. Elicit a thorough history in all cases of suspected osteomyelitis. Information such as the type of trauma, time since the initial trauma, and initial treatment are important to the outcome of the case.

B. A thorough physical examination of the entire animal is essential. Rule out pathology of other body systems. Physical examination of the affected part is important in order to assess stability, draining tracts, etc.

C. Radiographs are essential in order to identify the focus and extent of the problem. Plain films can demonstrate sequestered bone fragments, loose implants and fracture stability in the acute stages of osteomyelitis (10 to 14 days). Dye studies (disulphein blue) may delineate the extent of draining tracts. As the disease progresses, one may see radiographic evidence of soft tissue swelling, periosteal elevation, and bone lysis.

D. Bacterial culture and sensitivity are imperative in the treatment of osteomyelitis. However, culture of draining tracts is often unrewarding. Deep needle aspiration or tissue culture during debridement are more often diagnostic.

E. Necrotic, poorly vascularized bone constitutes the primary obstacle when treating osteomyelitis. Successful medical management can only be achieved in a well-vascularized milieu. Thorough debridement, lavage, and the establishment of drainage are probably of greater importance than is antibiotic selection. Excise all unstable necrotic bone, infected soft tissue, blood clots, and excess suture. Perform copious lavage with isotonic or antiseptic (0.05 percent chlorhexidine) fluids. In acute cases of post-traumatic osteomyelitis, adequate drainage can be established by a closed suction apparatus or by open drainage. Initial treatment of osteomyelitis is ideally based on sensitivity results. Presumptive antibiotic therapy should be instituted if the suspicion of a bacterial etiology is high or if septic arthritis is suspected. Utilize a broad-spectrum bacteriocidal antibiotic (e.g., cephalosporin).

F. If the fragments are stable, infected bone can unite and revascularize. However, instability hinders revascularization and favors continued infection. An unstable fracture fixation must be made stable at the time of surgery. Bone plates and external fixators have both been used successfully in the revision of previously unstable fixations. Any significant cortical defect would benefit from an autogenous cancellous graft. In osteomyelitis cases, the graft should be delayed (usually 1 to 2 weeks) in order to provide a more desirable recipient bed.

G. The same principles apply when treating an osteomyelitis of longer duration. Distinct sequestra may be more readily identified and should be removed. Resulting cortical defects can be treated by a delayed cancellous bone graft.

References

Bardet JF, Hohn RB, Basinger R. Open drainage and delayed autogenous cancellous bone grafting for treatment of chronic osteomyelitis in dogs and cats. JAVMA 1983; 183:312.

Daly WR. Orthopaedic infections. In: Slatter DH, ed. Textbook of small animal surgery. Philadelphia: WB Saunders, 1985:2020.

Holmberg DL. The use of prophylactic penicillin in orthopedic surgery: a clinical trial. Vet Surg 1985; 14:160.

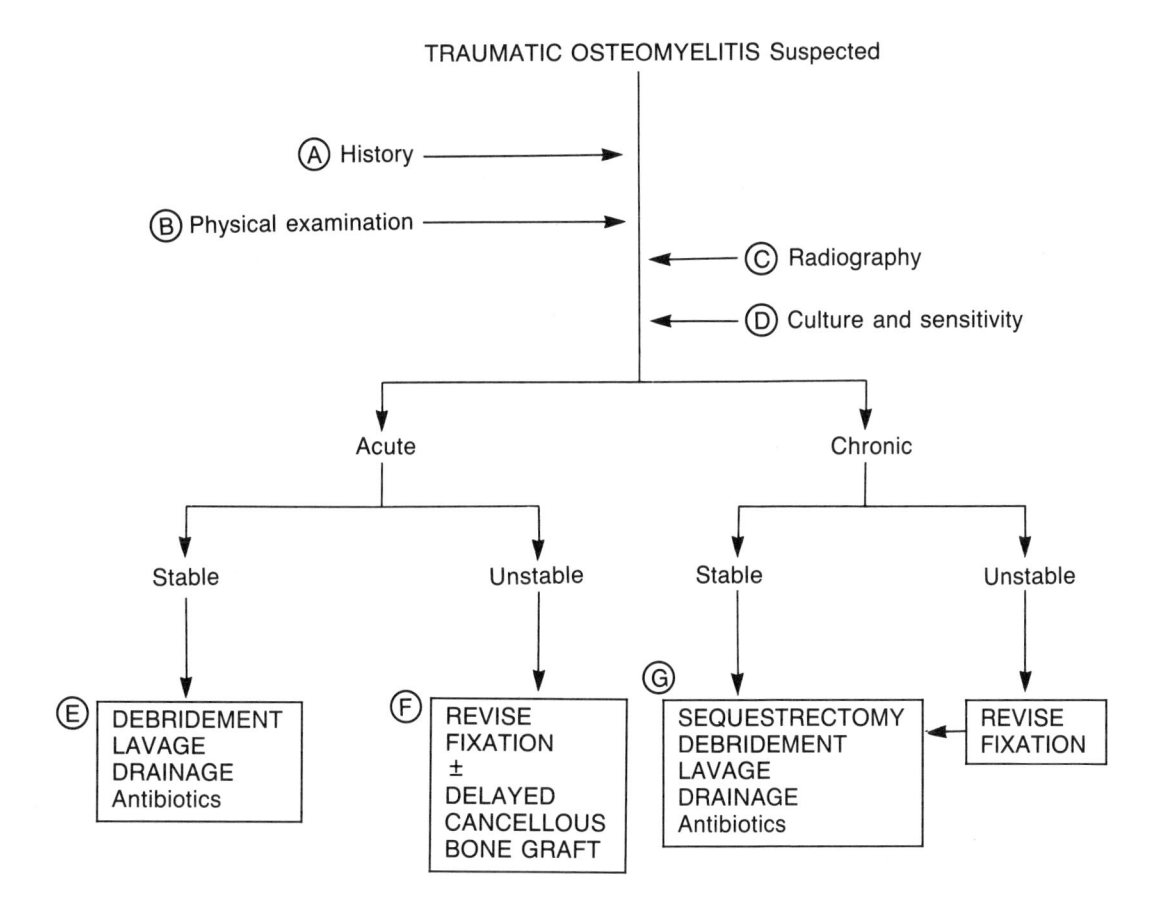

TRAUMATIC OSTEOMYELITIS Suspected

- (A) History
- (B) Physical examination
- (C) Radiography
- (D) Culture and sensitivity

Acute
- Stable → (E) DEBRIDEMENT / LAVAGE / DRAINAGE / Antibiotics
- Unstable → (F) REVISE FIXATION ± DELAYED CANCELLOUS BONE GRAFT

Chronic
- Stable → (G) SEQUESTRECTOMY / DEBRIDEMENT / LAVAGE / DRAINAGE / Antibiotics
- Unstable → REVISE FIXATION → (G)

SHOULDER PAIN

Craig W. Miller

A. Shoulder pain may be divided, somewhat artificially, into intrinsic and extrinsic mechanisms. Intrinsic mechanisms directly involve the articulating surfaces. Extrinsic mechanisms involve nearby structures, (e.g., infraspinatus contracture) or distal structures capable of initiating shoulder pain, (e.g., cervical discs).

B. Shoulder instability is relatively uncommon in the dog. Traumatic luxations and/or subluxations can be seen in all breeds, but some small breeds show a predisposition to medial luxation and/or subluxation without a history of trauma. In order to maintain stability, the shoulder is dependent upon surrounding ligamentous and tendinous structures. Disruption of these structures often results in chronic instability. Biplanal radiography is necessary because medial shoulder luxation may not be evident in the lateral projection (Fig. 1).

C. Acute traumatic luxations may be reduced under general anesthesia. If on palpation the reduction is stable, the limb should be immobilized in a Velpeau sling for 2 weeks, followed by restricted exercise for 4 to 6 weeks. Subsequent recurrent or chronic luxation and/or subluxation may ensue in these cases.

D. Open reduction and surgical stabilization are advocated for unstable, recurrent, or chronic shoulder luxation and/or subluxation. Techniques may be classified as: stabilization by prosthetic implants and stabilization by autogenous structures. Generally, the results of prosthetic stabilization are less successful than autogenous stabilization. Biceps tendon transposition and supraspinatus tendon transposition have been used successfully in cases of medial luxation.

E. Intrinsic causes of shoulder pain that does not present with instability, may be subclassified as: those with a mechanically normal range of motion and those with a mechanically restricted range of motion. Restriction of range of movement is caused by osteophyte impingement, impingement by fracture fragments and/or fibrosis, and contraction of surrounding joint capsule and supporting structures.

F. Some controversy exists regarding surgical intervention in osteochondritis dissecans of the humeral head. Spontaneous detachment and resorption of the cartilage flap seems to be the exception rather than the rule. Since cartilage discontinuity causes inflammation and eventual degenerating changes within the joint, surgical intervention is warranted in clinically affected animals. The cartilage flap should be removed and any undermined cartilage at the periphery of the lesion should be curretted. The joint should be thoroughly explored, and any loose bodies should be removed.

G. In the case of a clinically lame dog, early osteochondritis dissecans of the humerus usually warrants a favorable prognosis if surgical exploration and removal of flap and loose material is performed.

H. Arthrodesis of the shoulder is a successful salvage procedure for severely degenerative joints. A cranially applied plate and lag screw fixation is recommended. A cancellous bone graft is taken from the osteotomized humeral head (Fig. 2).

I. A multitude of chronic arthroses can affect the shoulder joint and cause pain. These may be classified as inflammatory and noninflammatory. Inflammatory arthropathies include those caused by infectious agents as well as immune-mediated arthropathies. The immune-mediated arthropathies may be divided into erosive (e.g., rheumatoid arthritis) and nonerosive (e.g., systemic lupus erythematosus and idiopathic immune-mediated arthritis). The treatment of these syndromes is usually medical and depends upon a definitive diagnosis.

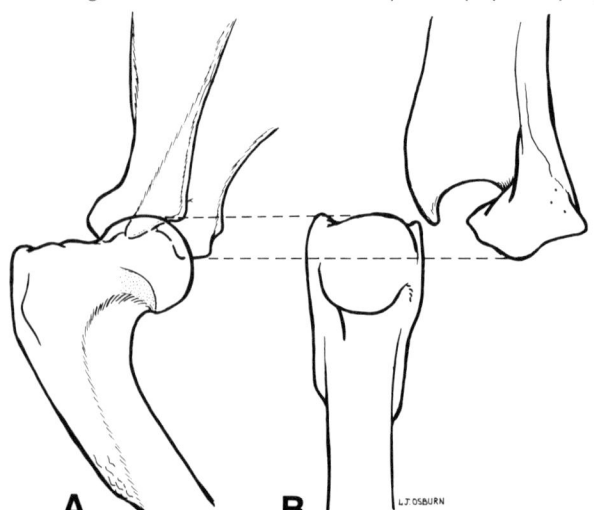

Figure 1 *A*, Lateral view of luxated shoulder; *B*, Cranial view of luxated shoulder. In the lateral view, superimposition of one bone on the other may not radiographically reveal the luxation until the second view is taken.

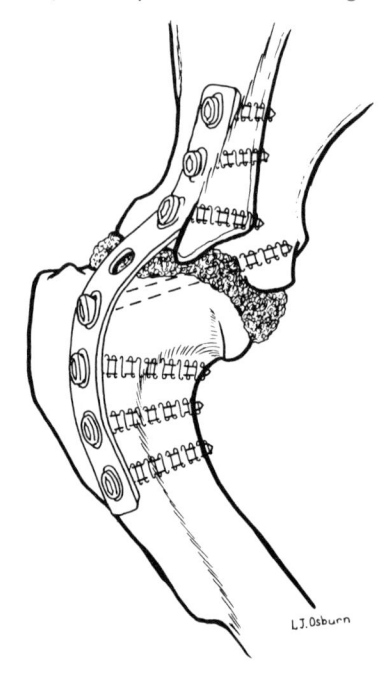

Figure 2 Arthrodesis of the shoulder joint. The joint cartilage is removed, and the resulting cavity is packed with cancellous bone.

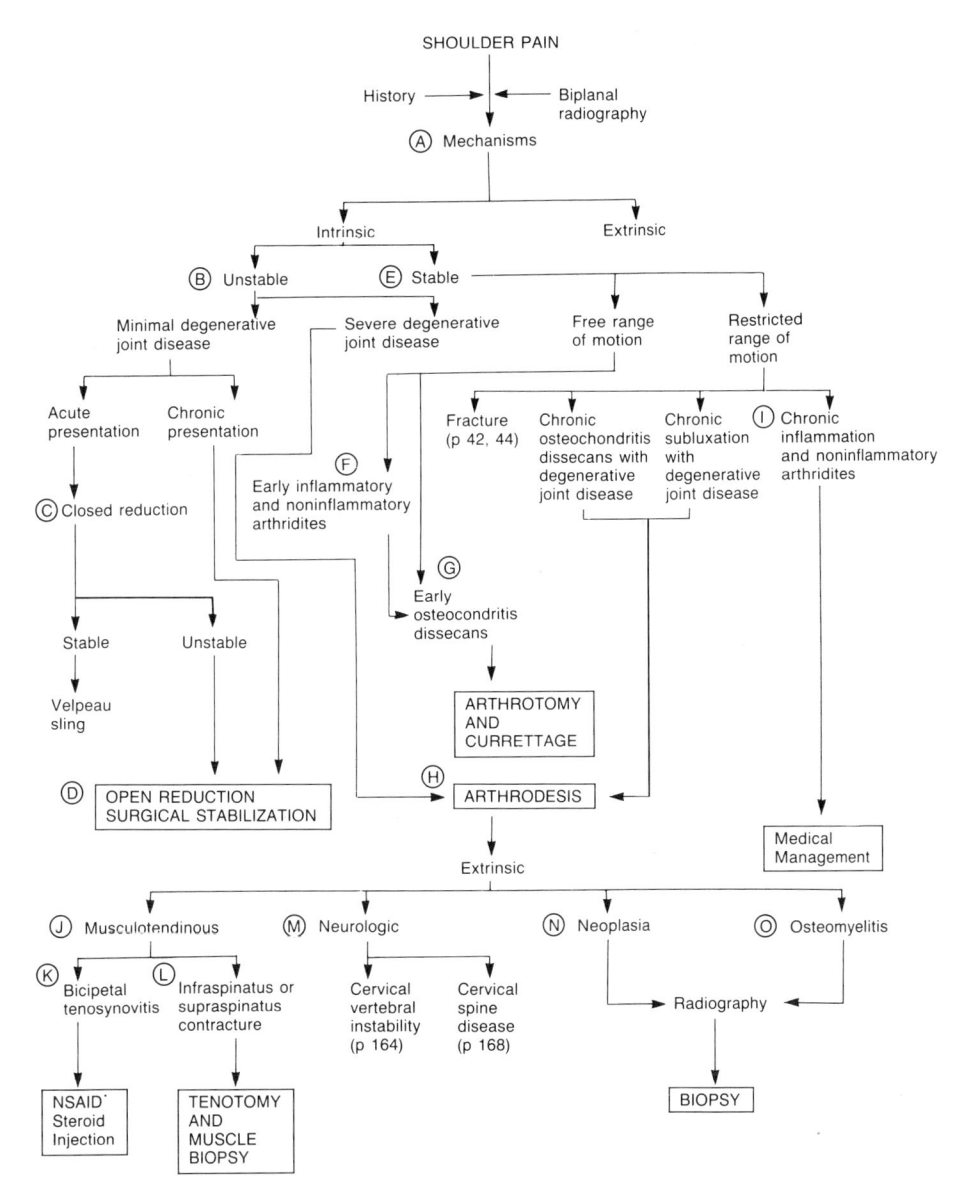

```
                        SHOULDER PAIN
                 History  →    ← Biplanal
                              radiography
                         ↓
                    Ⓐ Mechanisms
                         ↓
              ┌──────────┴──────────┐
           Intrinsic              Extrinsic
       ┌──────┴──────┐         ┌──────┴──────┐
     Ⓑ Unstable   Ⓔ Stable   Free range   Restricted
                              of motion    range of
                                            motion
```

Flowchart (Shoulder Pain) — key branches:

- Ⓐ Mechanisms → Intrinsic / Extrinsic
- Intrinsic → Ⓑ Unstable / Ⓔ Stable
  - Ⓑ Unstable → Minimal degenerative joint disease (Acute presentation → Ⓒ Closed reduction → Stable → Velpeau sling; Unstable → Ⓓ OPEN REDUCTION SURGICAL STABILIZATION) / Chronic presentation
  - Severe degenerative joint disease → Ⓗ ARTHRODESIS
  - Ⓕ Early inflammatory and noninflammatory arthrides
- Ⓔ Stable → Free range of motion → Fracture (p 42, 44) / Chronic osteochondritis dissecans with degenerative joint disease / Chronic subluxation with degenerative joint disease
  - Ⓖ Early osteochondritis dissecans → ARTHROTOMY AND CURRETTAGE
- Restricted range of motion → Ⓘ Chronic inflammation and noninflammatory arthridites → Medical Management

Extrinsic:
- Ⓙ Musculotendinous → Ⓚ Bicipetal tenosynovitis → NSAID* Steroid Injection; Ⓛ Infraspinatus or supraspinatus contracture → TENOTOMY AND MUSCLE BIOPSY
- Ⓜ Neurologic → Cervical vertebral instability (p 164) / Cervical spine disease (p 168)
- Ⓝ Neoplasia → Radiography → BIOPSY
- Ⓞ Osteomyelitis → Radiography

*Nonsteroidal anti-inflammatory drugs

J. Musculotendinous causes of extrinsic shoulder lameness are not common. Lameness is caused either by inflammation or mechanical restriction.

K. Bicipetal tenosynovitis is often a diagnosis of elimination. Other causes of shoulder lameness must be carefully investigated before a diagnosis of bicipetal tenosynovitis can be made. Aspirin or intra-articular steroids have been advocated.

L. Infraspinatus and supraspinatus contracture have been documented in active sporting breeds. The etiology is uncertain. Tenotomy of the insertion of the affected muscle has proven beneficial in the few reported cases. The limb is carried in a flexed position and, in the case of infraspinatus contracture, the antebrachium is turned outwards.

M. Neurologic conditions, especially with nerve root involvement, can mimic shoulder-caused lameness.

N. Neoplastic conditions of nearby bone or soft tissue can cause lameness attributable to the shoulder. Examples of primary neoplasms include synovial cell sarcoma and osteosarcoma. Examples of metastatic neoplasms include plasma cell myeloma and lymphosarcoma. Diagnosis is made by radiography and biopsy.

O. Osteomyelitis of the scapula or humerus may be confused with primary joint problems. Etiologic agents can be bacterial or fungal. Diagnosis is made by radiography, biopsy, and culture.

References

Brinker WO, Hohn RB, Prieur WD. Manual of internal fixation in small animals. Heidelberg: Springer-Verlag, 1984:127.

Brinker WO, Piermattei DL, Flo GL. Handbook of small animal orthopedics and fracture treatment. Philadelphia: WB Saunders, 1983; 134.

Olsson SE. Osteochondrosis in the dog. In: Kirk RW, ed. Current vet therapy VI. Philadelphia: WB Saunders, 1977:880.

Moore RW, Withrow SJ. Arthrodeses. Comp Cont Ed. 3rd ed. 1981:319.

Pettit GD, Chatburch DD, Hegreberg GA, Meyers KM. Studies on the pathophysiology of infraspinatus muscle contracture in the dog. Vet Surg 1978; 7:8.

SCAPULAR FRACTURE

Craig W. Miller

A. The possibility of concurrent thoracic trauma, i.e., pulmonary contusion, traumatic myocarditis, and pneumothorax, should be investigated when the animal is presented with trauma of the proximal forelimb. Thoracic radiography and electrocardiography are recommended in all suspected cases of automobile injury or similar trauma.

B. Most scapular body and spine fractures are treated conservatively with a Velpeau sling. Such fractures are often not severely displaced because of support from the surrounding musculature. Fractures with significant angular displacement can result in degenerative joint disease of the shoulder from nonphysiological loading. These fractures should be treated by open reduction and internal fixation (Fig. 1).

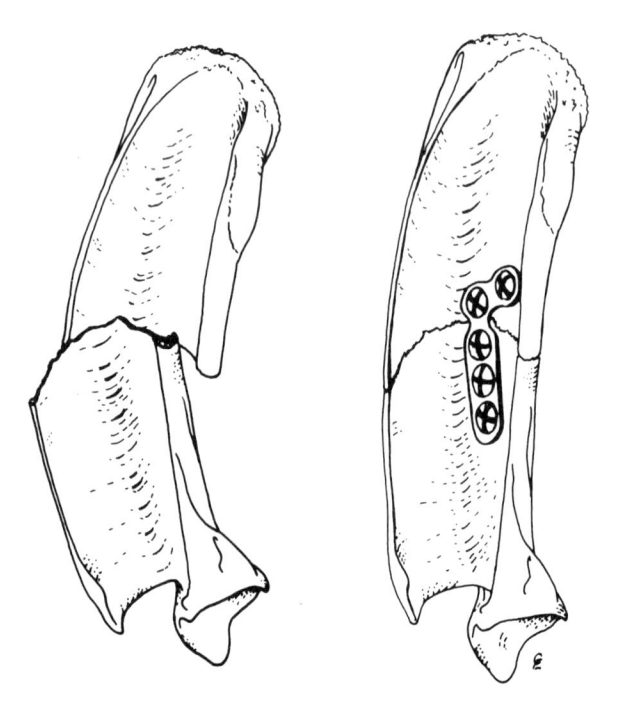

Figure 1 Displaced fracture of the blade of the scapula, reduced and stabilized by means of a fragment plate in the infraspinous fossa.

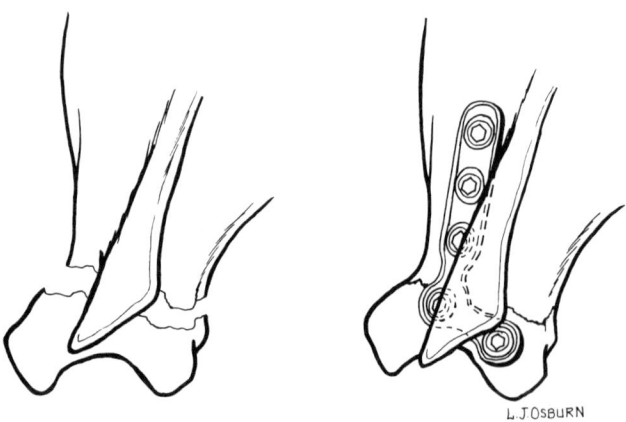

Figure 2 Scapula neck fracture stabilized by a fragment plate.

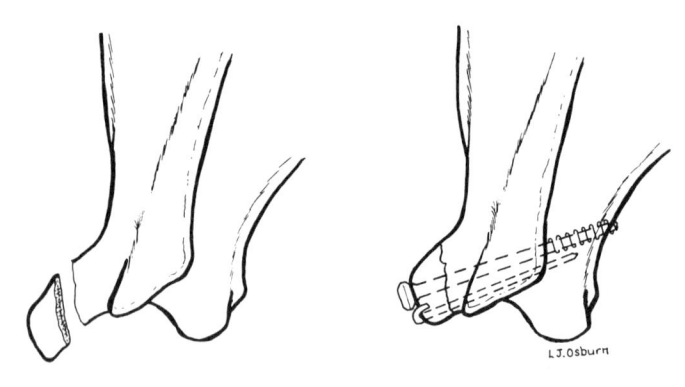

Figure 3 Fracture of the supraglenoid tubercle stabilized by a pin and lag screw.

C. Acromial fractures tend to distract from the pull of the acromial portion of the deltoid muscle. Although such fractures can be treated conservatively, quicker and more consistent healing is obtained by internal fixation. Interfragmentary wiring in small dogs, or pin and tension-band wiring in larger dogs, is usually satisfactory.

D. Fractures of the scapular neck tend to override so that the distal fragment is displaced dorsomedially. The suprascapular nerve is subject to laceration or entrapment. Fixation is achieved by cross-pins or T-plate (Fig. 2).

E. The goal of articular fracture repair is always anatomical reduction and interfragmentary compression. Glenoid fractures can often be repaired by lag screw(s) in combination with cross-pins or a plate.

F. Fractures of the supraglenoid tubercle displace distally because of the pull of the biceps brachii. Fixation can be accomplished by lag screw or pins and tension-band wire (Fig. 3).

G. Dorsal displacement of the scapula is caused by disruption of the attachment of the serratus ventralis muscle. Disruption of the trapezius, rhomboideus, teres major, and latissimus dorsi muscles may also be present. If possible, acute scapular displacements are best treated by surgical repair of the ruptured muscles. In cases of recurrent or chronic displacement, the scapula can be wired to an underlying rib.

References

Brinker WO, Hohn RB, Prieur WD. Manual of internal fixation in small animals. Heidelberg: Springer-Verlag, 1984:127.

Brinker WO, Piermattei DL, Flo GL. Handbook of small animal orthopedics and fracture treatment. Philadelphia: WB Saunders, 1983:134.

SCAPULAR FRACTURE OR DISPLACEMENT Suspected

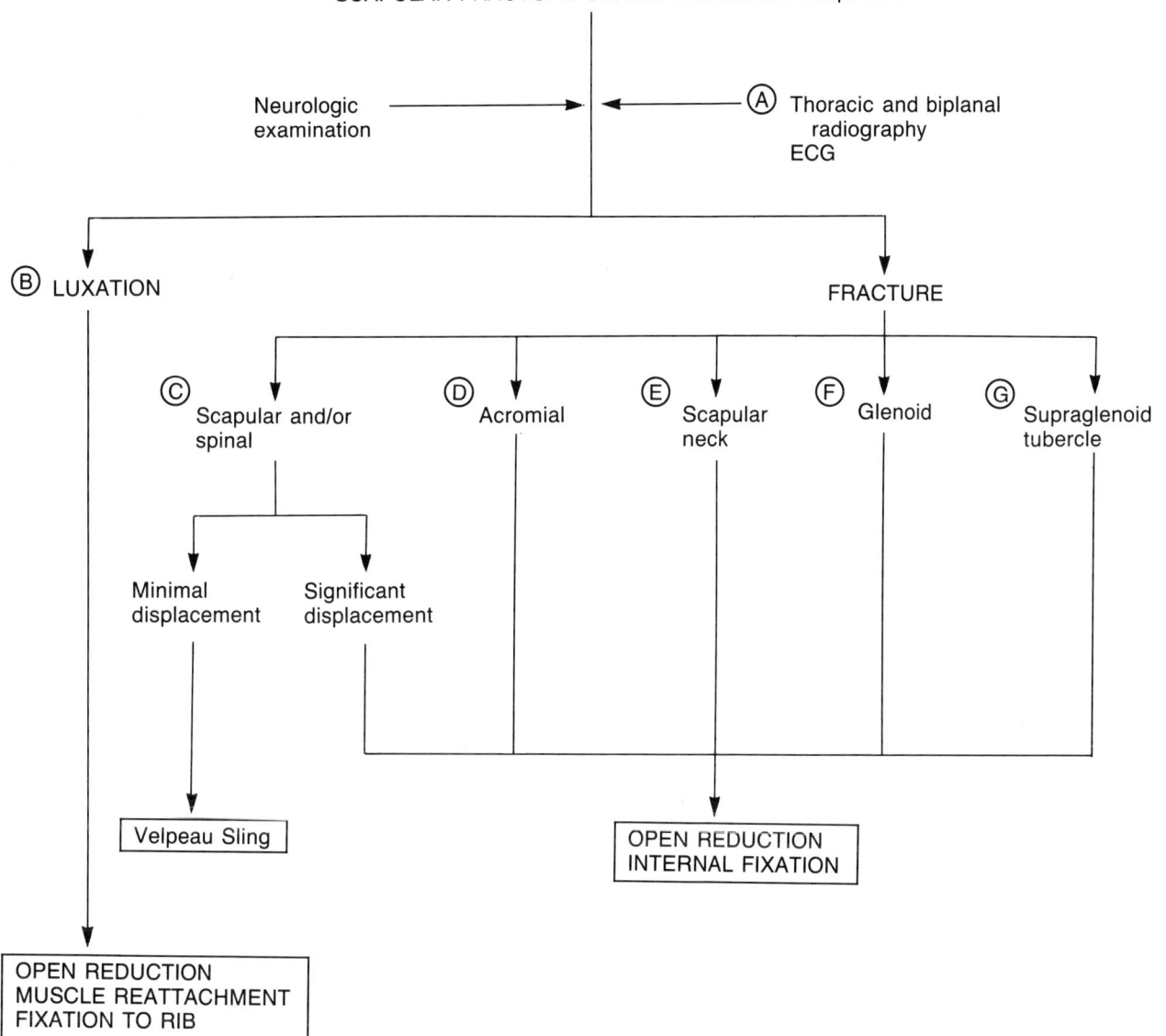

- Neurologic examination
- (A) Thoracic and biplanal radiography ECG

(B) LUXATION
→ **OPEN REDUCTION MUSCLE REATTACHMENT FIXATION TO RIB**

FRACTURE

- (C) Scapular and/or spinal
  - Minimal displacement → **Velpeau Sling**
  - Significant displacement → **OPEN REDUCTION INTERNAL FIXATION**
- (D) Acromial → **OPEN REDUCTION INTERNAL FIXATION**
- (E) Scapular neck → **OPEN REDUCTION INTERNAL FIXATION**
- (F) Glenoid → **OPEN REDUCTION INTERNAL FIXATION**
- (G) Supraglenoid tubercle → **OPEN REDUCTION INTERNAL FIXATION**

PROXIMAL HUMERAL FRACTURE

Craig W. Miller

A. The possibility of trauma should be investigated in cases of humeral fractures. Thoracic radiography and electrocardiography help to identify such life-threatening problems as pneumothorax, hemothorax, pulmonary contusion, collapsed lung lobe, and traumatic myocarditis. Decisions about the timing of humeral fracture repair depend upon a thorough presurgical work-up.

B. Growth plate fractures of the proximal humerus are encountered infrequently. The method of treatment depends upon the type of fracture, i.e., Salter-Harris classification (see p 30); the degree of displacement; and the duration of the injury.

C. Salter-Harris Type I or II fractures that are acute and minimally displaced can often be repaired by closed reduction and internal fixation. The fixation can be provided by two or more Steinmann pins or Kirschner wires.

D. Growth plate fractures that are over 24 hours old or are significantly displaced necessitate open reduction. Care should be taken to preserve the germinal cell layer attached to the epiphyseal fragment.

E. Articular fractures, fractures at the base of the humeral head, and chronic or displaced growth plate fractures necessitate open reduction. Fixation of growth plate fractures can be accomplished with multiple pin fixation. One or more lag screws can be used in dogs approaching skeletal maturity. Proximal articular fractures are uncommon and should be repaired by interfragmentary compression when possible. Reducible fractures at the base of the humeral head can also be repaired by one or more lag screws (Fig. 1).

F. Fractures of the humeral head that are so comminuted as to preclude anatomical reduction (e.g., gunshot wounds) should be treated by primary shoulder arthrodesis. This method results in good quality, pain-free ambulation.

G. Fractures of the greater tubercle of the humerus are prone to distractive forces and, therefore, should be treated by lag-screw or tension-band wiring (Fig. 2).

References

Brinker WO, Hohn RB, Prieur WD. Manual of internal fixation in small animals. Heidelberg: Spinger-Verlag, 1984:127.

Brinker WO, Piermattei DL, Flo GL. Handbook of small animal orthopedics and fracture treatment. Philadelphia: WB Saunders, 1983:134.

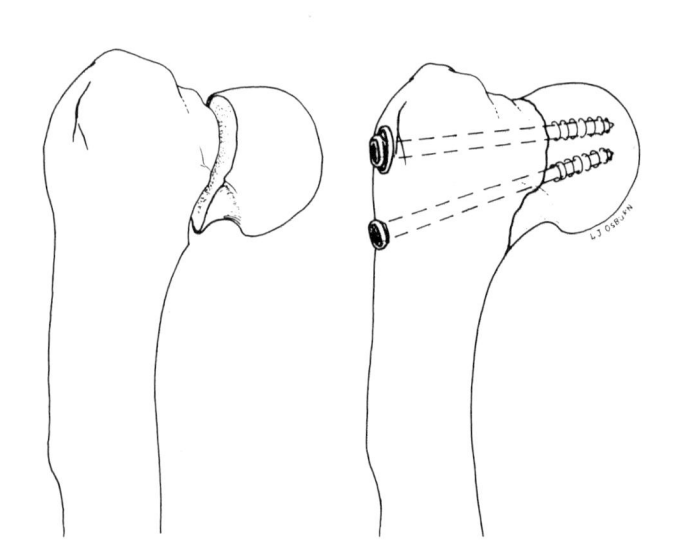

Figure 1 Lag screw fixation of the humeral head.

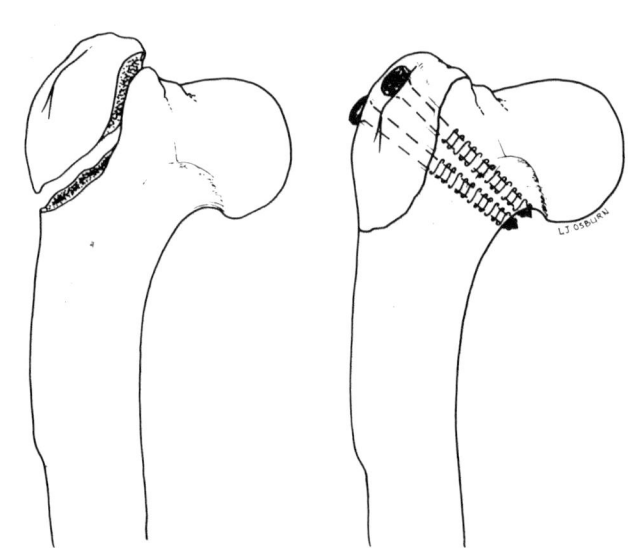

Figure 2 A displaced fracture of the greater tubercle stabilized by two lag screws.

PROXIMAL HUMERAL FRACTURE

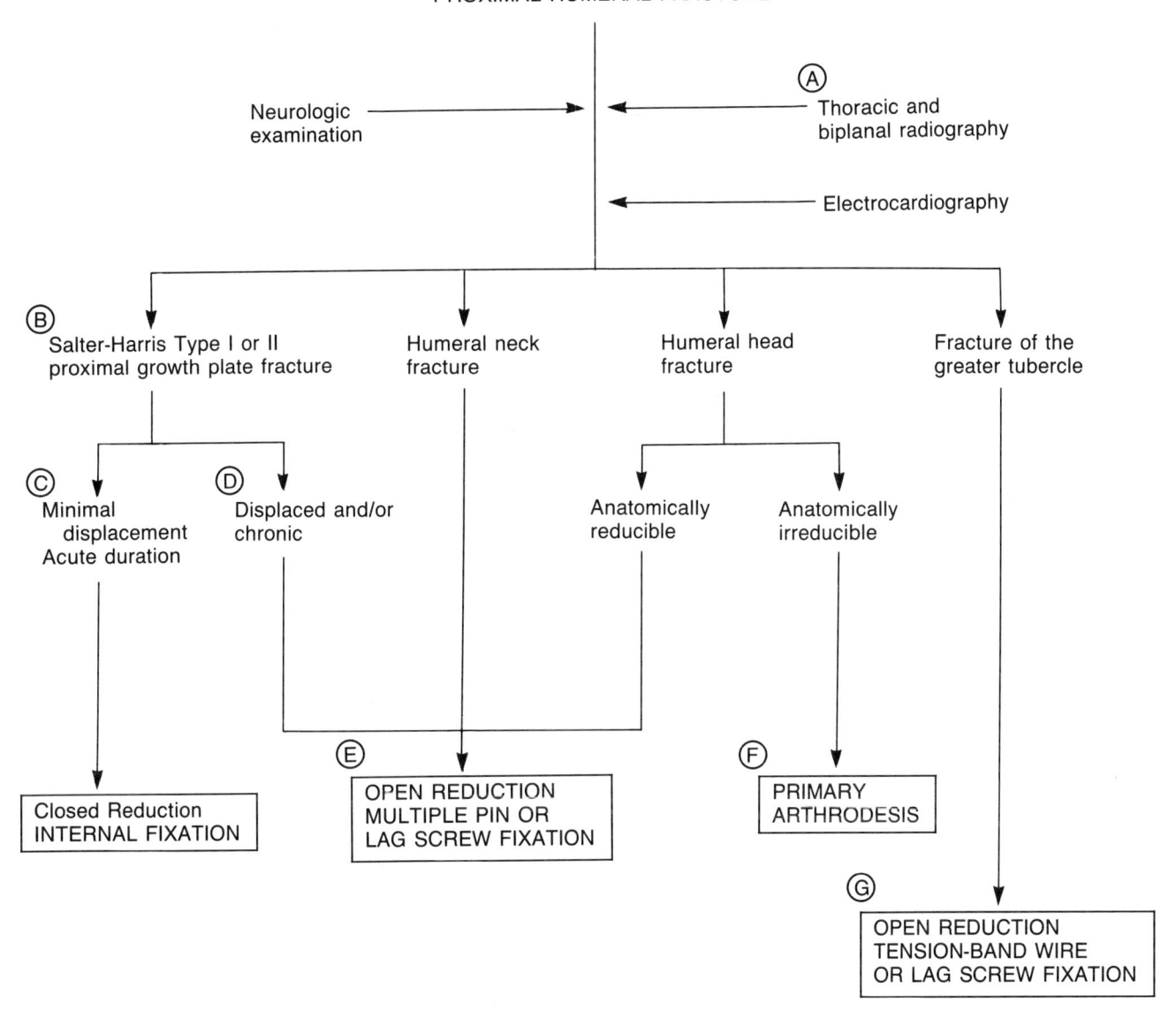

Ⓐ Thoracic and biplanal radiography
Neurologic examination
Electrocardiography

Ⓑ Salter-Harris Type I or II proximal growth plate fracture

Humeral neck fracture

Humeral head fracture

Fracture of the greater tubercle

Ⓒ Minimal displacement Acute duration

Ⓓ Displaced and/or chronic

Anatomically reducible

Anatomically irreducible

Closed Reduction INTERNAL FIXATION

Ⓔ **OPEN REDUCTION MULTIPLE PIN OR LAG SCREW FIXATION**

Ⓕ **PRIMARY ARTHRODESIS**

Ⓖ **OPEN REDUCTION TENSION-BAND WIRE OR LAG SCREW FIXATION**

45

HUMERUS SHAFT FRACTURE

Craig W. Miller

A. A neurologic examination must be done in order to rule out peripheral nerve and brachial plexus damage. Particular attention is paid to radial nerve function since it is at risk as it passes laterally over the humerus.

B. The possibility of concurrent thoracic trauma must be investigated by electrocardiography and thoracic radiography. Biplanal radiographs are imperative to accurately assess and plan the treatment of shaft fractures.

C. In fracture management of the young (skeletally immature) dog, there are several anatomic and physiologic differences: the open growth plates must be considered during fracture management; iatrogenic damage to the germinal cells may result in a functional disaster even though the shaft fracture is healed; and the young dog also has a more active periosteum, which can be used to the surgeon's advantage in some cases.

D. Fractures presented soon after injury, especially in small dogs and cats, may be amenable to closed reduction. Because the humerus is difficult to immobilize by coaptation, casting or splinting of humeral fractures is not effective. The closed reduction can be maintained by an external fixator. A Type I configuration with a single or double bar is usually satisfactory, but more complex configurations can be used in larger animals with unstable fractures. Care must be taken to avoid the growth plates when placing the pins for the fixator.

E. Fractures that are not amenable to closed reduction must be surgically approached and reduced. Reduction can be maintained by compression plating in transverse fractures. If plating instrumentation is not available, the external fixator can be used effectively after open reduction.

F. Long oblique fractures are subject to shear forces as well as bending and rotation. Fixation must be planned to counteract these three forces. Interfragmentary compression of such fractures prevents fracture collapse from shear forces (Fig. 1).

G. Anatomic reduction and rigid internal fixation of comminuted humeral fractures is desirable. Interfragmentary compression and rigid stabilization is provided in a similar manner to that used with long oblique fractures.

H. Unfortunately not all comminuted fractures of the humeral shaft can be reduced anatomically. Severely comminuted fractures or fractures with segmental bone loss are a difficult challenge for the veterinary surgeon. Closed reduction of the fracture and application of an external fixator may be effective, especially in smaller patients. Intermediate fragments should be incorporated in the pin configuration when possible. An extension plate is useful in bridging comminuted humeral fractures in larger animals. A cancellous bone graft is mandatory in such cases. Cortical allografts have also been advocated for bridging large segmental defects. This procedure must be technically precise and strict asepsis must be maintained. The technical difficulties involved in handling and storing allografts make this procedure useful only in a large referral-type setting.

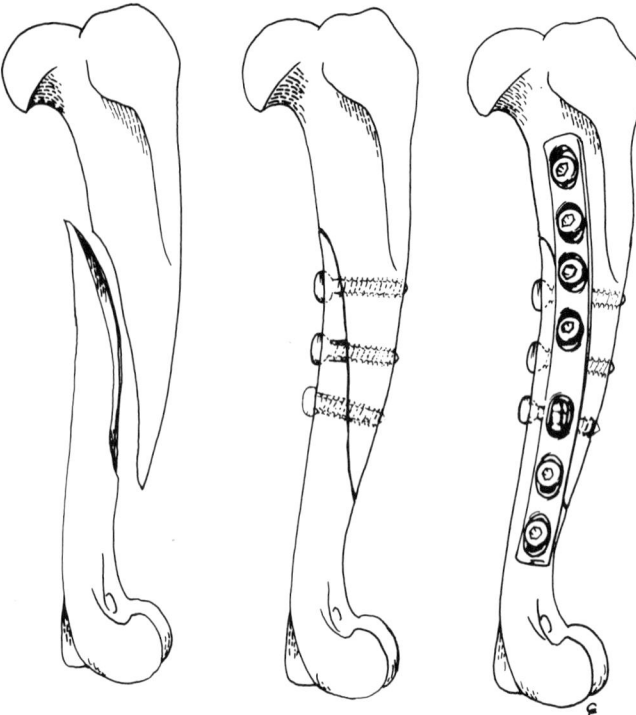

Figure 1 Spiral fracture of the humeral shaft that is stabilized from the posterior aspect by means of three lag screws and on the lateral aspect by a neutralizing plate.

References

Braden T. Surgical correction of humeral fractures. In: Bojrab MJ, ed. Current techniques in small animal surgery, 2nd ed. Philadelphia: Lea & Febiger, 1975:676.

Brinker WO, Hohn RB, Prieur WD. Manual of internal fixation in small animals. Heidelberg: Springer-Verlag, 1986:138.

Brinker WO, Piermatti DL, Flo GL. Handbook of small animal orthopedics and fractures treatment. Philadelphia: WB Saunders, 1983:140.

Withrow SJ. Principles of intramedullary pinning and cerclage wiring. Proceedings of the 47th Annual Meeting of the American Animal Hospital Association, 1980.

HUMERUS SHAFT FRACTURE Suspected

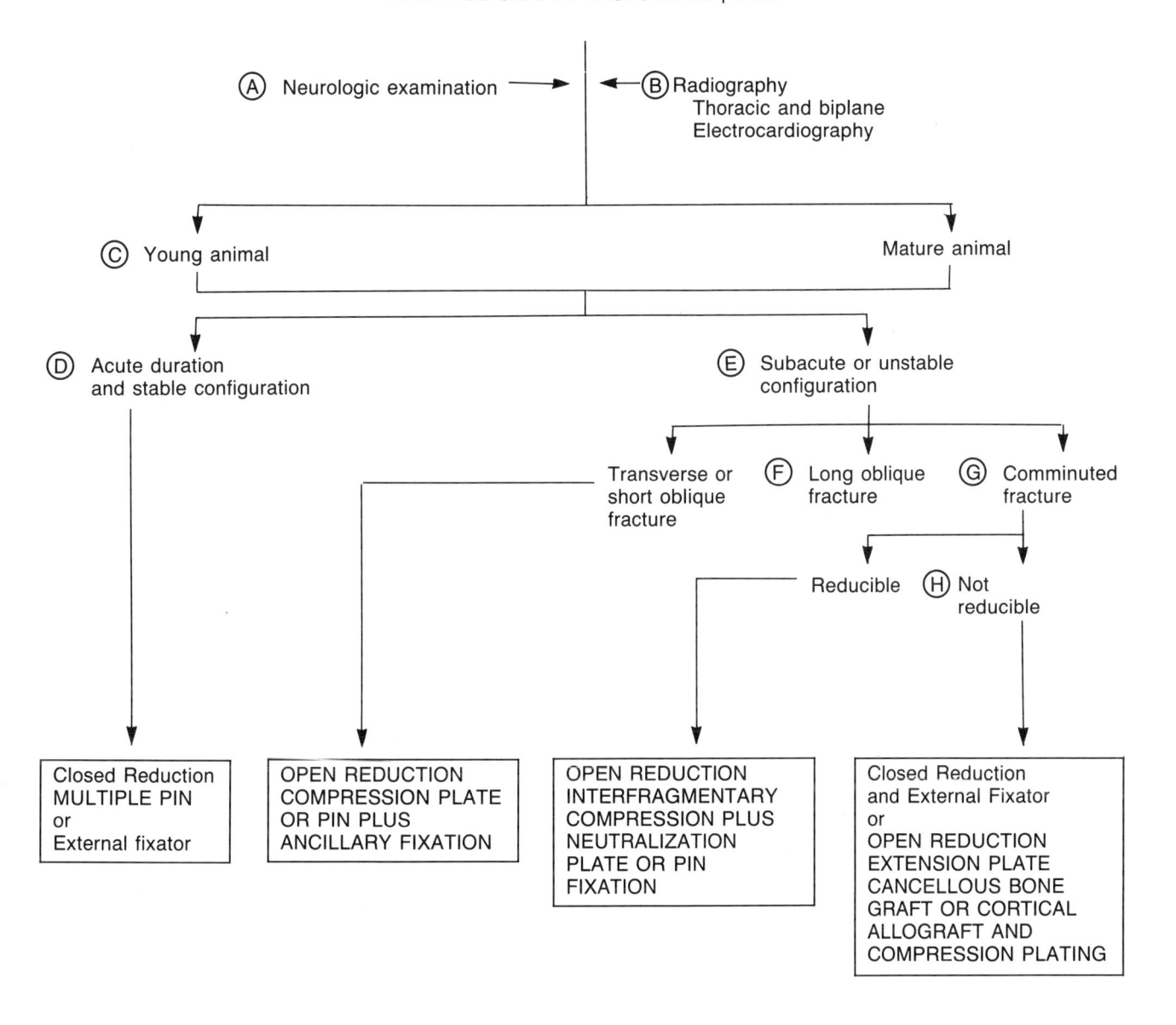

- (A) Neurologic examination
- (B) Radiography
  Thoracic and biplane
  Electrocardiography

- (C) Young animal
- Mature animal

- (D) Acute duration and stable configuration
- (E) Subacute or unstable configuration

- Transverse or short oblique fracture
- (F) Long oblique fracture
- (G) Comminuted fracture

- Reducible
- (H) Not reducible

Closed Reduction
MULTIPLE PIN
or
External fixator

OPEN REDUCTION
COMPRESSION PLATE
OR PIN PLUS
ANCILLARY FIXATION

OPEN REDUCTION
INTERFRAGMENTARY
COMPRESSION PLUS
NEUTRALIZATION
PLATE OR PIN
FIXATION

Closed Reduction
and External Fixator
or
OPEN REDUCTION
EXTENSION PLATE
CANCELLOUS BONE
GRAFT OR CORTICAL
ALLOGRAFT AND
COMPRESSION PLATING

DISTAL HUMERAL FRACTURE

Craig W. Miller

A. As with all humeral fractures, special care is taken to rule out concurrent thoracic and peripheral nerve trauma by means of careful neurologic and radiologic examination.

B. Supracondylar fractures usually involve the supratrochlear foramen. Salter-Harris I fractures of the distal humeral growth plate occur infrequently. Supracondylar fractures are best treated by open reduction and internal fixation with plate, screw, and pins (Figs. 1 and 2).

C. Transverse supracondylar fractures are less susceptible to shear forces than oblique or multiple fractures. Bending and rotational forces must be counteracted to allow healing to occur. An intramedullary pin seated into the medial condyle and a laterally placed K-wire is a commonly used fixation technique, but affords rather poor stability. Cross pins may also be used in distal fractures. Rush pins or plating can be used in large dogs.

D. Interfragmentary compression can be applied to oblique supracondylar fractures by cerclage wires or, preferably, lag screws. The fracture can be further stabilized by intramedullary pins, Kirschner wires or, for good stability, a neutralization plate may be used.

E. Multiple supracondylar fractures can be treated by external fixator in small dogs and cats. This can be supplemented by an intramedullary pin in selected cases. Larger dogs are best stabilized by single or double plates. A cancellous bone graft is used to fill defects if the fracture cannot be anatomically reconstructed.

F. Condylar fractures of the distal humerus most often involve the lateral condyle. Most of the weight borne on the foreleg is transferred through the radial head to the lateral humeral condyle. The eccentric position of the condyle makes it vulnerable to rotational shearing forces when excessive load is transmitted up the limb, such as happens when landing on an outstretched foreleg after falling or jumping from a height.

G. Closed reduction of lateral condylar fractures is possible in acute cases (less than 24 to 36 hours) with minimal swelling. Reduction can be maintained with a condyle clamp while the fracture is fixed by pins and/or screws placed through a stab incision. In cases treated by either open or closed techniques, anatomic reduction and interfragmentary compression are the goals of any articular fracture repair. This is most commonly achieved by lag screw fixation across the condylar fracture and lateral Kirschner wire placement to counteract rotation. Multiple Kirschner wire fixation may be successfully employed in treating small young animals (see Fig. 1).

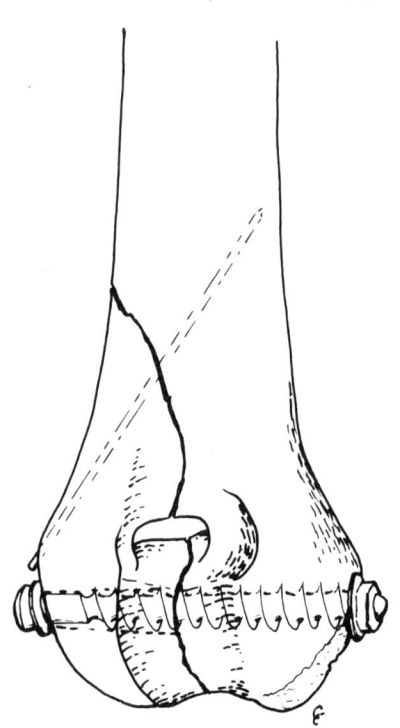

Figure 1 Lateral condylar fracture stabilized by means of Kirschner wire, and lag screw fixation of the condyles supported by a medial nut.

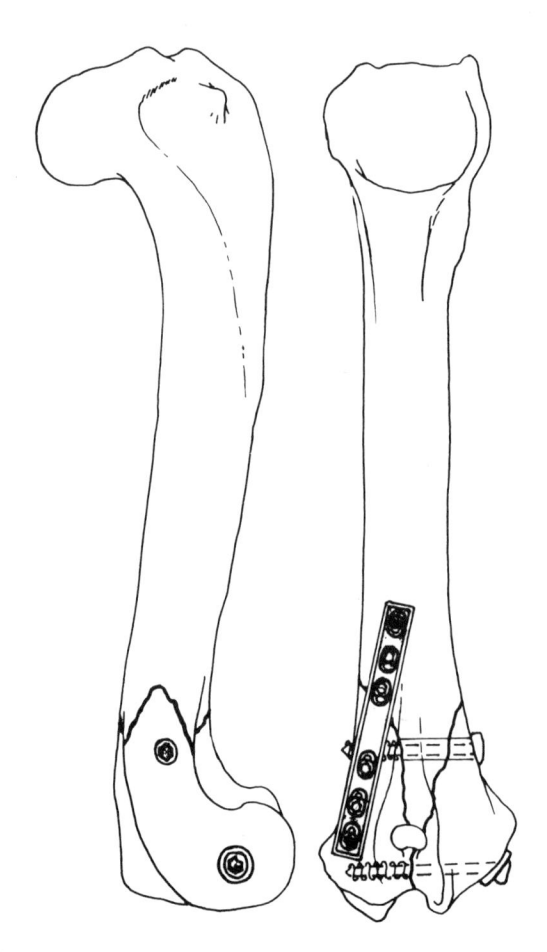

Figure 2 A supracondylar "Y" fracture of the distal humerus stabilized by means of two lag screws (the distal one is a cancellous screw) and a posteriorly placed dynamic compression plate.

```
                          DISTAL HUMERAL FRACTURE Suspected
                                         │
                          Ⓐ Neurologic examination ────────►
                                         ◄──────── Biplanal radiography
                                         ◄──────── Electrocardiography
                                         │
        ┌────────────────────────────────┼────────────────────────────────┐
     Ⓑ Supracondylar                  Ⓕ Condylar                      Intercondylar
        fracture                         fracture                        fractures
```

Supracondylar fracture branch

- **Salter Harris I** → CROSS PINNING
- Ⓒ **Simple transverse**
  - Small dog or cat → CROSS PINS OR INTRAMEDULLARY PIN WITH ANCILLARY SUPPORT
  - Large dog → RUSH PIN OR PLATE
- Ⓓ **Simple oblique**
  - Small dog or cat → CROSS PINS OR INTRAMEDULLARY PIN WITH ANCILLARY SUPPORT
  - Large dog → UNILATERAL PLATE
- Ⓔ **Comminuted**
  - Small dog → EXTERNAL FIXATOR
  - Large dog → SINGLE OR DOUBLE PLATES AND CANCELLOUS BONE GRAFT

Condylar fracture branch

- Ⓖ **Closed reduction possible**
  - Young small dog → MULTIPLE KIRSCHNER WIRE FIXATION
  - Large or older dog → PERCUTANEOUS LAG SCREW AND KIRSCHNER WIRE FIXATION
- Ⓗ **Closed reduction not possible** → Open reduction → LAG SCREW AND KIRSCHNER WIRE FIXATION

Intercondylar fractures branch

- Ⓘ **Simple T or Y fractures**
  - Small to mid-sized animal → TRANSCONDYLAR LAG SCREW WITH RUSH PIN OR CROSS PIN FIXATION
  - Large dog → TRANSCONDYLAR LAG SCREW WITH SINGLE OR DOUBLE PLATE FIXATION
- Ⓙ **Comminuted T or Y fractures**
  - Reduction possible → TRANSCONDYLAR LAG SCREW WITH DOUBLE PLATE FIXATION AND CANCELLOUS BONE GRAFT
  - Reduction impossible → PRIMARY ELBOW ARTHRODESIS OR AMPUTATION

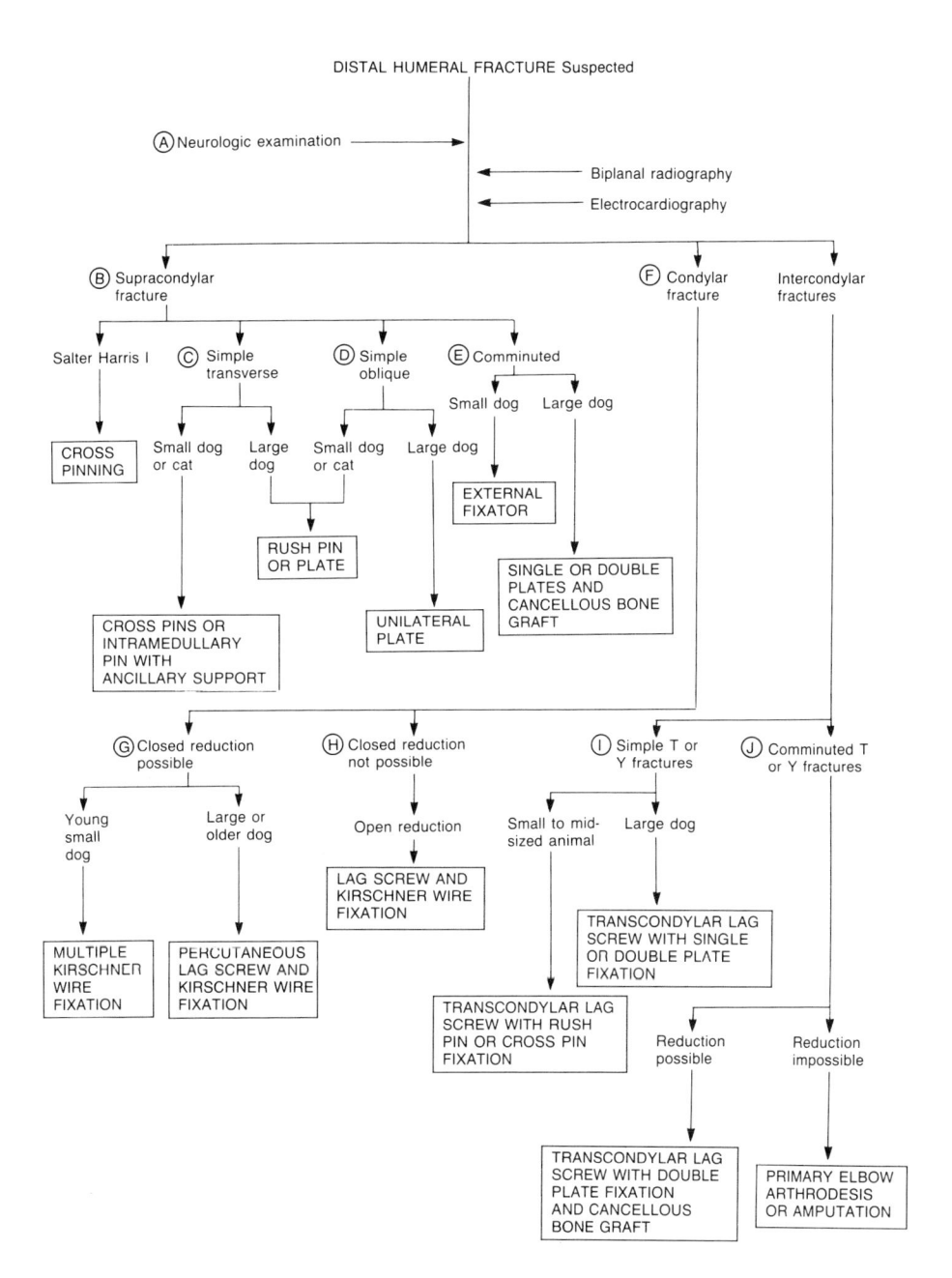

H. If closed reduction is not possible, open reduction by a lateral approach is performed in order to reduce lateral condylar fractures. Olecranon osteotomy or triceps tenotomy (in young animals) can be used for the reduction of recalcitrant fractures. Fixation is essentially the same as for closed reduction in which practical osteotomy approach is preferred.

I. Anatomical reduction and interfragmentary compression are the goals of any articular fracture repair. These are especially important in the elbow joint where decreased range of motion and osteoarthrosis are common sequelae to fractures. A transolecranon approach (or triceps tenotomy) provides adequate exposure of the articular surfaces. A "T" fracture follows the line of the distal and intercondylar growth plates whereas a "Y" fracture occurs through the intercondylar growth plate, but continues proximally through the arches of both medial and lateral condyles.

J. Comminuted intercondylar fractures of the distal humerus are a difficult challenge for the veterinary surgeon. Decreased elbow range-of-motion is common following such fractures even though they are adequately repaired. A cancellous bone graft should be used to fill defects when anatomical reduction is not possible. In severely fragmented fractures, such as those resulting from gunshot wounds, primary elbow arthrodesis or amputation may have to be considered.

References

Brinker WO, Hohn RB, and Prieur WD. Manual of internal fixation in small animals. Heidelberg: Springer-Verlag, 1984; 140.

Brinker WO, Piermattei DL, Flo GL. Handbook of small animal orthopedics and fracture treatment, Philadelphia: WB Saunders, 1983; 145.

Dingwall JS. Management of elbow fractures in the dog. Mod Vet Pract 1970; Feb:37.

Rudy RR. Management of limb fractures in small animals. Vet Clin North Am 1975; 5:197.

ELBOW PAIN

Geoff Sumner-Smith

In animals the most common causes of pain originate from the elbow joint rather than from associated soft tissue structures. Ligaments and tendons are more rarely injured than is the joint which, it must be remembered, forms articulations among three bones.

A. A history of either an acute accident or chronic pain may indicate a problem relating to the joint. Consequently, unless soft-tissue damage is obvious, this possibility must be eliminated before a diagnosis of intrinsic pain (pain within the joint itself) is made. Examine the joint in flexion and extension, noticing any alteration of the normal range of movement (ROM). Palpate the joint to ascertain if there is displacement of bones and segments. Enlargement of the joint capsule can be seen by placing the joint in flexion. Palpate the soft tissue to aid in the diagnosis of rupture, perfusion, or fibrosis.

B. Routine lateral and A-P radiography demonstrates luxations, fractures, degeneration, and productive changes, but oblique and flexed views are required to demonstrate the more subtle changes seen in the various forms of osteochondrosis and early arthritis.

C. Degenerative joint disease results in loss of normal articular congruence and may result from cartilage degeneration, osteophyte impingement, chronic luxation, intra-articular fractures, or loose bodies ("joint mice") from osteochondritis dissecans.

D. Inflammatory joint disease results in the destruction of the joint surface. Articular crepitus, concomitant with inflammation or fibrosis of the synovial capsule as well as ligament laxity is common. Instability of the joint or, in contrast, contracture of all soft tissues and a marked decrease in the ROM may occur.

E. Extrinsic pain originates in the soft tissue adjacent to the joint. Referral of pain from the shoulder or spine is rarely diagnosed in animals, although it may occur more commonly than is realized.

F. Injury to surrounding musculotendinous structures is not as common in small animals as it is in large, but sprain of the triceps tendon may result in a later fibrosis of the structure, and in very athletic animals the tendon may rupture. The gap may be palpated if the animal is examined before diffusion occurs.

G. The radial nerve may be damaged when the distal humerus is fractured or during surgery to correct conditions close to or in the joint.

References

Alexander JW. Leonard's orthopaedics surgery of the dog & cat. 3rd ed. Philadelphia: WB Saunders, 1985:86.

Olsson SE. Pathophysiology, morphology and clinical signs of osteochondrosis in the dog. In: Bojrab MJ, ed. Pathophysiology in small animal surgery. 2nd ed. Philadelphia: Lea & Febiger, 1981.

Olsson SE. Morphology and physiology of the growth cartilage under normal and pathological conditions. In: Sumner-Smith G, ed. Bone in clinical orthopaedics. Philadelphia: WB Saunders, 1982:159.

Puglisi TA. Canine humeral joint instability. Part 1. Comp Cont Ed 1986; 8(9):593.

Puglisi TA. Canine humeral joint instability. Part 2. Comp Cont Ed 1986; 8(10):741.

ELBOW PAIN

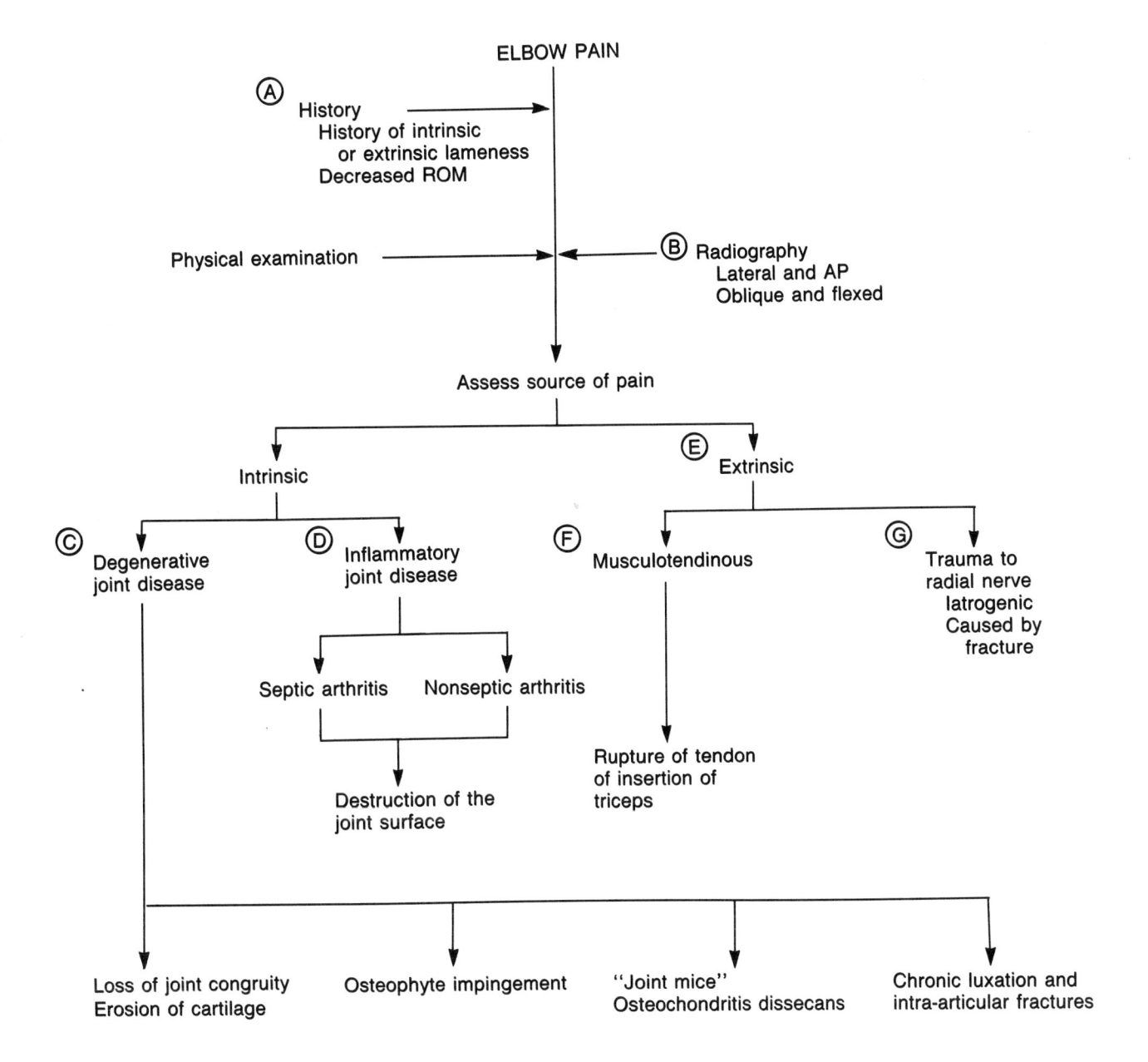

Ⓐ History
History of intrinsic or extrinsic lameness
Decreased ROM

Physical examination → ← **Ⓑ Radiography**
Lateral and AP
Oblique and flexed

Assess source of pain

- Intrinsic
  - **Ⓒ** Degenerative joint disease
  - **Ⓓ** Inflammatory joint disease
    - Septic arthritis
    - Nonseptic arthritis
    - → Destruction of the joint surface
- **Ⓔ** Extrinsic
  - **Ⓕ** Musculotendinous
    - Rupture of tendon of insertion of triceps
  - **Ⓖ** Trauma to radial nerve
    Iatrogenic
    Caused by fracture

- Loss of joint congruity / Erosion of cartilage
- Osteophyte impingement
- "Joint mice" / Osteochondritis dissecans
- Chronic luxation and intra-articular fractures

ARTHRITIS OF THE ELBOW

Geoff Sumner-Smith

A. Inflammation within the elbow joint is usually clearly of sudden onset (acute) or the pain has been slow and insidious in onset (chronic).

B. Luxation of the joint follows trauma, except in cases of congenital luxation seen in chondrodystrophy. The ligaments and capsules are invariably torn. If it is possible to perform closed reduction, the joint is supported for a few days, but if manipulation is not successful, open reduction is required and at that time an attempt should be made to repair torn ligaments and the synovial capsule.

C. Inflammatory joint disease may be either septic or sterile, and is differentiated by aspiration and culture (see p 20). Septic disease is treated with systemic antibiotics (AB) and nonseptic disease with nonsteroidal anti-inflammatory drugs (NSAIDs).

D. Inflammatory joint disease which follows fracture luxation of components of the joint invariably requires open surgery and internal fixation of the element. Early surgery is mandatory; otherwise thickening of the synovial membrane impairs reduction and prejudices full recovery of function. In chronic cases of luxation of the radial head, excision of the head may be necessary.

E. Chronic arthritis may be divided into rheumatoid arthritis, in which more than one joint will be affected, and degenerative joint disease, consequent upon unnatural wear of the joint surfaces.

F. Systemic lupus erythematosus (SLE) is a nonerosive arthritis that is accompanied by serological abnormalities (LE cell and antinuclear antibody positive). Treatment with cytotoxic drugs and steroids is preferred.

G. In young animals, degenerative joint disease is usually a facet of osteochondritis dissecans; surgery is recommended in all but mild cases and when the patient is approaching the age of skeletal maturity (14 mo).

H. Chronic degenerative arthritis may follow any of the previous conditions, particularly the osteochondrosis complex. NSAIDs may help in many cases, but intractible and very painful joints should be arthrodesed.

References

Pederson NC, Pool RR. Canine joint disease. Vet Clin North Am 1978; 8:465.

Sawyer DC. Synovial fluid analysis of canine joints. JAVMA 1963; 43:609.

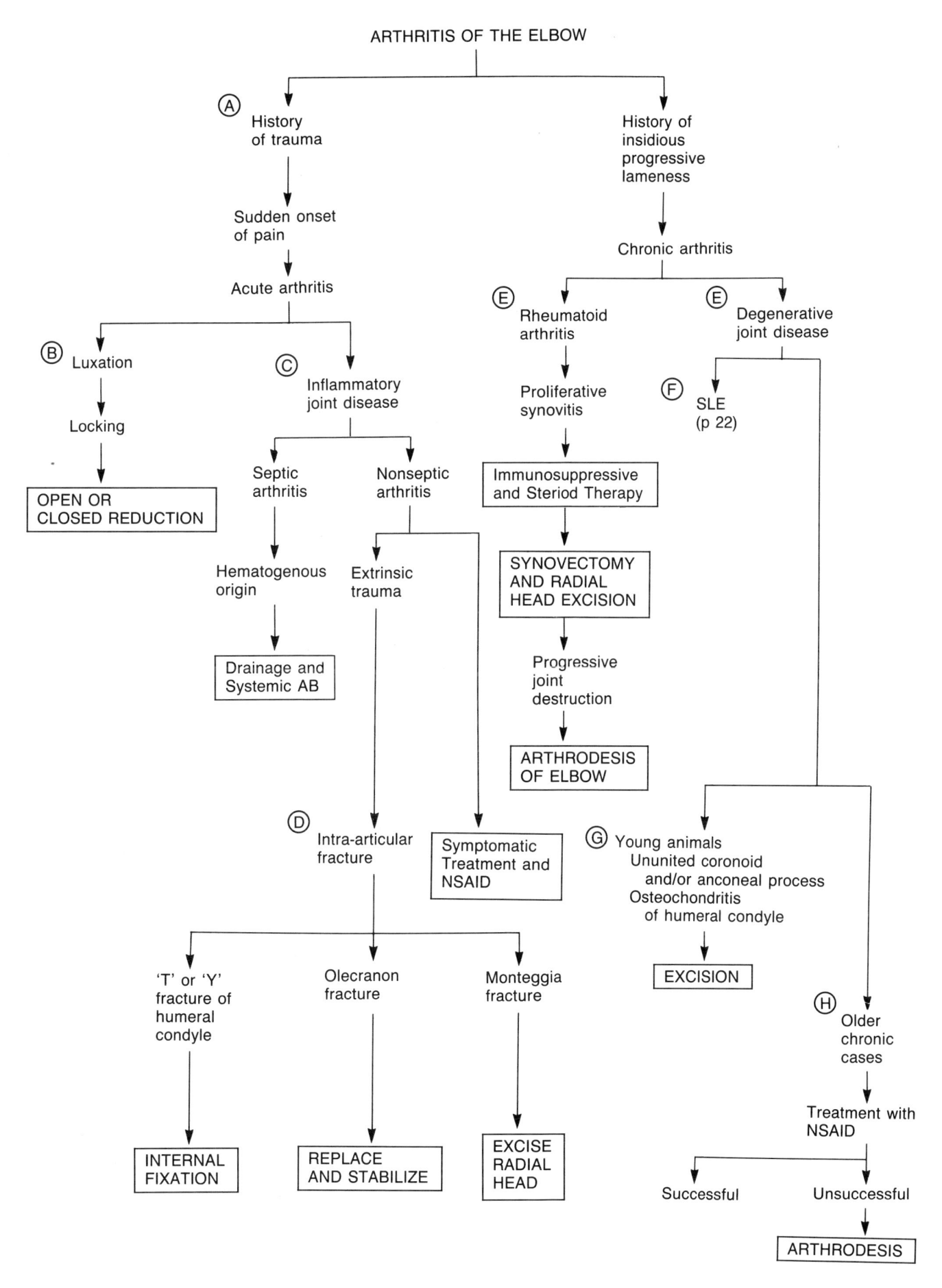

ARTHRITIS OF THE ELBOW

- Ⓐ History of trauma
  - Sudden onset of pain
  - Acute arthritis
    - Ⓑ Luxation
      - Locking
        - **OPEN OR CLOSED REDUCTION**
    - Ⓒ Inflammatory joint disease
      - Septic arthritis
        - Hematogenous origin
          - **Drainage and Systemic AB**
      - Nonseptic arthritis
        - Extrinsic trauma
          - Ⓓ Intra-articular fracture
            - 'T' or 'Y' fracture of humeral condyle
              - **INTERNAL FIXATION**
            - Olecranon fracture
              - **REPLACE AND STABILIZE**
            - Monteggia fracture
              - **EXCISE RADIAL HEAD**
          - **Symptomatic Treatment and NSAID**

- History of insidious progressive lameness
  - Chronic arthritis
    - Ⓔ Rheumatoid arthritis
      - Proliferative synovitis
        - **Immunosuppressive and Steriod Therapy**
        - **SYNOVECTOMY AND RADIAL HEAD EXCISION**
        - Progressive joint destruction
          - **ARTHRODESIS OF ELBOW**
    - Ⓔ Degenerative joint disease
      - Ⓕ SLE (p 22)
      - Ⓖ Young animals
        - Ununited coronoid and/or anconeal process
        - Osteochondritis of humeral condyle
          - **EXCISION**
      - Ⓗ Older chronic cases
        - Treatment with NSAID
          - Successful
          - Unsuccessful
            - **ARTHRODESIS**

53

ELBOW DISLOCATION

Geoff Sumner-Smith

In small animals, most cases of elbow luxation involve dislocation of both the radial head and the ulna from the articulation with the humerus. The ulna or the radius rarely luxate without the other bone being involved. The lateral condyle of the humerus is rounded, and the medial condyle is square; consequently, luxations are almost invariably lateral. The occasional medial luxation is accompanied by severe damage to the collateral ligaments.

A. If closed reduction is not carried out within a few days of the trauma, considerable difficulty in achieving this may be experienced because of contraction of soft tissues. With the patient under general anesthesia, the joint is flexed; medial pressure is applied while the antebrachium is pronated or an extension device may be employed (Fig. 1).

B. Postreduction radiograph should confirm that all joint surfaces have been returned to their proper positions. If the head of the radius remains slightly luxated, further manipulation should be attempted.

C. Unless a full range of motion is achieved without any loss of stability, the joint should be considered unstable and treated as such.

D. Unstable joints should be supported by conform bandaging of the forelimbs and exercise restricted for 3 weeks. Stable reductions need only be supported in a bandage for 4 to 5 days.

References

Campbell JR. Luxation and ligamentous injuries of the elbow of the dog. Vet Clin North Am 1971; 1:429.

Johnson RG, Hampel NL. Elbow luxation. In: Slatter DH, ed. Textbook of small animal surgery. Philadelphia: WB Saunders, 1985:2092.

Stevens DR, Sande RD. An elbow dysplasia syndrome in the dog. JAVMA 1974; 165:1065.

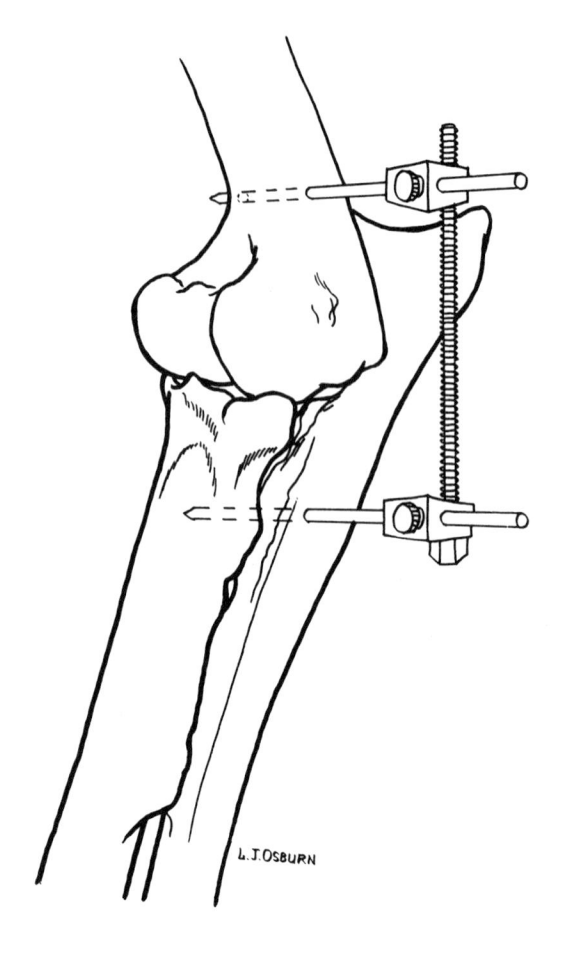

Figure 1 External fixator device used to reduce chronic luxation of the elbow joint. In employing this system, the tissues should be stretched slowly in order that they are not torn unnecessarily. If fine judgement is employed, otherwise irreducible luxations may be successfully replaced.

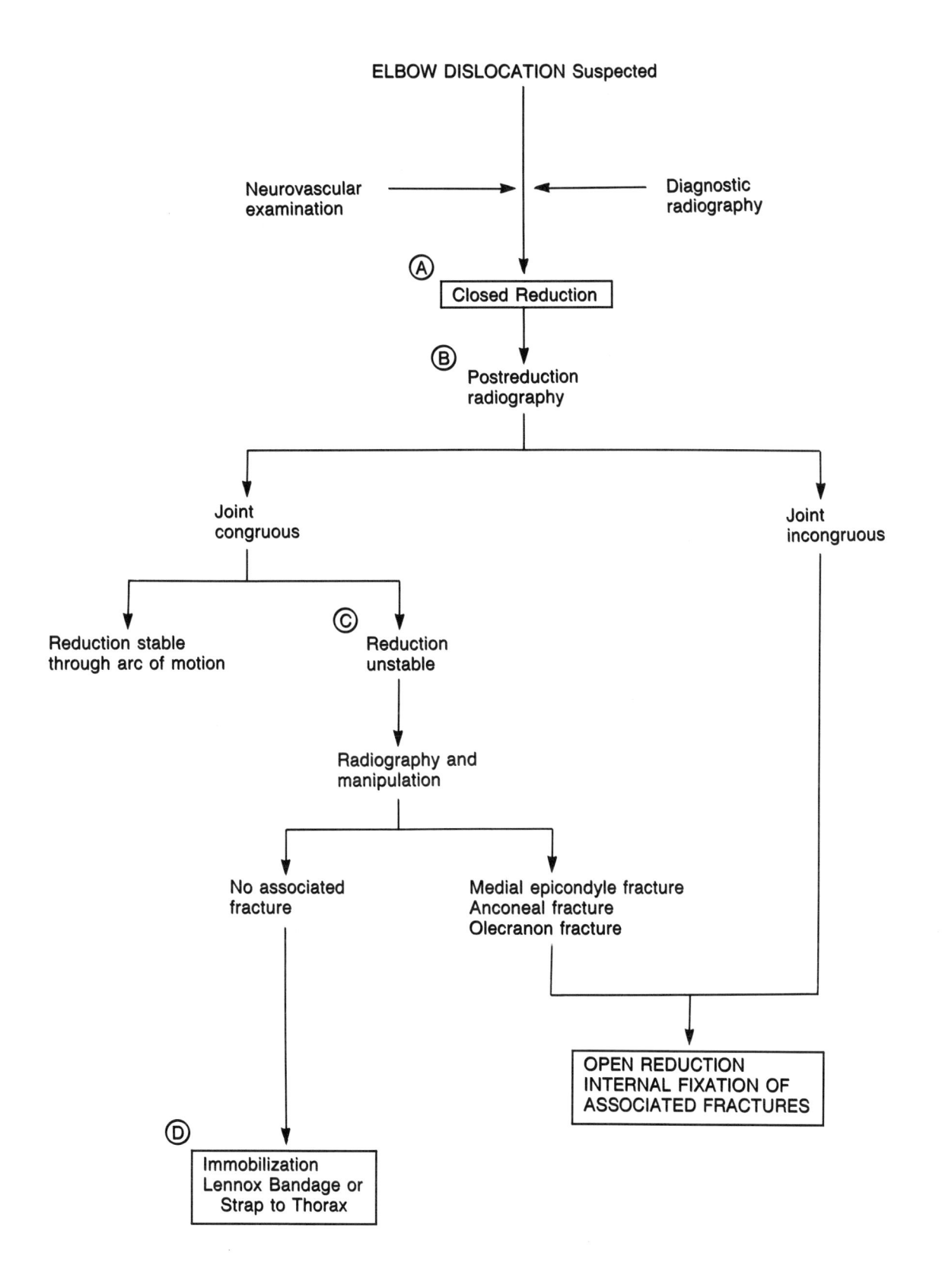

```
                    ELBOW DISLOCATION Suspected

        Neurovascular  ────────→  ←──────── Diagnostic
        examination                          radiography
                                    │
                              Ⓐ     ▼
                            ┌─────────────────┐
                            │ Closed Reduction │
                            └─────────────────┘
                              Ⓑ     │
                                    ▼
                              Postreduction
                               radiography
                                    │
                ┌───────────────────┴───────────────────┐
                ▼                                       ▼
            Joint                                    Joint
          congruous                               incongruous
            │                                        │
    ┌───────┴───────┐                                │
    ▼          Ⓒ   ▼                                │
Reduction stable   Reduction                         │
through arc of    unstable                           │
   motion            │                               │
                     ▼                               │
               Radiography and                       │
                manipulation                         │
                     │                               │
            ┌────────┴────────┐                      │
            ▼                 ▼                      │
        No associated    Medial epicondyle fracture  │
          fracture       Anconeal fracture           │
            │            Olecranon fracture          │
            │                 │                      │
            │                 └──────────┬───────────┘
            │                            ▼
            │                  ┌──────────────────────┐
     Ⓓ     ▼                  │  OPEN REDUCTION      │
    ┌──────────────┐           │  INTERNAL FIXATION OF │
    │ Immobilization│          │  ASSOCIATED FRACTURES │
    │ Lennox Bandage or│       └──────────────────────┘
    │ Strap to Thorax │
    └──────────────┘
```

ANTEBRACHIAL FRACTURES

Geoff Sumner-Smith

A. The integrity of the radial and ulnar nerves is essential to the determination of subsequent treatment of fractures of the forearm.

B. Routine anteroposterior (A-P) and lateral radiography reveals any associated luxations or fractures not diagnosed at the physical examination.

C. Fractures of the olecranon process should be treated by internal fixation employing the tension-band principal (Fig. 1); they should not be treated conservatively. Even immature patients may be treated in this manner, since the associated growth plate does not add to the overall length of the forelimb. If conservative treatment is employed, it may result in contracture of the triceps muscle group and the development of fibrosis.

D. Shaft fractures with more than 50 percent of alignment, in young dogs, respond well to plaster walking casts. When apposition is poor, internal fixation, employing plates is preferred (Fig. 2) because many cases treated with intramedullary pinning respond poorly, and the technique is to be deprecated. Fractures of the distal shaft, in the toy dog, should never be treated conservatively. A high incidence of nonunion occurs in such cases.

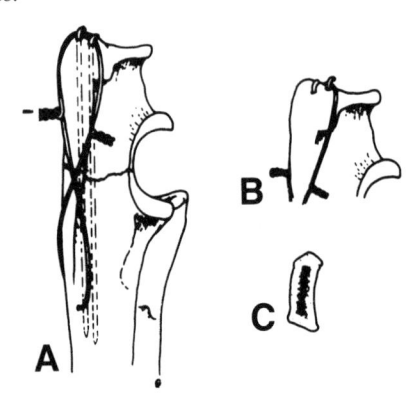

Figure 1 Tension-band fixation of the olecranon process.

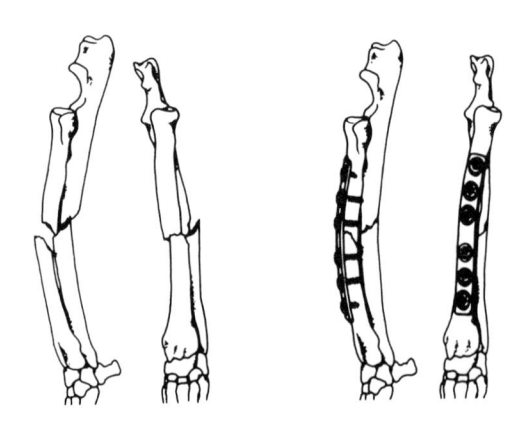

Figure 2 Plating of a fracture of the radius and ulna.

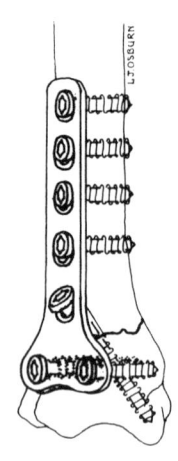

Figure 3 Fracture of the distal radius stabilized by a special canine T-plate. One screw may be lagged across the fracture.

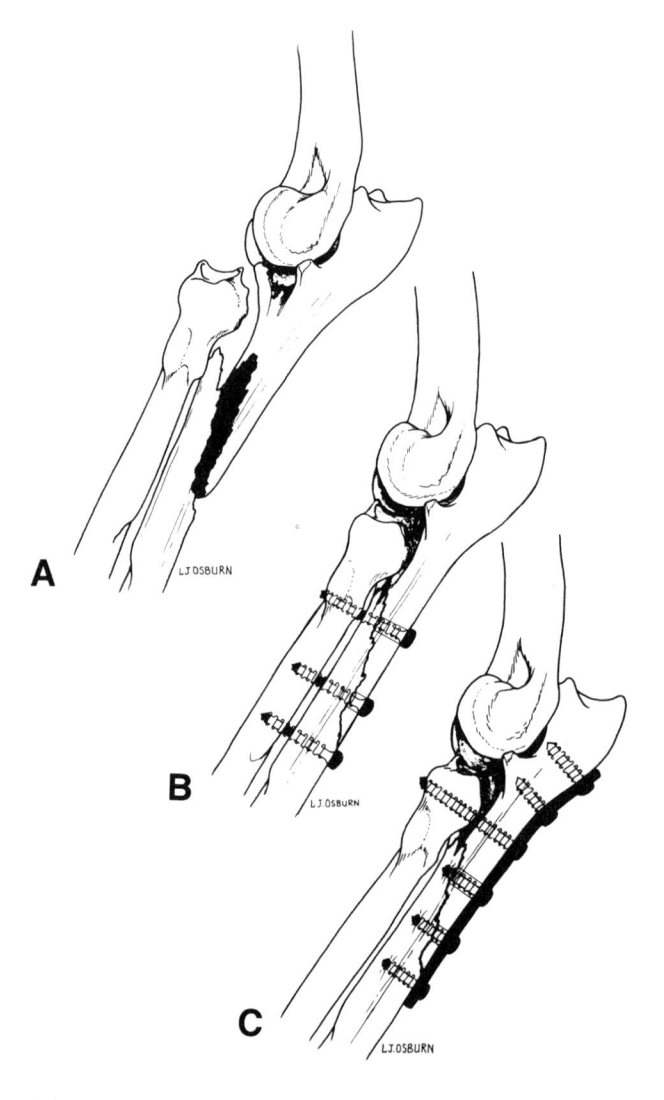

Figure 4 Monteggia fracture: *A*, radiohumeral luxation and fracture of the ulna; *B*, stabilization with screws following reduction; *C*, stabilization with screws and a plate following reduction.

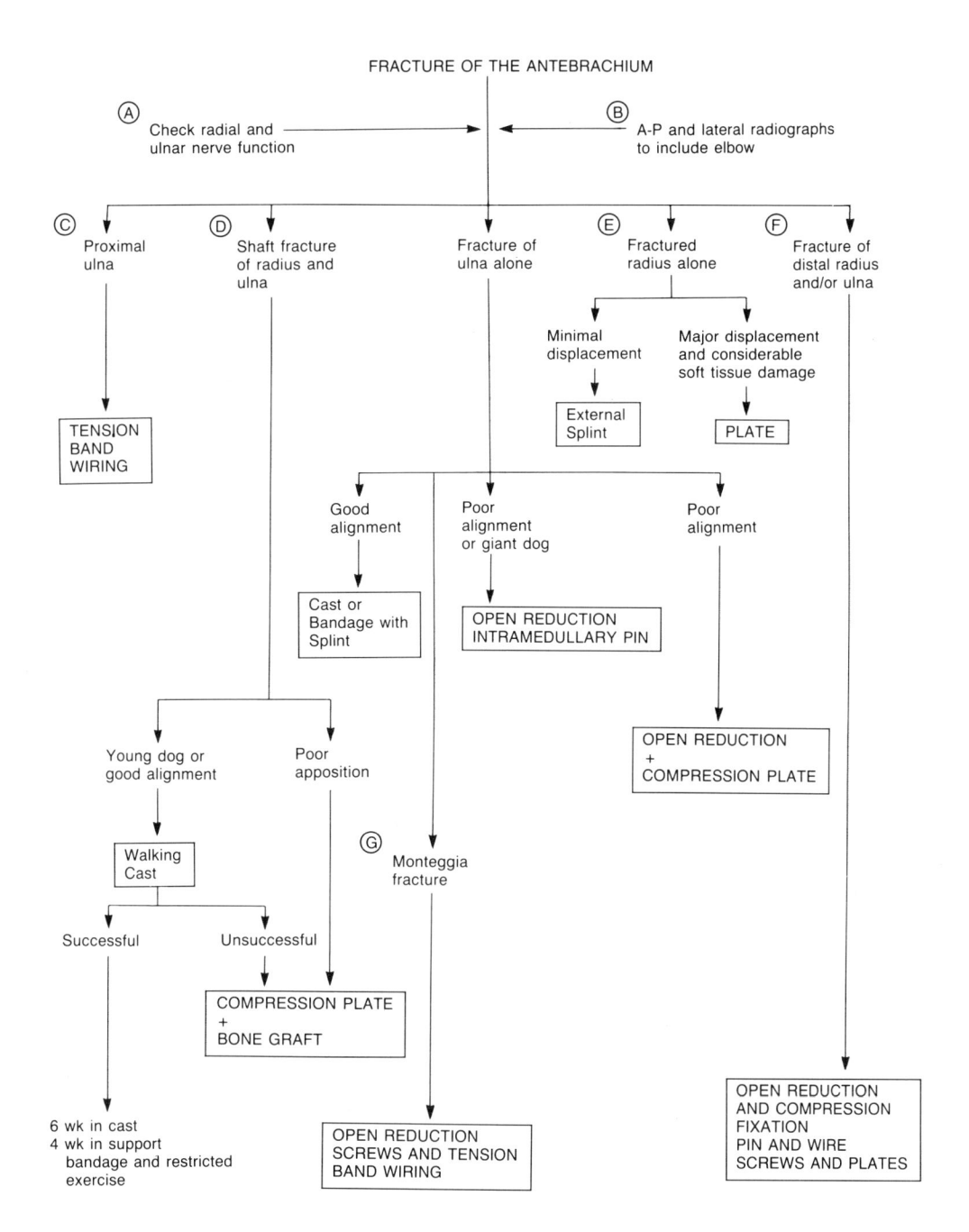

```
                    FRACTURE OF THE ANTEBRACHIUM
                              │
    (A) Check radial and ─────┼───── (B) A-P and lateral radiographs
        ulnar nerve function  │          to include elbow
                              │
    ┌────────┬────────────┬───┴────────┬──────────────┬─────────────┐
   (C)      (D)           │           (E)            (F)
   Proximal  Shaft fracture Fracture of  Fractured     Fracture of
   ulna      of radius and  ulna alone   radius alone  distal radius
             ulna                                      and/or ulna
```

Flowchart (reading-order summary):

- C. Proximal ulna → TENSION BAND WIRING
- D. Shaft fracture of radius and ulna
- E. Fractured radius alone
  - Minimal displacement → External Splint
  - Major displacement and considerable soft tissue damage → PLATE
- Fracture of ulna alone:
  - Good alignment → Cast or Bandage with Splint
    - Young dog or good alignment → Walking Cast
      - Successful → 6 wk in cast, 4 wk in support bandage and restricted exercise
      - Unsuccessful → COMPRESSION PLATE + BONE GRAFT
    - Poor apposition → COMPRESSION PLATE + BONE GRAFT
  - Poor alignment or giant dog → OPEN REDUCTION INTRAMEDULLARY PIN
  - Poor alignment → OPEN REDUCTION + COMPRESSION PLATE
- (G) Monteggia fracture → OPEN REDUCTION SCREWS AND TENSION BAND WIRING
- F. Fracture of distal radius and/or ulna → OPEN REDUCTION AND COMPRESSION FIXATION PIN AND WIRE SCREWS AND PLATES

E. Fracture of the distal radius alone is uncommon. Usually it may be treated following reduction by external support, but if the fracture is severely displaced and associated with major soft tissue damage, plating is recommended (Fig. 3).

F. Valgus displacement of fractures of the distal radius and ulna is the rule. In adult dogs, casting with the paw in varus and the carpus flexed is satisfactory in the hands of skilled surgeons. More satisfactory results may be obtained employing internal fixation, following exact reduction of the distal segment, particularly if that segment is small. The techniques are specialized, and a number have been described in the literature.

G. Monteggia fractures (cranial luxation of the head of the radius associated with fracture of the proximal ulna) (Fig. 4A) are crippling to the function of the elbow joint and require internal fixation (Fig. 4B, C), following reduction of the luxated radius. The radius must be secured to the ulna and the fracture of the latter treated by tension band fixation.

References

Bloombert MS. Fractures of the radius ulna. In: Bojrab MJ, ed. Current techniques in small animal surgery. Philadelphia: Lea & Febiger, 1983:694.

Harrison JS. In: Brinker WO, Hohn RB, Prieur WD, eds. Manual of internal fixation in small animals. New York: Springer-Verlag, 1984:144.

Reidy RL. Symposia management of limb fractures in small animals. Vet Clin North Am 1975; 5:145.

ACUTE ANTEBRACHIOCARPAL LUXATION–SUBLUXATION

Jon F. Dee

A. Typically, antebrachiocarpal luxations occur with the limb in the dorsiflexed position while severely loaded. On occasion, a good physical examination may be hindered by a significant amount of soft tissue swelling. In these instances, facilitate the examination by using a combination of rest, ice, and compression, followed by reexamination in 24 to 48 hours when the swelling has subsided. It is imperative that the joint be examined thoroughly and stressed throughout its full range of motion; this should include medial, lateral, dorsal, and palmar stress.

B. Take standard anteroposterior (A-P), lateral, and stressed radiographs, and compare these with similar views of the opposite limb.

C. The standard components of these antebrachiocarpal luxations are (1) palmar radiocarpal (ulnocarpal) ligament tears or avulsions and (2) short collateral ligament tears or styloid fractures, which include fractures of the distalmost portion of the ulna.

D. To date, the palmar component of these injuries has been primarily managed by coaptation. Utilize countersunk K-wires or lag screws for avulsions.

E. To assess the extent of the short radial collateral ligamentous injury, it is critical that the medial aspect of the joint be stressed during both extension and flexion in order to evaluate the oblique component of the short radial collateral ligament, as well as to assess the straight component of the short collateral ligament, which is stressed during extension. Because of the size of these ligaments, suture reconstruction is difficult at best. Attempt autogenous reconstruction by using a portion of the flexor carpi radialis tendon as described by Earley. Use synthetic material to attempt reconstruction of the components of the short radial collateral ligament. Autogenous reconstruction of the short ulna collateral ligament may be attempted by using a portion of the ulnaris lateralis tendon as described by Roe and Dee.

F. Styloid fractures of the radius or the ulna are generally best repaired by using a pin and figure-of-eight tension band wire technique.

G. Not uncommonly, these instabilities include a fracture of the distal one-fifth of the ulna. These are best managed by a bone-plating technique.

H. After these various components have been managed by some form of reduction and repair, the carpus is cast in approximately 20 degrees of palmar flexion for approximately 4 to 6 weeks, then splinted in decreasing amounts of flexion. This is followed by a soft roll dressing and gradual rehabilitation.

I. Clinical failures are salvaged by an arthrodesis. A partial arthrodesis fo the antebrachiocarpal joint alone may be attempted, but most commonly a panarthrodesis is the method of choice.

References

Dee JF. Injuries to the distal radius and ulna, carpus and metacarpus. Proc AAHA 1984:349.

Earley TD. Canine carpal ligament injuries. Vet Clin North Am 1978; 8:183.

Miller MF, Christensen GC, Evans HE. Anatomy of the dog. Philadelphia: WB Saunders, 1964:225.

Roe SC, Dee JF. Lateral ligamentous injury to the carpus of a racing greyhound. JAVMA 1986; 1189:453.

ACUTE ANTEBRACHIOCARPAL LUXATION–SUBLUXATION Suspected

- (A) Physical examination
- (B) A-P, lateral, and "stressed" radiographic views based upon the physical examination

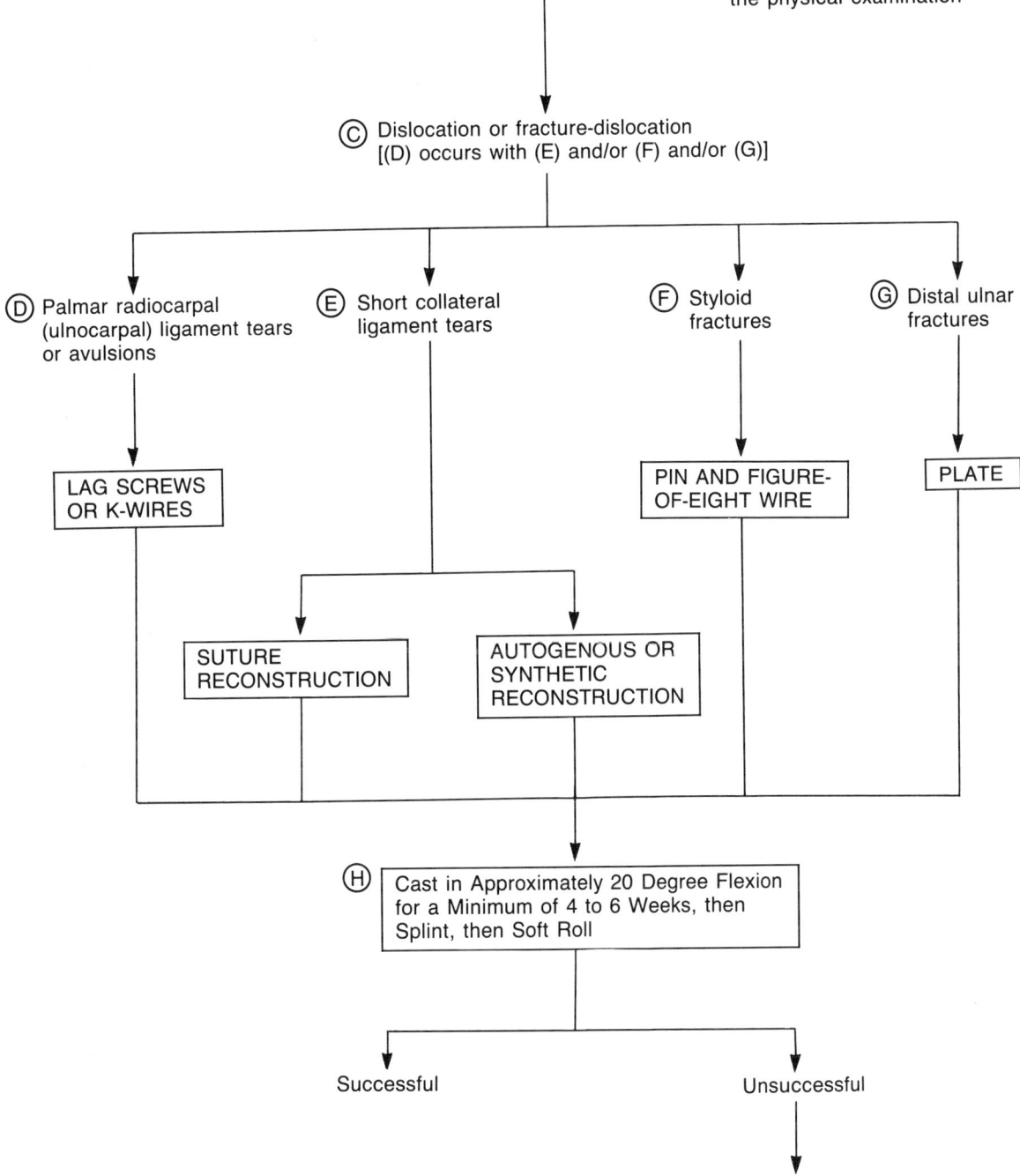

(C) Dislocation or fracture-dislocation [(D) occurs with (E) and/or (F) and/or (G)]

- (D) Palmar radiocarpal (ulnocarpal) ligament tears or avulsions → **LAG SCREWS OR K-WIRES**
- (E) Short collateral ligament tears → **SUTURE RECONSTRUCTION** or **AUTOGENOUS OR SYNTHETIC RECONSTRUCTION**
- (F) Styloid fractures → **PIN AND FIGURE-OF-EIGHT WIRE**
- (G) Distal ulnar fractures → **PLATE**

(H) Cast in Approximately 20 Degree Flexion for a Minimum of 4 to 6 Weeks, then Splint, then Soft Roll

- Successful
- Unsuccessful → (I) **ARTHRODESIS**

STYLOID FRACTURE

Jon F. Dee

The lateral surface of the styloid process of the radius articulates with the radiocarpal bone. The styloid process of the ulna articulates with the ulna carpal bone and with the accessory carpal bone. The radial and ulnar styloid processes are the attachments of the origins of the short radial and short ulnar collateral ligaments, respectively. Styloid fractures are avulsion sprain fractures that affect joint surfaces and, therefore, require repair by open reduction and rigid internal fixation in order to achieve optimal long-term results.

A. The amount of swelling and instability depends on the severity and number of other associated injuries. Varying degrees of subluxation or luxation of the antebrachiocarpal joint are often seen in conjunction with styloid fractures.

B. Small styloid fractures are best stabilized with pin(s) and figure-of-eight tension band wire repair (Fig. 1A).

C. Larger fractures of the radial styloid process may require a lag screw for compression in conjunction with a Kirschner wire for additional rotary stability (Fig. 1B).

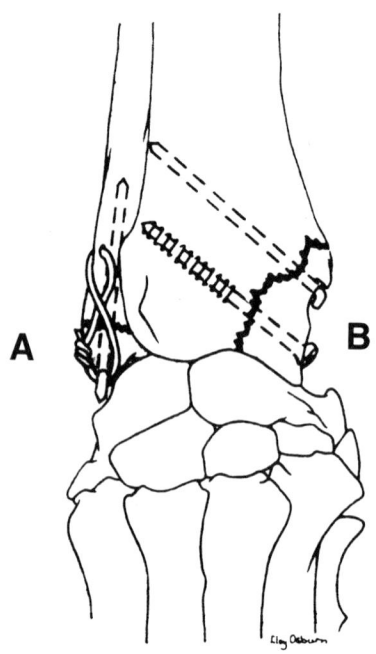

Figure 1 Styloid fractures. *A*, fracture of the ulnar styloid stabilized with a pin and figure-of-eight tension band wire. *B*, pin and lag screw fixation of a large radial styloid process fracture.

References

Brinker WO, Piermattei DL, Flo GL. Handbook of small animal orthopedics and fracture treatment. Philadelphia: WB Saunders, 1983:164.

Dee JF. Injuries to the distal radius and ulna, carpus and metacarpus. Proc AAHA 1984:349.

Dee JF, Dee LG, Earley TD. Fractures of carpus, tarsus, metacarpus and phalanges. In: Brinker WO, Hohn RB, Prieur WD, eds. Manual of internal fixation in small animals. Heidelberg: Springer-Verlag, 1983:190.

STYLOID FRACTURE Suspected

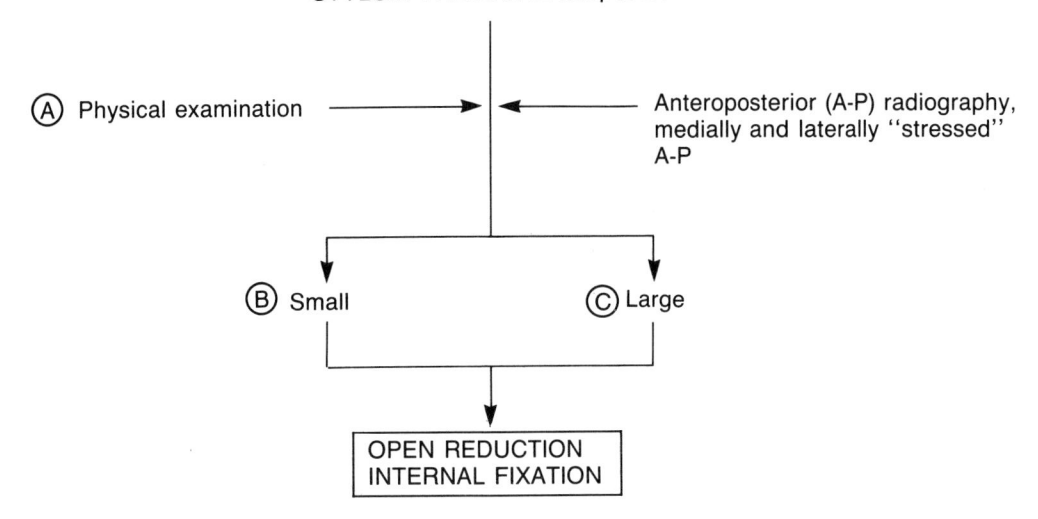

(A) Physical examination → ← Anteroposterior (A-P) radiography, medially and laterally "stressed" A-P

(B) Small   (C) Large

OPEN REDUCTION
INTERNAL FIXATION

ACCESSORY CARPAL BONE FRACTURE

Jon F. Dee

Fractures of the accessory carpal bone, whether they are of a ligamentous or a tendinous nature, are primarily hyperextension injuries.

A. As revealed by physical examination of the carpus, ligamentous avulsion fractures of the accessory carpal bone are characterized by a decreased range of motion, with pain on flexion. Tendinous avulsion fractures of the accessory carpal bone have a normal range of motion and increased soft tissue swelling; any pain present is present on extension.

B. Lateral radiographs in the extended position tend to distract the fracture fragments and enhance visualization. Repair may be achieved by pinning and a figure-of-eight wire (Fig. 1).

C. Ventral avulsion fractures of the accessory carpal bone are Type III sprain injuries that result in an intra-articular fragment, which is produced by the avulsion of the accessory carpal ulnar ligament from the base of the accessory carpal bone. This intra-articular fracture leads to degenerative joint disease. Small fragments are excised; larger fragments are fixed in the normal anatomic position by means of a small positional or lag screw (depending on the size of the fragment) (Fig. 2). The surgical approach is from the palmar aspect of the carpus between the paired accessory carpal-metacarpal ligaments. Postoperatively, the carpus is cast in decreasing amounts of palmar flexion for 6 to 8 weeks.

D. Dorsal avulsion fractures of the accessory carpal bone may be either sprain or strain-type injuries. Tendinous strain injuries involve avulsions of the flexor carpi ulnaris tendon from the dorsal aspect of the accessory carpal bone. These are repaired by small fragment excision and tendinous reconstruction via a dorsoventral transosseous tunnel in the accessory carpal bone. Dorsal avulsion sprains involve the dorsolateral basilar aspect of the accessory carpal bone. Avulsions of the small ligament located there are excised. Both of these lesions are postoperatively cast in decreasing degrees of palmar flexion for 6 to 8 weeks.

E. Severely comminuted fractures of the accessory carpal bone are uncommon injuries that are best managed by casting the carpus in a moderate degree of palmar flexion, with gradual return to normal position.

References

Brinker WO, Piermattei DL, Flo GL. Handbook of small animal orthopedics and fracture treatment. Philadelphia: WB Saunders, 1983:171.

Dee JF, Dee LG, Eaton-Wells RW. Injuries of high performance

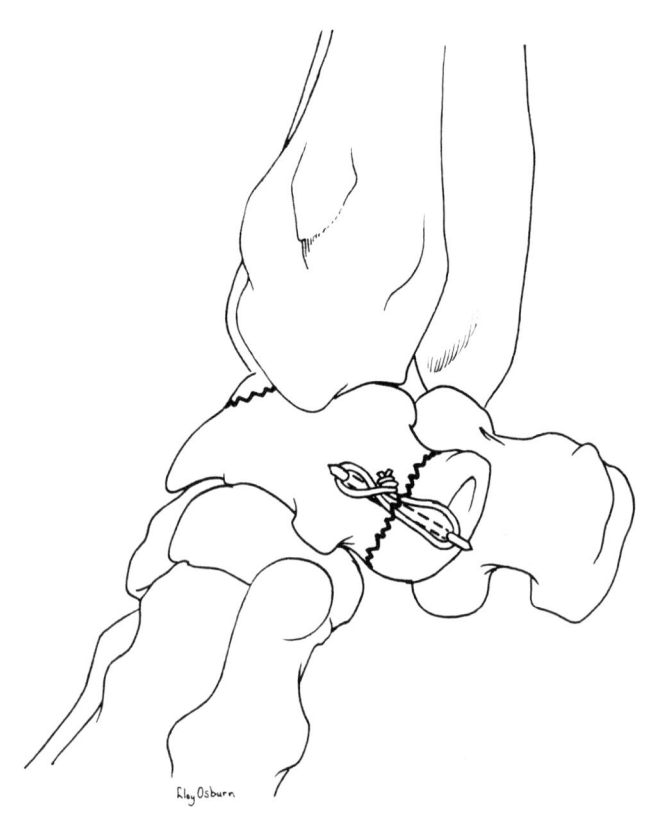

Figure 1 Accessory carpal fracture—lateral component, stabilized with a single pin and a figure-of-eight wire.

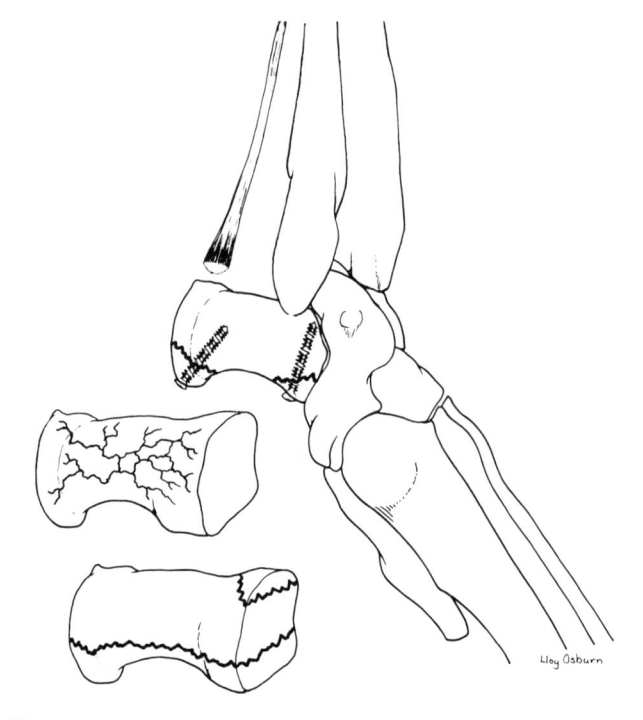

Figure 2 Fractures of the accessory carpal bone stabilized with miniscrews. Avulsion of the tendon is treated by suturing through the bone.

ACCESSORY CARPAL BONE FRACTURE Suspected

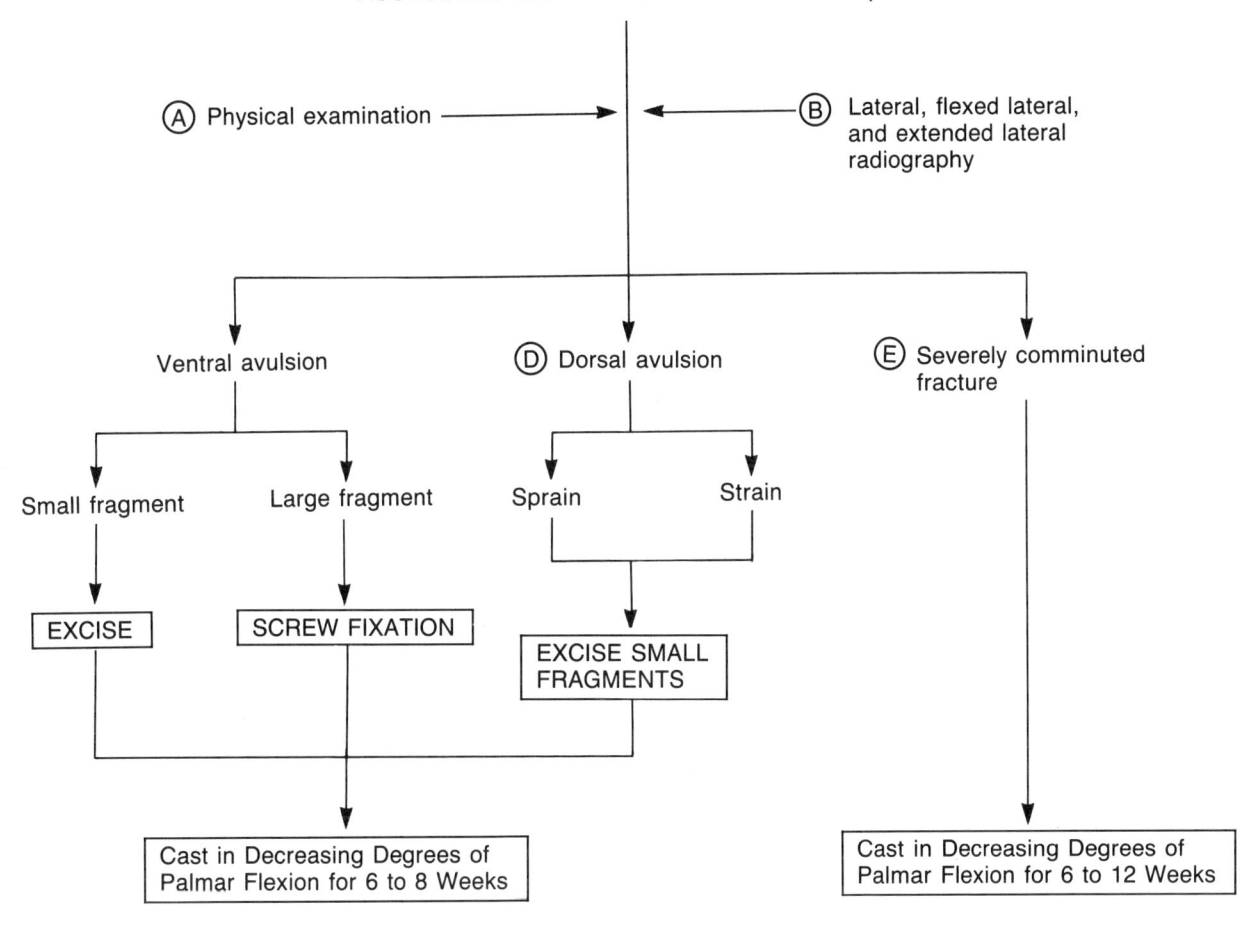

```
                    |
    (A) Physical examination ——→   ←—— (B) Lateral, flexed lateral,
                                         and extended lateral
                                         radiography
                    |
    ┌───────────────┼───────────────┐
    ↓               ↓               ↓
Ventral avulsion  (D) Dorsal      (E) Severely comminuted
                      avulsion         fracture
   ┌──┴──┐         ┌───┴───┐
   ↓     ↓         ↓       ↓
 Small  Large    Sprain  Strain
 frag.  frag.
   ↓     ↓         └───┬───┘
 EXCISE SCREW          ↓
        FIXATION   EXCISE SMALL
                   FRAGMENTS
         ↓
   Cast in Decreasing Degrees of       Cast in Decreasing Degrees of
   Palmar Flexion for 6 to 8 Weeks     Palmar Flexion for 6 to 12 Weeks
```

dogs. In: Whittick WG, ed. Canine orthopedics II. Philadelphia: Lea & Febiger, in press.

Dee JF, Dee LG. Fractures and dislocations associated with the racing greyhound. In: Newton CW, Nunamaker DW, eds. Textbook of small animal orthopaedics. Philadelphia: JB Lippincott, 1985:467.

Johnson KH. Accessory carpal bone fractures in the racing greyhound. Vet Surg 1987; 16:60.

RADIAL CARPAL BONE FRACTURE AND LUXATION

Jon F. Dee

Radial carpal bone fractures and luxations are uncommon injuries in dogs and cats.

A. Hairline fractures of the radial carpal bone may be characterized only by some decreased range of motion with slight pain or flexion. More severe fractures and fracture luxations of the radial carpal bone may present a great deal of soft tissue swelling, pain, and some crepitation of bony fragments.

B. Routine anteroposterior (A-P) lateral, flexed lateral, and in some cases, oblique radiographs can aid in the appreciation of the extent of the fractures and/or luxations not diagnosed on physical examination.

C. Oblique sagittal fractures of the body of the radial carpal bone originate midway beneath the distal end of the radius, extend obliquely in a medial direction, and end above the second carpal bone. Some of these fractures do not extend through both cortices and have minimal displacement; these may be successfully coapted. Others with more severe displacement are repaired by lag screw fixation, starting extra-articularly on the palmar prominence of the radial carpal bone and directing the screw dorsolaterally (Fig. 1A, 1B).

D. Avulsions of the palmar prominence of the radial carpal bone are caused by distraction of the origin of the palmar radial carpal-metacarpal ligament or the insertion of the oblique component of the short radial collateral ligament on the palmar prominence of the radial carpal bone, or both. This avulsion is stabilized by either lag screw or pin and wire fixation (Fig. 1C).

E. Small dorsal or palmar chips of the radial carpal bone are best visualized on lateral and flexed views. These small chips are excised.

F. Repair luxations of the radial carpal bone and frequently found associated fractures by open reduction. Repair associated fractures of the palmar prominence, and also occasionally of the radial styloid, by pin and figure-of-eight tension wire band. Excise small chips. Occasionally the flexor carpi radialis muscle may be torn. Repair it and other damaged soft tissues by suturing. Protect the carpus in a neutral position.

References

Brinker WO, Piermattei DL, Flo GL. Handbook of small animal orthopedics and fracture treatment. Philadelphia: WB Saunders, 1983:167.

Dee JF. Injuries to the distal radius and ulna, carpus and metacarpus. Proc AAHA 1984:349.

Dee JF, Dee LG, Earley TD. Fractures of carpus, tarsus, metacar-

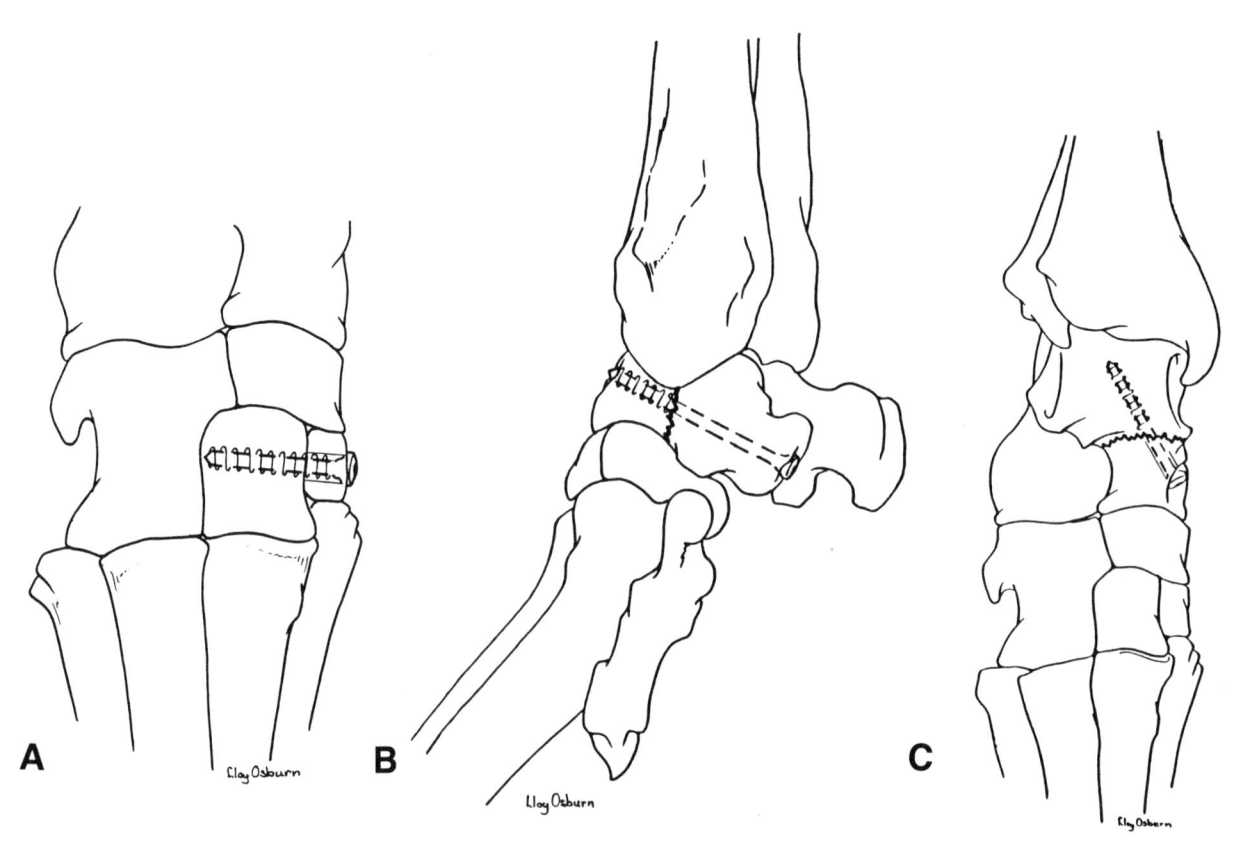

Figure 1 Lag screw fixation of various radial carpal bone fractures.

RADIAL CARPAL BONE FRACTURE AND LUXATION Suspected

- **A** Physical examination
- **B** A-P, lateral, flexed lateral, and oblique radiography

- **C** Sagittal (oblique) fracture of the body
  - Minimal displacement → Cast → Successful / Unsuccessful
  - Major displacement → LAG SCREW
- **D** Palmar prominence avulsions → K-WIRE AND CERCLAGE, OR LAG SCREW, OR PIN AND FIGURE-OF-EIGHT WIRE
- **E** Dorsal chips / Palmar chips → EXCISE SMALL CHIPS
- **F** Luxations with fractures → OPEN REDUCTION → EXCISE SMALL CHIPS

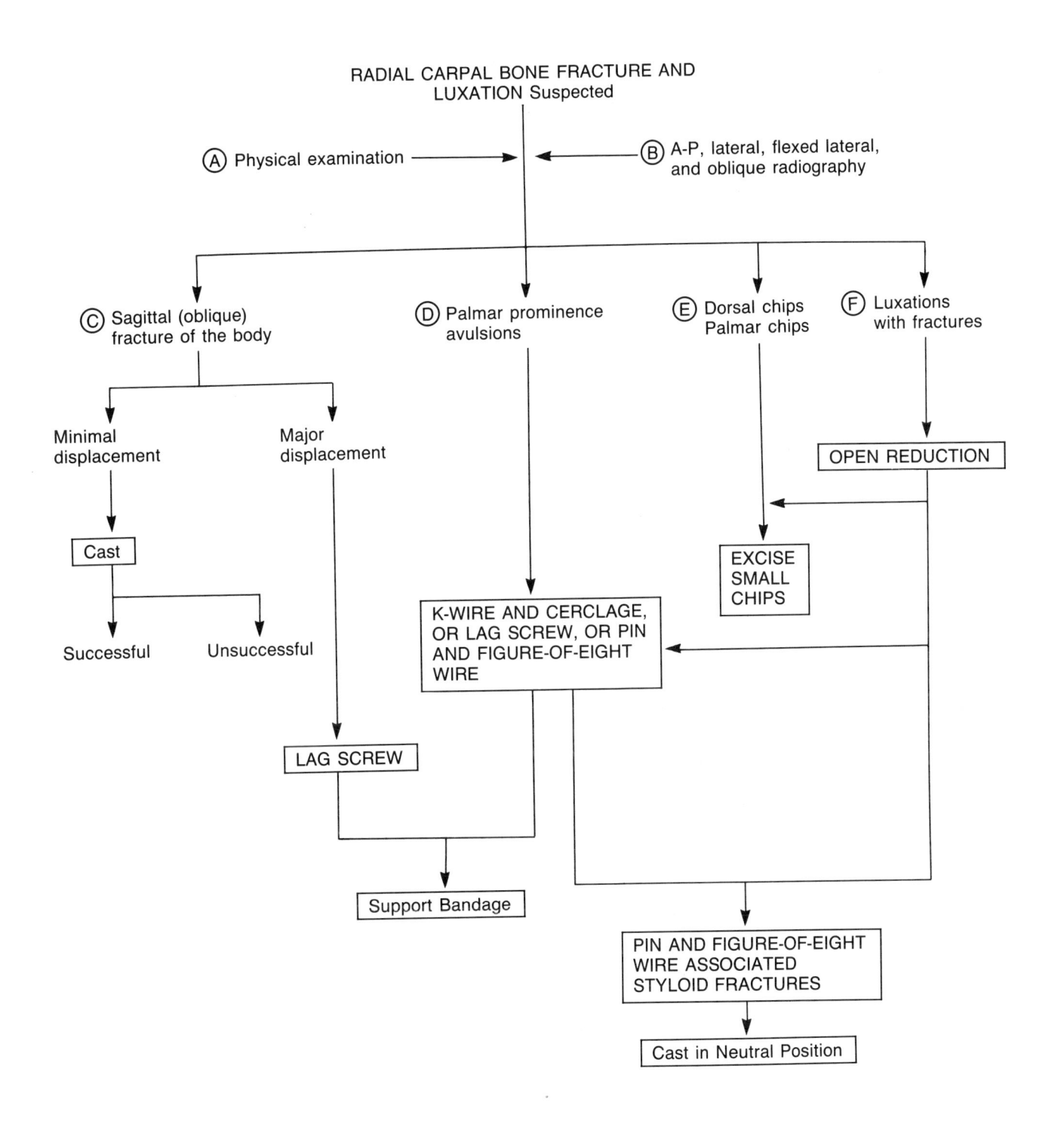

→ Support Bandage

PIN AND FIGURE-OF-EIGHT WIRE ASSOCIATED STYLOID FRACTURES → Cast in Neutral Position

pus and phalanges. In: Brinker WO, Hohn RB, Prieur WD, eds. Manual of internal fixation in small animals. Heidelberg: Springer-Verlag, 1983:190.

Earley TD, Dee JF. Trauma to the carpus, tarsus and phalanges of dogs and cats. Vet Clin North Am 1980; 10:717.

Miller MF, Christensen GC, Evans HE. Anatomy of the dog. Philadelphia: WB Saunders, 1964:225.

CARPAL ARTHRODESIS
Jon F. Dee

Arthrodesis is reserved as a surgical salvage procedure for joints when other medical and surgical methods have failed or have little chance of success. It is an attempt to eliminate motion and pain and therefore improve overall limb function.

A. Physical examination of the carpus consists of evaluating range of motion and stressing the various joints in all planes.

B. Take stress radiographs in order to asses which joint level or levels are involved.

C. The indications for carpal arthrodesis include hyperextension injuries and other carpal instabilities in which primary surgical repair and/or appropriate casting methods have failed. Other indications include polytrauma, unmanageable degenerative joint disease, and flexion deformity from distal radial nerve injury.

D. Generally when speaking of panarthrodesis versus partial (subtotal) arthrodesis, we are referring to an arthrodesis (fusion) of all of the joints of an area rather than one less than the total, which is partial arthrodesis. For example, in the carpus, a panarthrodesis includes the antebrachial carpal, the middle carpal, and the carpometacarpal joints.

E. A partial arthrodesis of the carpus most commonly refers to an arthrodesis that includes both the middle carpal and the carpometacarpal joint levels.

F. The less commonly performed arthrodesis of the antebrachial carpal joint only is simply referred to as an arthrodesis of the antebrachial carpal joint. In the tarsus, a panarthrodesis is the exception rather than the rule. In fact, partial arthrodesis in the tarsus frequently involves only one section of a joint level. For example, one may perform an arthrodesis of the calcaneoquartal joint and leave the talocalcaneocentral joint essentially intact. For these reasons, it may eliminate confusion to anatomically name the fused components of the arthrodesis.

G. An arthrodesis of all three carpal joint levels may be obtained by the application of a plate on either the dorsal or the palmar surface of the carpus. In either case, an attempt should be made to obtain screw fixation in the radial carpal bone. Dorsal plating is easier to accomplish (Fig. 1), but palmar plating has the mechanical advantage of being on the tension side of the carpus.

H. Cross pins have been utilized from the medial aspect of the distal radius to the lateral aspect of the base of metacarpal (MC) V and from the lateral aspect of the ulnal to the medial aspect of the base of metacarpal II.

I. External fixators have been reserved primarily for the arthrodesis of open injuries.

J. Perform partial arthrodesis in order to provide stability to the middle and carpometacarpal joints, while sparing range of motion of the antebrachiocarpal joint. Caution must be exercised in the placement of a T-plate, lest it impinge on the distal aspect of the radius during extension.

K. More commonly these joints are immobilized by intramedullary pins that are inserted via slots cut in the dorsal cortex of the metacarpal bones. The pins are then run up the canals, across the carpometacarpal and middle carpal joints, to seat in the radial- and ulnocarpal bones. Pack the denuded joints with cancellous bone, and cast for 6 to 8 weeks (Fig. 2).

L. Isolated arthrodesis of the antebrachiocarpal joint is the least frequently performed. An upside down T-plate with screws in the radial- and ulnocarpal bones may be utilized.

M. A cross-pin technique may also be utilized to arthrodese the antebrachiocarpal joint. Pins are driven from the medial aspect of the distal radius to seat in the ulnocarpal bone and from the lateral aspect of the distal ulna to seat in the radial carpal bone (Fig. 3).

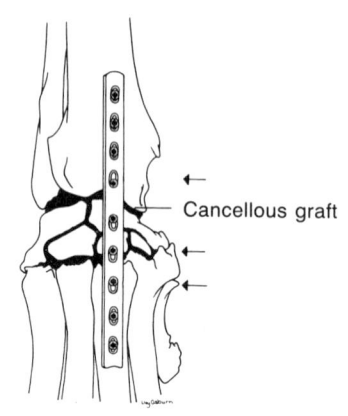

Figure 1 Pan-arthrodesis of the carpal joint with DC plate and associated grafts.

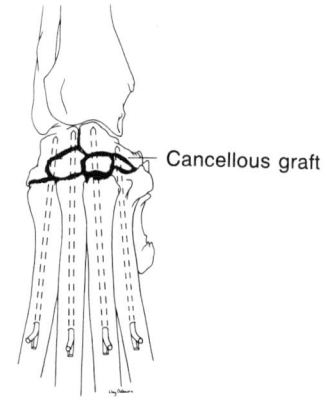

Figure 2 Distal arthrodesis with intramedullary pins and grafts.

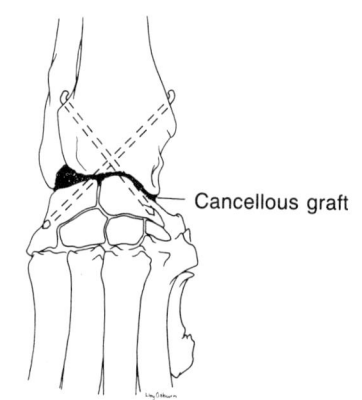

Figure 3 Antebranchial joint arthrodesis with crossed-pins and associated graft.

CARPAL ARTHRODESIS

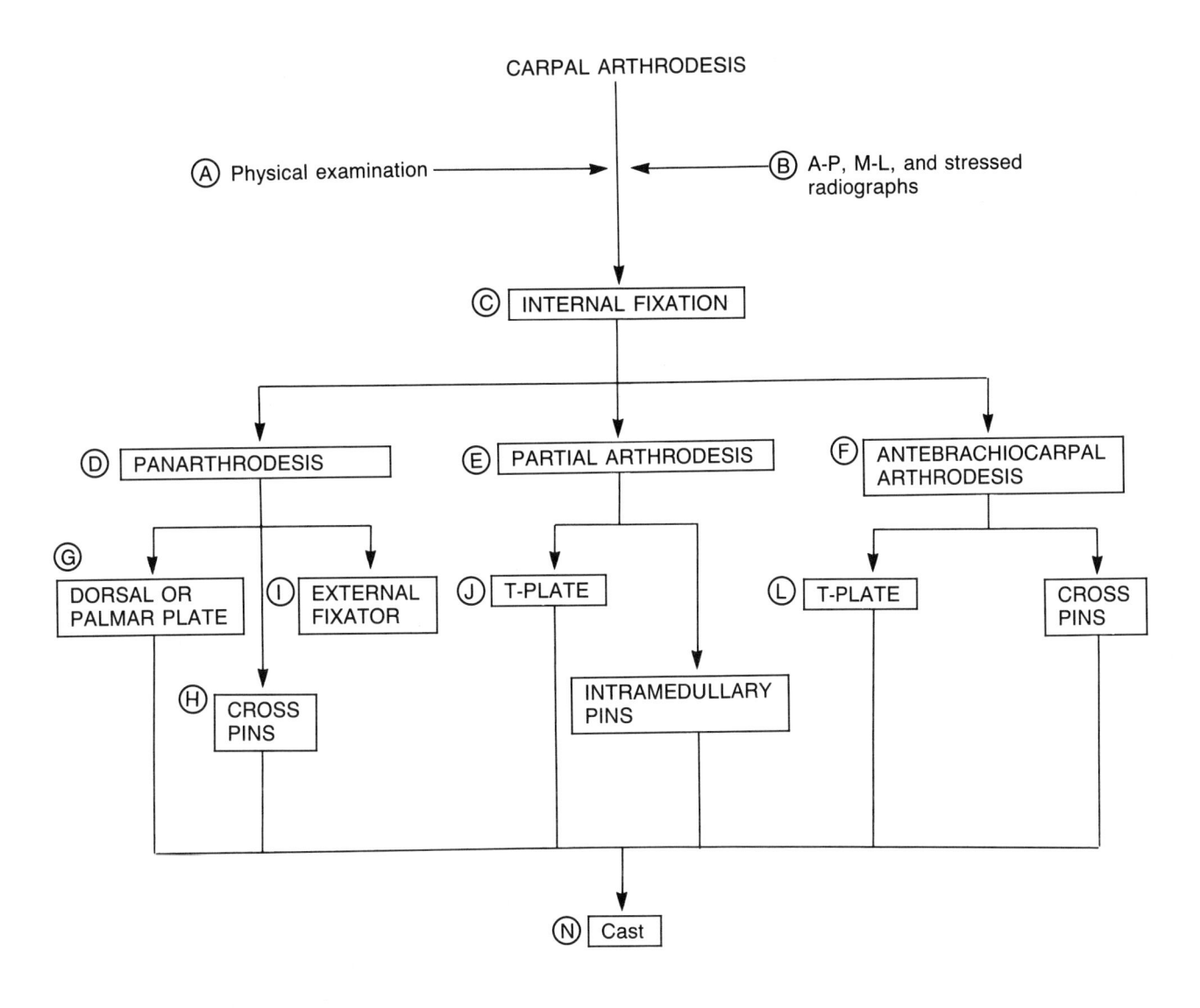

```
                    CARPAL ARTHRODESIS
                             │
   (A) Physical examination ──→ ←── (B) A-P, M-L, and stressed
                             │           radiographs
                             ↓
                    (C) INTERNAL FIXATION
                    ┌────────┼────────┐
                    ↓        ↓        ↓
            (D) PANARTHRODESIS  (E) PARTIAL   (F) ANTEBRACHIOCARPAL
                                ARTHRODESIS    ARTHRODESIS
           ┌────┬────┐            │          ┌────┬────┐
           ↓    ↓    ↓            ↓          ↓         ↓
      (G) DORSAL OR  (I) EXTERNAL (J) T-PLATE  (L) T-PLATE  CROSS
      PALMAR PLATE   FIXATOR                               PINS
              ↓    ↓                ↓
           (H) CROSS         INTRAMEDULLARY
              PINS                PINS
                             │
                          (N) Cast
```

N. Critical features of all cases are adequate removal of cartilage, ample cancellous bone graft, and rigid immobilization. All cases are placed in the approximate amount of extension normal for the individual or breed. Plated or pinned cases are cast until radiographic evidence of union is apparent.

References

Brinker WO, Piermattei DL, Flo GL. Handbook of small animal orthopedics and fracture treatment. Philadelphia: WB Saunders, 1983.

Earley TD. Canine carpal ligament injuries. Vet Clin North Am 1978;8:183.

Earley TD, Piermattei DL, Dee JF, Weigel JP. Canine carpus and tarsus short course. Proceedings. Knoxville, Tennessee: University of Tennessee, 1981:1.

Newton CD, Nunamaker DM. Textbook of small animal orthopaedics. Philadelphia: JB Lippincott, 1985:567.

Slocum B. Partial carpal fusion in the dog. Presented at fifth annual meeting. Snowmass, Colorado: Vet Orth Soc 1978.

METACARPAL (METATARSAL) FRACTURE

Jon F. Dee

A. Metacarpal (metatarsal) fractures usually present as an acute nonweight-bearing lameness with extensive swelling, crepitation, and pain. There is history of direct trauma. In contrast, the acute hairline stress fracture is also nonweight-bearing, but has significant local pain and swelling, no crepitation, and no history of direct trauma.

B. Anteroposterior (A-P), lateral, and oblique radiographs are routinely taken. Take stressed medial and lateral A-P radiographs for suspected acute fatigue fractures that are not demonstrated on routine projections. Detail film and cassettes are utilized.

C. Coapt nondisplaced fractures and displaced fractures that can be anatomically reduced.

D. Avulsion fractures of the base of metacarpals (MC) II and V are usually the result of hyperextension injuries and are very unstable. Fractures of the base of metacarpal II tend to be small and are therefore managed by pin and figure-of-eight tension band wire. Lag screw fixation may be utilized to repair larger, more oblique fractures that may occur to the base of metacarpal V. Avulsions of the base of metatarsal (MT) II are uncommon. Avulsions of the lateral aspect of the base of metatarsal V do not lead to instability and may routinely be coapted.

E. Optimum results are obtained in long, oblique fractures of the shaft of the metacarpal (metatarsal) bones by open reduction and internal fixation with two or more small cortical bone screws, used in a lag fashion. The fracture is then coapted until the fracture is healed. An alternate method of repair is the use of a Kirschner pin and cerclage wires.

F. Manage solitary or multiple unstable transverse shaft fractures by the insertion of intramedullary Kirschner wires via slots made in the dorsal cortex just proximal to the metacarpal (metatarsal)-phalangeal joint. The extra effort made to keep the free ends of the wires away from the metacarpal (metatarsal)-phalangeal extensor mechanism is worthwhile; it enhances long-term joint range of motion (Fig. 1A).

G. Manage comminuted fractures by a combination of plates and lag screws. Plates are placed on the medial side of the bone for metacarpal (metatarsal) II fractures and on the lateral side for metacarpal (metatarsal) V fractures. Metacarpal (tarsal) III and IV fractures are plated on their dorsal surface (Fig. 1B).

H. Metacarpal (metatarsal) neck fractures are highly unstable and are best managed in a Rush pin fashion, starting the pin medial and distal for metacarpal (metatarsal) II fractures and lateral and distal for metacarpal (metatarsal) V fractures. This avoids the extensor mechanism (Fig. 1C).

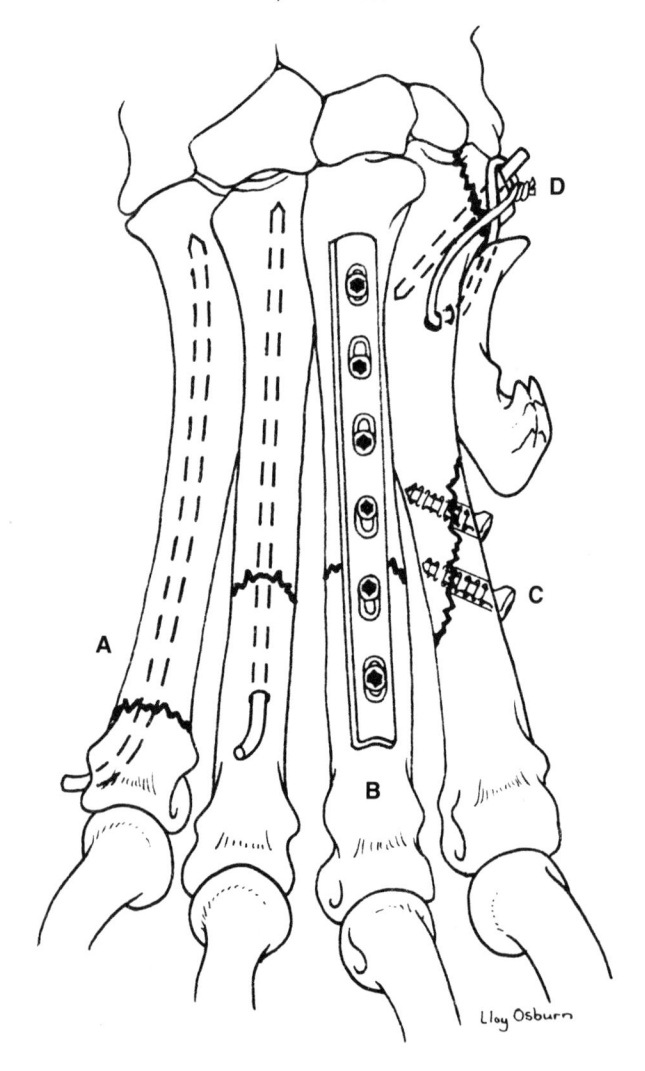

Figure 1 Various fractures of the metacarpal (or metatarsal) bones stabilized by *A*, intramedullar pins, *B*, DC plate, *C*, screw and *D*, pin with figure-of-eight wire.

References

Dee JF. Fractures in the racing greyhound. In: Bojrab MJ, ed. Patho-physiology in small animal surgery. Philadelphia: Lea and Febiger, 1981.

Dee JF, Dee LG. Fractures and dislocations associated with the racing greyhound. In: Newton CW, Nunamaker DW, eds. Textbook of small animal orthopaedics. Philadelphia: JB Lippincott, 1985:467.

Dee JF, Dee LG, Earley TD. Fractures of carpus, tarsus, metacarpus and phalanges. In: Brinker WO, Hohn RB, Prieur WD, eds. Manual of internal fixation in small animals. Heidelberg: Springer-Verlag, 1983:190.

Dee JF, Dee LG, Eaton-Wells RW. Injuries of high performance dogs. In: Whittick WG, ed. Canine orthopedics II. Philadelphia: Lea and Febiger, in press.

METACARPAL (METATARSAL) FRACTURE Suspected

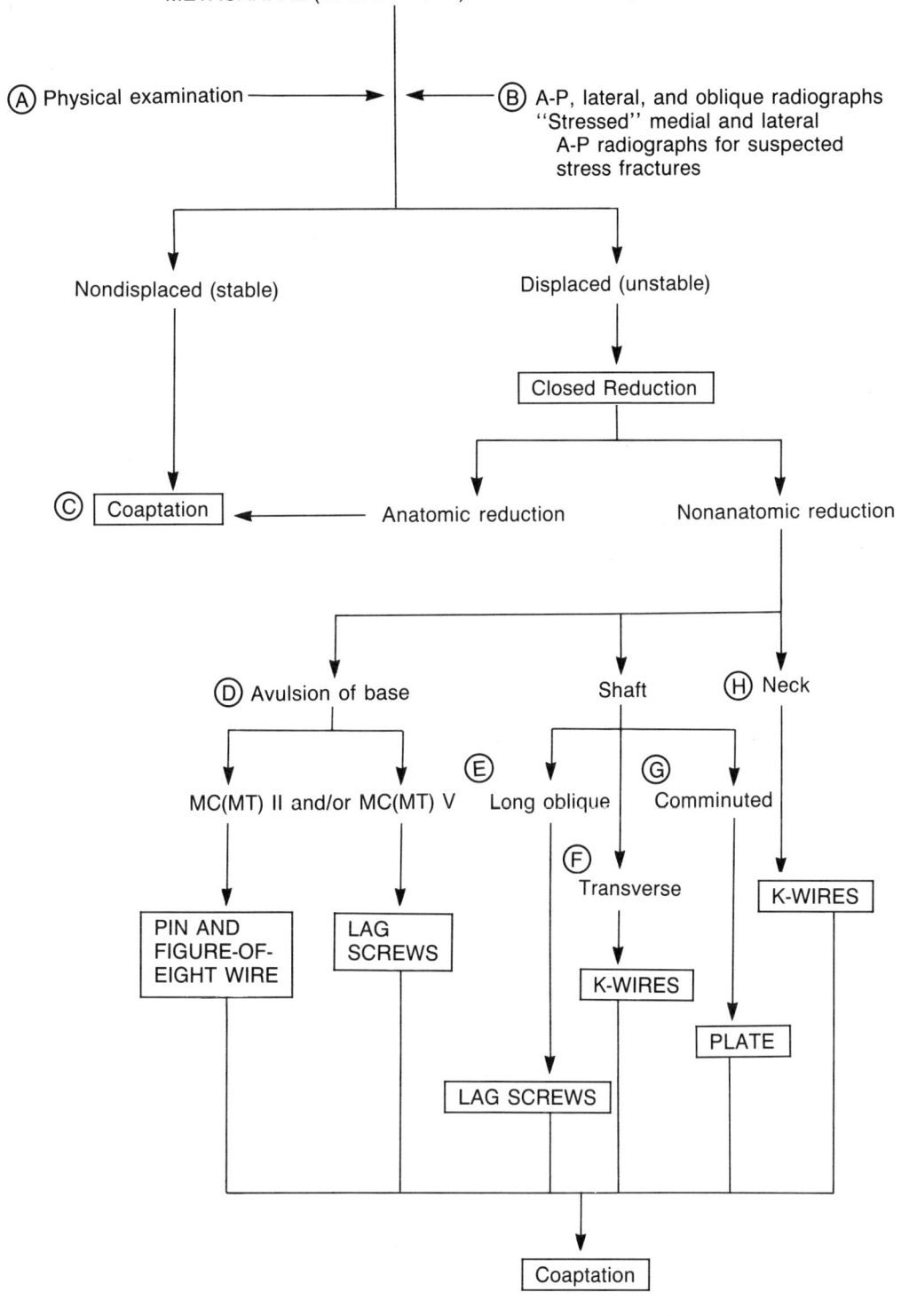

(A) Physical examination → ← (B) A-P, lateral, and oblique radiographs "Stressed" medial and lateral A-P radiographs for suspected stress fractures

Nondisplaced (stable) | Displaced (unstable)

Closed Reduction

Anatomic reduction → (C) Coaptation

Nonanatomic reduction

(D) Avulsion of base | Shaft | (H) Neck

MC(MT) II and/or MC(MT) V

PIN AND FIGURE-OF-EIGHT WIRE | LAG SCREWS

(E) Long oblique | (G) Comminuted

(F) Transverse

K-WIRES

LAG SCREWS

PLATE

K-WIRES

Coaptation

METACARPAL OR METATARSAL-PHALANGEAL SUBLUXATION, LUXATION

Larry G. Dee

A. Type I is characterized by a second degree sprain or stretching of one collateral ligament.

B. Use external coaptation with a splint for 1 week. Splinting for a longer period may result in joint stiffness, pain, and lameness.

C. Use elastic bandage (Elasticon or Vetwrap) to brace the affected digit against the other digits. Maintain strapping for a minimum of 3 weeks. The purpose of strapping is to permit anterior-posterior joint motion while preventing lateral and medial joint instability.

D. Keep the toe nail trimmed short. Allow walking on a leash, preferably in sand or on a soft surface. Allow swimming or whirlpool therapy.

E. Imbricate the affected ligament with a synthetic absorbable suture that has sustained strength, such as polydioxanone.

F. If complete unilateral collateral ligament disruption has occurred, the inner collateral ligament on digits II and V are usually affected. The sesamoidean ligament and the sesamoidean-phalangeal ligaments may be damaged.

G. The affected ligaments are exposed via a posterior approach. It may be necessary to preplace sutures before reducing the luxation. Small diameter nylon (3-0 or 4-0) and synthetic absorbable suture have been used successfully. Polydioxanone is currently favored.

H. If complete joint dislocation has occurred, the joint is preserved if closed reduction or surgical intervention results in a stable joint. If it is estimated that reasonable joint stability cannot be achieved, amputation is usually required in order to prevent chronic pain, lameness, and loss of function.

I. If seen early, the joint may be treated by closed reduction; this can result in relative stability because of the support of the sesamoids.

J. Chronic dislocations may require open reduction. The dislocated bones may become trapped and require sharp dissection of the entrapping ligaments to effect reduction.

K. Sutures are usually preplaced after reduction has been achieved.

L. Amputation usually includes the removal of the distal MC or MT cartilage and the sesamoids. The MC and/or MT condyles are smoothed to blend into the shaft. The pad is not saved.

M. A padded bandage is used for 2 weeks in order to protect the suture line.

References

Dee JF, Dee LG, Eaton-Wells RW. Injuries of high performance dogs. In: Whittick WG, ed. Canine orthopedics II. Philadelphia: Lea and Febiger, in press.

Earley TD, Dee JF. Trauma to the carpus, tarsus and phalanges of dogs and cats. Vet Clin North Am 1980; 10:717.

Miller MF, Christensen GC, Evans HE. Anatomy of the dog. Philadelphia: WB Saunders, 1964:191.

METACARPAL-
OR
METATARSAL–PHALANGEAL
SUBLUXATIONS OR LUXATIONS Suspected

Physical examination → ← Radiographs

- (A) Type I
  - (E) SUTURE
  - (B) Splint
  - (C) Strap
  - (D) Physical Therapy
- (F) Type II
  - (G) SUTURE
- (H) Type III
  - Stable
    - (I) Closed Reduction
    - (J) OPEN REDUCTION
      - (K) SUTURE
  - Unstable
    - (L) AMPUTATE
    - (M) Padded Bandage

PHALANGEAL LUXATION

Larry G. Dee

A. On examination of Type I first (P1) and second phalangeal (P2) luxations, these are small tears or stretching of one collateral ligament.

B. Apply a support wrap for 3 to 4 weeks. The nail should be trimmed short in order to reduce leverage on the affected joint.

C. Imbricate the affected ligament with one to three synthetic absorbable sutures (polydioxanone).

D. In Type II P1 to P2 luxations, one of the collateral ligaments is completely disrupted accompanied by varying amounts of capsular damage. Avulsion chips may be present.

E. Open the joint capsule, and flush with saline. Excise small avulsion chips.

F. Suture the torn collateral ligament and adjacent tissue with several horizontal mattress sutures. Either nonabsorbable or polydioxanone sutures are preferred.

G. Coaptation should be maintained for 6 weeks.

H. A splint may be preferred for the first 2 to 3 weeks with a support wrap for the remainder of the 6-week period.

I. Arthrodesis may be accomplished with a small bone plate or with a pin and figure-of-eight wire.

J. The articular cartilage of P1 is removed to prevent chondrosis. The pad is saved to cushion the stump.

K. The suture line is protected for 2 weeks with a padded bandage.

L. In P1 to P2 Type III luxations, bilateral collateral ligament damage has occurred. The joint is often completely unstable, and avulsion chips may be present.

M. Same classification as with P1 to P2 luxations. The treatment is usually amputation because of chronic instability and pain associated with severe injury to this joint in spite of surgical repair.

N. Type I or II luxations of P2 to P3 are treated by closed reduction.

O. This treatment may result in later amputation on account of chronic pain.

References

Dee JF, Dee LG, Eaton-Wells RW. Injuries of high performance dogs. In: Whittick WG, ed. Canine orthopedics II. Philadelphia: Lea and Febiger, in press.

Earley TD, Dee JF. Trauma to the carpus, tarsus and phalanges of dogs and cats. Vet Clin North Am 1980; 10:717.

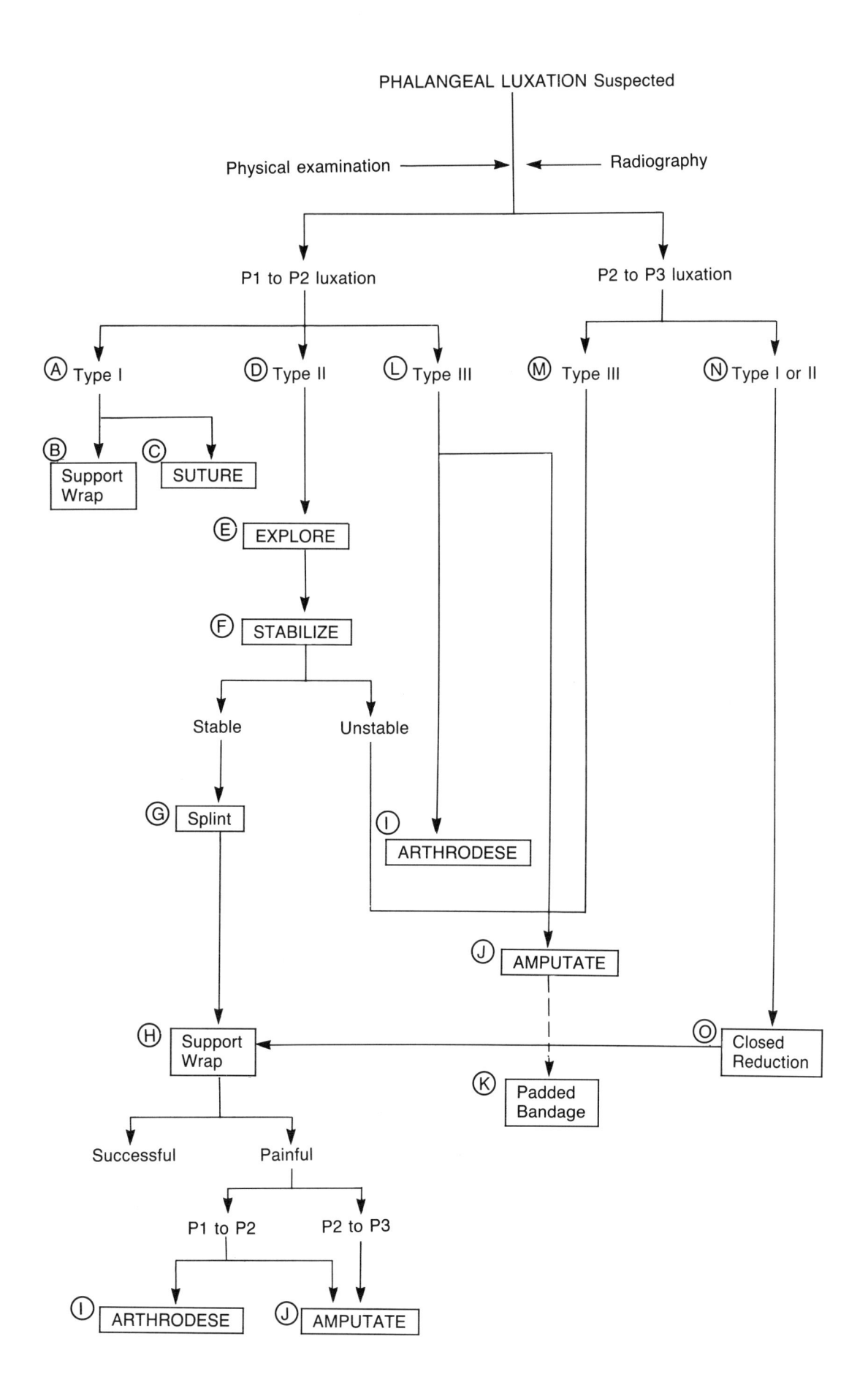

PHALANGEAL LUXATION Suspected

Physical examination → ← Radiography

- P1 to P2 luxation
  - Ⓐ Type I
    - Ⓑ Support Wrap
    - Ⓒ SUTURE
  - Ⓓ Type II
    - Ⓔ EXPLORE
    - Ⓕ STABILIZE
      - Stable → Ⓖ Splint
      - Unstable → Ⓘ ARTHRODESE
  - Ⓛ Type III → Ⓘ ARTHRODESE
- P2 to P3 luxation
  - Ⓜ Type III → Ⓙ AMPUTATE
  - Ⓝ Type I or II → Ⓞ Closed Reduction

Ⓗ Support Wrap
- Successful
- Painful
  - P1 to P2 → Ⓘ ARTHRODESE
  - P2 to P3 → Ⓙ AMPUTATE

Ⓚ Padded Bandage

PHALANGEAL FRACTURE

Jon F. Dee

A. Phalangeal fracture(s) are characterized by pain, swelling, and crepitation.

B. The addition of oblique views to the customary radiographic views is often of value in assessing the fracture.

C. Many shaft fractures of the first or second phalanx may be successsfully coapted.

D. On occasion, mini plates may be utilized in order to maintain reduction of unstable shaft fractures (Fig. 1A).

E. Oblique fractures of the first (P1) and second phalanges (P2) may be repaired by the use of mini 1.5 and 2.0 mm cortical bone screws used in a lag fashion or by the use of cerclage wire (Fig. 1B).

F. Articular fractures of the first and second phalanges may sometimes be managed by lag screws. Avulsion fractures of the insertion of the superficial digital flexor tendon from the proximal palmar aspect of the second phalanx may be held in reduction by the placement of paired dorsal to palmar transosseous tunnels through which a suture is passed in order to capture the avulsed fragment (Fig. 1C).

G. Irreparable articular phalangeal fractures may be arthrodesed by either mini plates or pin and figure-of-eight wire fixation (Fig. 2), but as a practical matter are more often amputated in order to yield a more predictable and timely result. Fractures of the third phalanx (P3) are routinely amputated.

References

Brinker WO, Piermattei DL, Flo GL. Handbook of small animal orthopedics and fracture treatment. Philadelphia: WB Saunders, 1983:181.

Earley TD, Piermattei DL, Dee JF, Weigel JP. Canine carpus and tarsus short course. Proceedings. Knoxville, Tennessee: University of Tennessee, 1981:1.

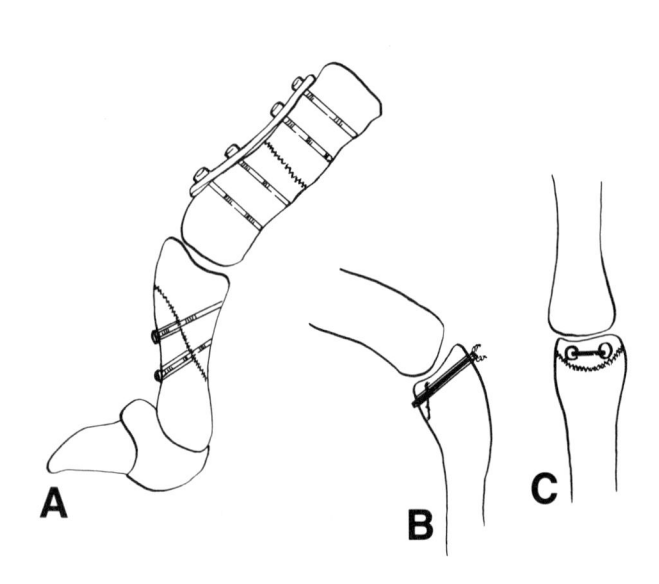

Figure 1 *A*, Fixation of shaft fracture with a mini plate in P1. *B*, Lag screw fixation of oblique fracture of P2. *C*, Tunneling and wiring of avulsed fragment.

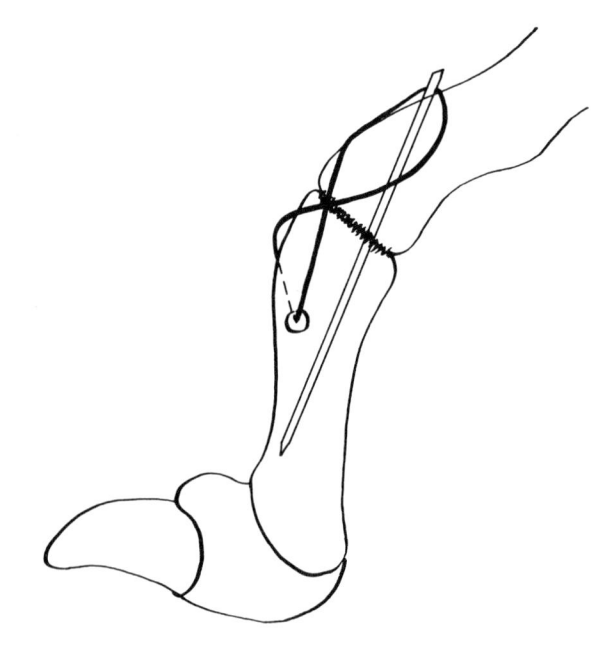

Figure 2 Arthrodesis P1–P2 with intramedullary pin and figure-of-eight wire.

PHALANGEAL FRACTURE Suspected

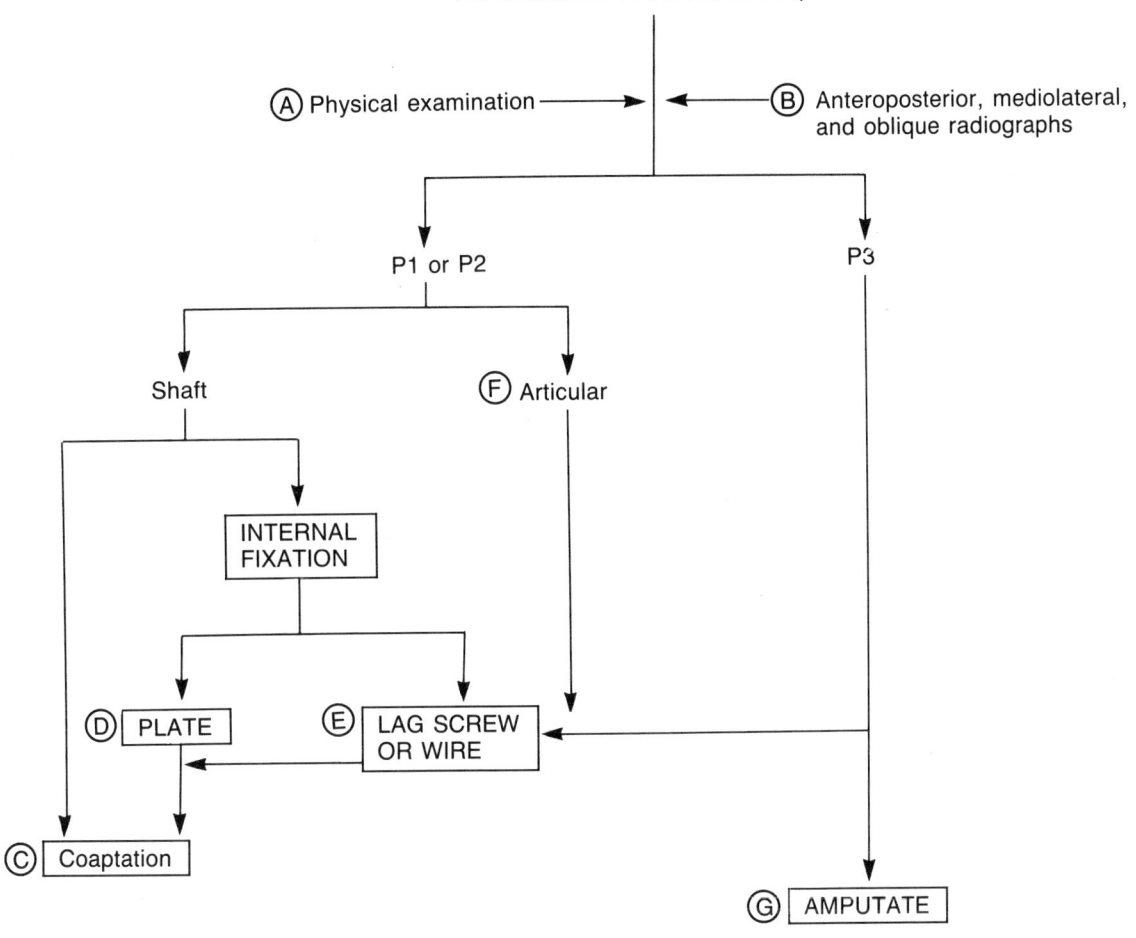

- (A) Physical examination
- (B) Anteroposterior, mediolateral, and oblique radiographs

P1 or P2
- Shaft
- (F) Articular

P3

INTERNAL FIXATION

(D) PLATE

(E) LAG SCREW OR WIRE

(C) Coaptation

(G) AMPUTATE

HIP PAIN

Geoff Sumner-Smith

Commonly animals are presented by an owner who states that the patient appears to have "a sore hip," and they are unable to add anything to that opinion. Pain in the area of the hip joint may originate from many conditions that are directly or indirectly related to the hip joint itself. It behooves a clinician to carry out a full examination instead of assuming that because the patient is of a breed that has a predisposition for a particular condition, it is necessarily suffering from same (e.g., German Shepherds—hip dysplasia, Greyhounds—injured gracilis muscle).

A. The history is very useful in coming to a final diagnosis. The length of time that signs have existed is extremely important to know. Hip dysplasia pain develops slowly, whereas the pain of hip luxation is acute in onset. Contracted muscles from fibrosis cause signs that are gradual in onset, whereas rupture of a muscle belly or tendon shows signs that are acute in onset. The history of a previously treated condition should be borne in mind; a luxation that occurred some months or years previously and was successfully treated may lead to degenerative joint disease. Spinal disc disease may recur despite previous fenestration of the lumbar discs. Healed fractures may produce heterotopic bone, which may impinge on nerves, as may scar tissue from old soft tissue injuries.

B. A general physical examination assists in deciding whether hip pain is a result of a generalized condition or is entirely related to the area of the hip. Prior to a physical elucidation of the exact area of pain, the patient's gait should be analysed (p 6, 8). This order of events cannot be too strongly stressed, as a critical analysis may be prejudiced if the previous evincement of pain indicates a local source when in fact the pain may be referred.

C. Radiographs are essential to diagnosis. All too frequently they are the first procedures to be undertaken, as an easy way to make a diagnosis that may well be fallacious: changes seen on the radiographs may have no relation to the cause of hip pain. Standard radiographs of the pelvis as well as the lumbar spine lateral and ventrodorsal (VD) positions are required.

D. Routine laboratory tests play an essential part in the diagnosis by assisting in differentiating pain that may originate from muscle disease, joints, or osseous skeleton. The more sophisticated tests for rheumatoid arthritis or systemic lupus erythematosus factors are not required at this stage, but should be borne in mind for use as the diagnosis is narrowed.

E. Pulled and ruptured muscles are common injuries in working dogs and those used in athletic sports. Particular functions of the activity may lead one towards a diagnosis. For example, sled dogs may injure the quadriceps group, Greyhounds the gracilis muscle—particularly the right muscle when racing on a left-hand tract.

F. If the animal is presented soon after the accident, early surgical intervention is necessary in order to prevent chronic changes. The area is invaded surgically, clots are removed and hemorrhage controlled, dead space is closed, and ruptured muscle fibers and tendons are apposed by suturing. Although exercise is permitted, it should be gentle and controlled.

G. When the muscle injury is chronic in nature, surgical invasion is required to sever and release the contracted fibers. Following surgery, the exercise should, although controlled, be quite positive and vigorous to prevent further adhesion and muscle tie-down.

H. When analgesics are selected as a method of treatment, they should be used judiciously and discontinued if and when signs subside. Care should be taken in prescribing nonsteroidal anti-inflammatory drugs, as dogs do not metabolize them as readily as do humans; some liver damage may be a consequence.

References

Dee JF, Eaton-Wels RD. Injuries of high performance dogs. In: Whittick WG, ed. Canine orthopaedics. 2nd ed. Philadelphia: Lea & Febiger, in press.

Vaughan LC. Muscle and tendon injuries in dogs. J small Anim Pract 1979; 20:711.

Vaughan LC. Tendon injuries in dogs. Calif Vet 1980; 34:15.

Vaughan LC, Edwards GB. The carbon fibers (Grafil) for tendon repairs in animals. Vet Rec 1978; 102:287.

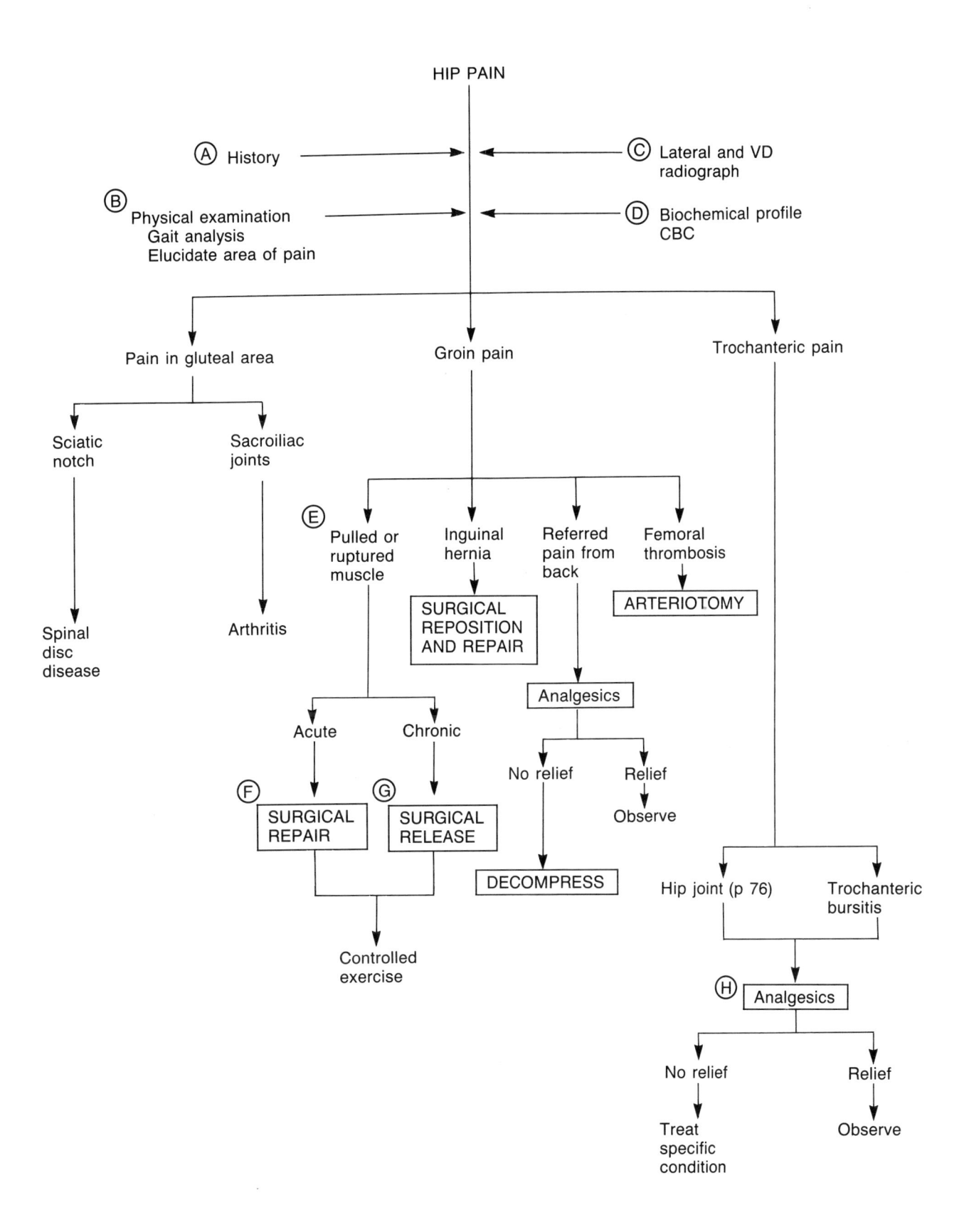

HIP PAIN

- Ⓐ History
- Ⓑ Physical examination
  - Gait analysis
  - Elucidate area of pain
- Ⓒ Lateral and VD radiograph
- Ⓓ Biochemical profile CBC

Pain in gluteal area
- Sciatic notch → Spinal disc disease
- Sacroiliac joints → Arthritis

Groin pain
- Ⓔ Pulled or ruptured muscle
  - Acute → Ⓕ **SURGICAL REPAIR** → Controlled exercise
  - Chronic → Ⓖ **SURGICAL RELEASE** → Controlled exercise
- Inguinal hernia → **SURGICAL REPOSITION AND REPAIR**
- Referred pain from back → Analgesics
  - No relief → **DECOMPRESS**
  - Relief → Observe
- Femoral thrombosis → **ARTERIOTOMY**

Trochanteric pain
- Hip joint (p 76)
- Trochanteric bursitis
- Ⓗ Analgesics
  - No relief → Treat specific condition
  - Relief → Observe

77

PELVIC TRAUMA

Allen G. Binnington

A. Even though a pelvic fracture or dislocation may be suspected from the history of acute trauma and nonuse of one or both of the hindlimbs, the vital signs should be monitored and treatment initiated immediately for such life-threatening conditions as shock, pneumothorax, and upper airway obstruction. Any bleeding should be controlled, and fluids or whole blood should be administered as necessary.

B. Once the vital signs have been stabilized, a complete physical examination of the hind quarters, plus diagnostic radiographs, confirms the presence of a pelvic fracture or coxofemoral dislocation and rules out fractures or dislocations involving other bones and joints.

C. The status of associated soft tissue injuries has a direct bearing on the proposed treatment of any pelvic injury. Some injuries may be of little consequence and are allowed to heal on their own; others may require repair at the time of the pelvic repair or warrant the postponement of pelvic surgery until healing is complete. Thoracic examination, to rule out cardiac arrythmias related to myocardial contusions and hemo- or pneumothorax, is essential. Evaluate the abdomen in order to detect multiple system injuries that can arise from abdominal or thoracic cavity trauma. Hemoperitoneum from liver, spleen, kidney, or mesenteric damage and uroperitoneum from urinary tract trauma can be detected on palpation and by abdominal tap and lavage. Abdominal lavage may also allow detection of injury to the gastrointestinal tract and pancreas. Special radiographic techniques, using constant media, may be necessary to detect injury to the urinary or reproductive system. A digital examination of the rectum allows assessment of the rectal wall and pelvic canal diameter. Evaluation of integumentary wounds and an assessment of whether fractures are compound or not is essential. As with all trauma cases, a thorough neurologic examination is necessary and, in the case of pelvic trauma, special attention is paid to lower vertebral injury, ischiatic and femoral nerve damage, and the status of innervation to the tail, rectal sphincter, and urinary bladder.

D. Life-threatening soft tissue injuries should be corrected immediately. Progressive hemo- or pneumothorax or hemoperitoneum require aggressive treatment as does rupture of the gastrointestinal system. Integumentary wounds and urinary tract injuries may be corrected as soon as the patient's status is compatible with a general anesthetic. Neurologic injuries may require either aggressive medical or surgical therapy or a "wait and see" attitude.

E. When major soft tissue complications are not present or have been corrected, repair of the pelvic fracture or coxofemoral luxation may then be undertaken.

References

Aron DN. Emergency management of the musculo-skeletal trauma patient. Comp Cont Ed 1982; 4(3):220.

Kirk RW, Bistner SI. Handbook of veterinary procedures and emergency treatment. 4th ed. Philadelphia: WB Saunders, 1985:2.

Zaslow IM, ed. Primary assessment and management of the injured patient in veterinary trauma and critical care. New York: Lea & Febiger, 1984:106.

PELVIC TRAUMA Suspected

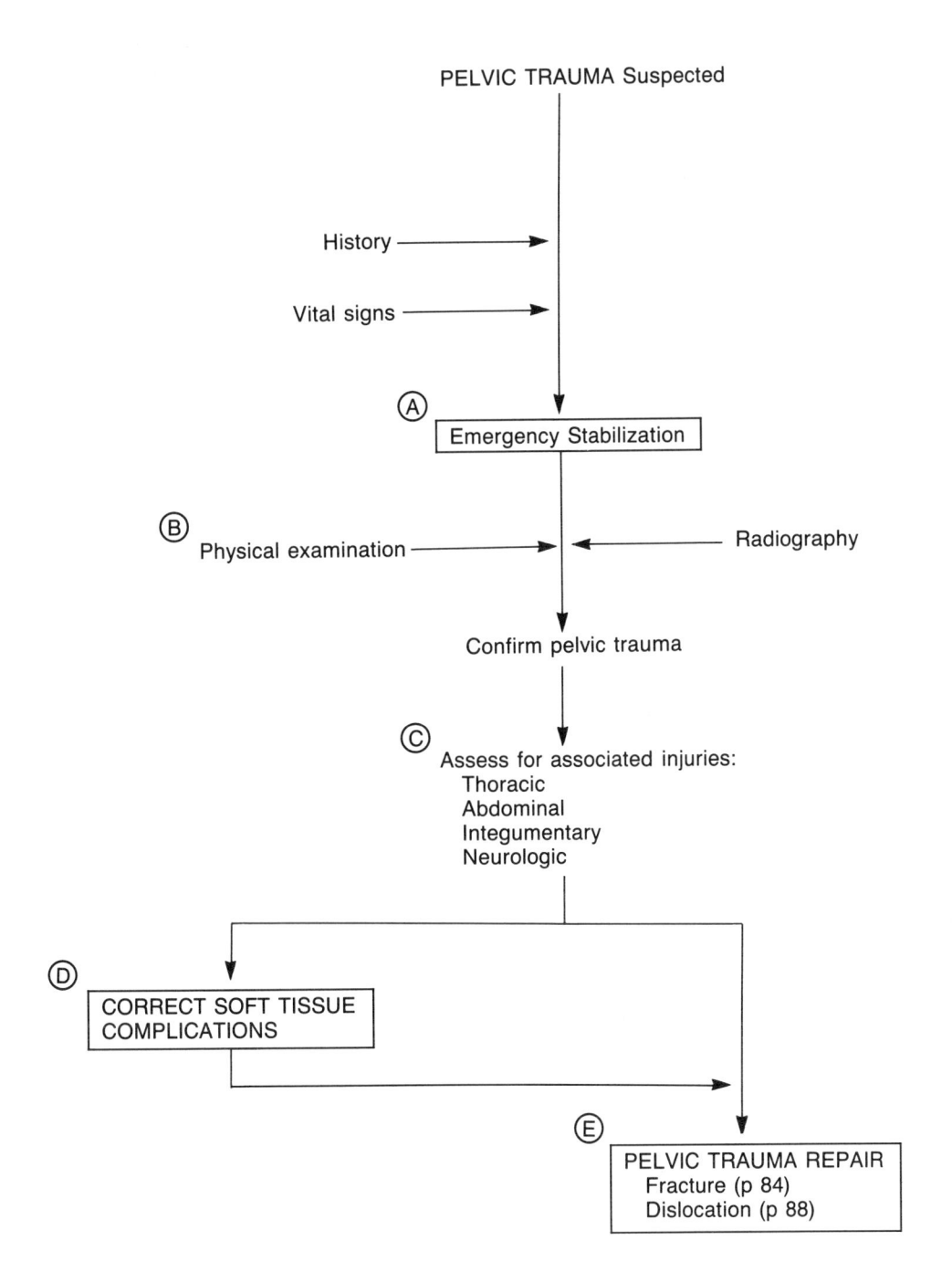

History →

Vital signs →

Ⓐ Emergency Stabilization

Ⓑ Physical examination → ← Radiography

Confirm pelvic trauma

Ⓒ Assess for associated injuries:
   Thoracic
   Abdominal
   Integumentary
   Neurologic

Ⓓ CORRECT SOFT TISSUE COMPLICATIONS

Ⓔ PELVIC TRAUMA REPAIR
   Fracture (p 84)
   Dislocation (p 88)

PELVIC FRACTURE

Joanne R. Cockshutt

A. Pelvic fractures are usually the result of traumatic injury, and a complete physical examination is mandatory to rule out the existence of complicating injuries (see p 78). Fractures of the pelvis are almost invariably multiple, but rarely compound. Palpation of the pelvis should include a gentle rectal examination to establish the integrity of the rectal wall. This also permits assessment of pelvic canal width.

B. Both ventrodorsal and lateral radiographic views are required. An oblique view, which separates the ilial shafts, may be valuable. An enema can be given to improve visualization of the pelvis. The sacroiliac joints should be checked for luxation.

C. The treatment chosen for pelvic fracture depends upon many factors. Conservative management is preferable in those animals with little or no displacement of the fracture and minimal soft tissue injury. Immature dogs, dogs weighing under 25 kg, and quiet, cooperative dogs all respond better to conservative treatment than do older, larger, or more active animals. Surgical repair is indicated in circumstances in which displacement of the fracture has significantly reduced the diameter of the pelvic canal. This is particularly important in the breeding female. Males and spayed females can tolerate a 50 percent reduction of the canal. Animals with gross pelvic instability, with compound fractures, or with other orthopaedic or soft tissue injuries that hinder ambulation are also candidates for surgical repair. Fractures involving the weight-bearing articular surface of the hip should be treated surgically (see p 82). In most cases, show-dogs, working dogs, and giant breed dogs benefit from surgical intervention.

D. Conservative treatment requires good nursing care to maintain satisfactory bowel function and to prevent skin ulceration during a 3- to 6-week period of close confinement. A nonweight-bearing sling may be required to prevent limb use during the initial 1 to 2 weeks of cage rest. Tape hobbles during the confinement period may provide support once the dog starts to ambulate. Physiotherapy by passive hip flexion, extension, and massage should be performed. After 1 month, a limited exercise program can be started and gradually increased.

E. Surgical reduction is best accomplished within 5 days of injury. Closed reduction and fixation by means of intramedullary pins or Kirschner–Ehmer fixator may suffice for rare fractures of the ischium, tuber ischii, or tuber coxae that require repair. Some oblique ilial fractures may also be repaired in this fashion. Open reduction and fixation are not without risk. Many methods of fixation have been described, but bone plates and screws provide the best results for fractures of the ilium and acetabulum (Fig. 1). Ischial fractures frequently accompany ilial fractures. Repair of the ilium commonly results in realignment of the ischium so that no additional treatment is required. Sacroiliac separation can cause prolonged discomfort. Reduction and fixation with screws or pins allows earlier ambulation. Similarly wiring the pelvic symphysis speeds recovery in cases of symphyseal fracture and/or separation (see p 86).

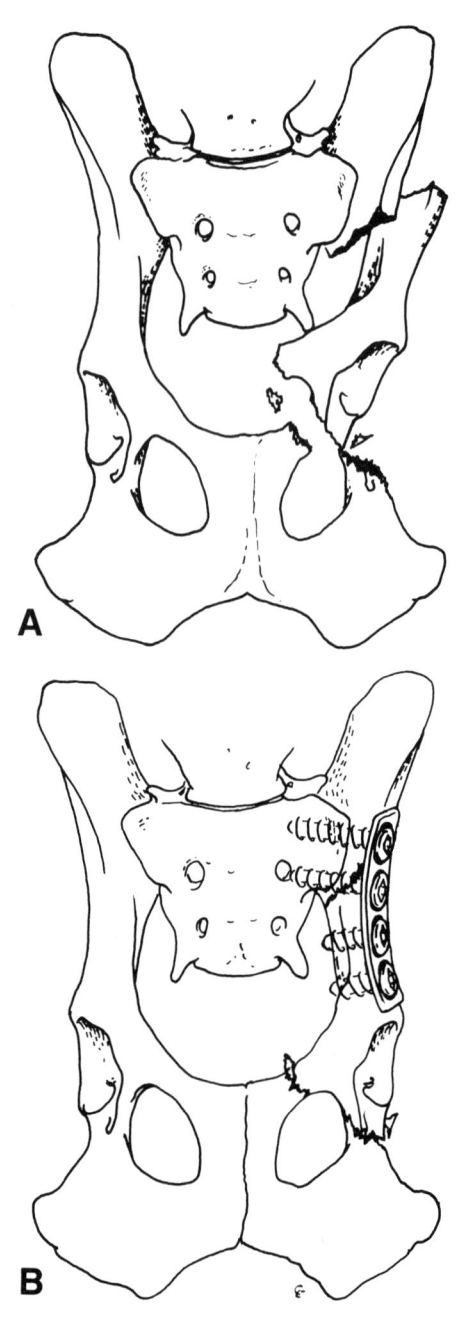

Figure 1 Fractures of the ilial shaft, pubis, and ischium (*A*) stabilized by means of a plate on the ilial shaft (*B*). The length of the plate and the number of screw holes varies according to the particular case. Fractures of the pubis and ischeum are usually sufficiently reduced so that individual attention is not required.

F. Degenerative joint disease is the major late complication and results from inadequate reduction of acetabular fractures. Gross fracture malunion causing pelvic

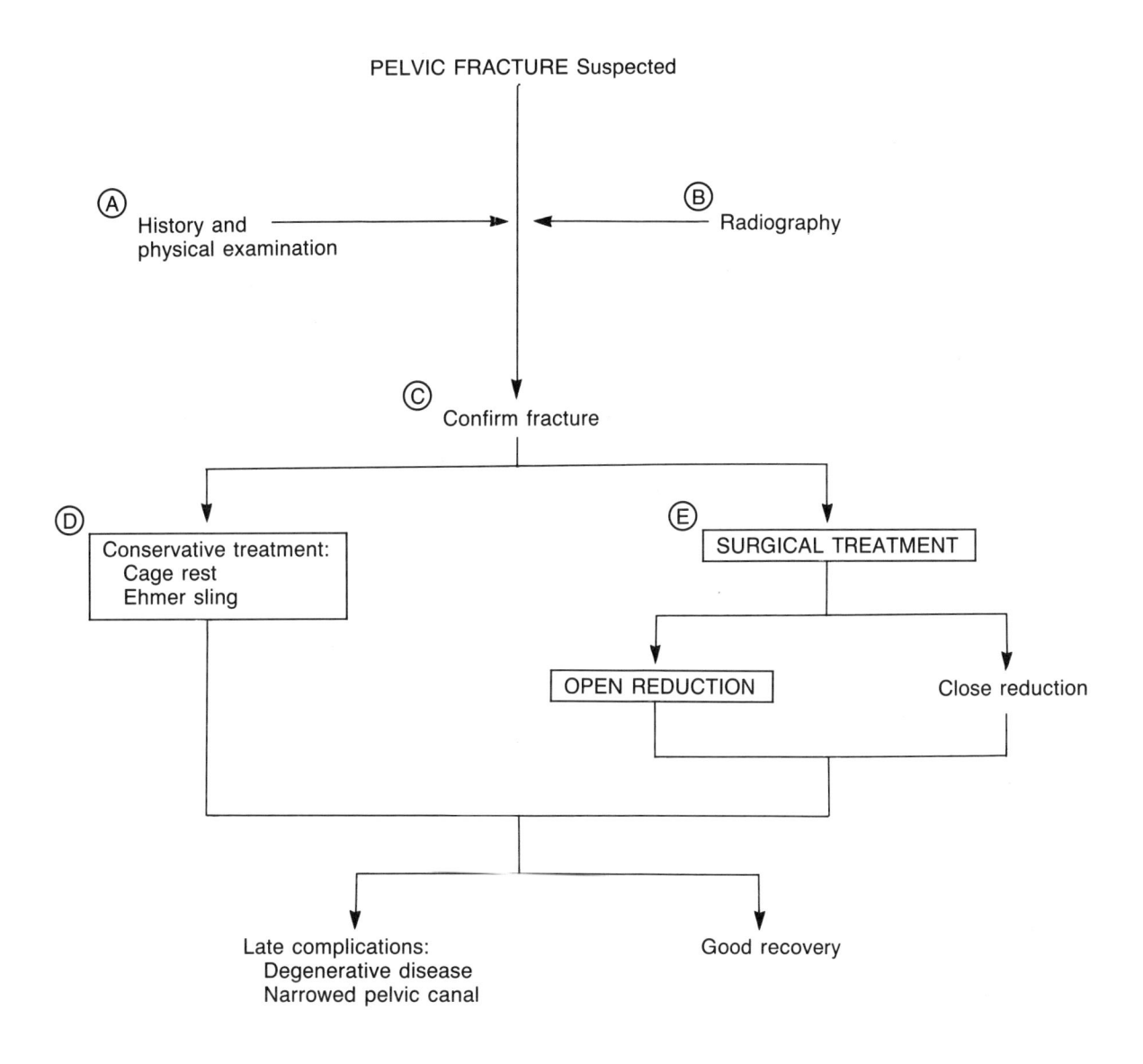

```
                    PELVIC FRACTURE Suspected
                              │
          Ⓐ                   │                   Ⓑ
    History and ──────────────┼────────────── Radiography
    physical examination      │
                              │
                             Ⓒ
                        Confirm fracture
                              │
                ┌─────────────┴─────────────┐
               Ⓓ                           Ⓔ
        ┌──────────────┐            ┌──────────────────┐
        │ Conservative │            │ SURGICAL TREATMENT│
        │ treatment:   │            └──────────────────┘
        │  Cage rest   │              │              │
        │  Ehmer sling │       ┌──────────────┐      │
        └──────────────┘       │ OPEN REDUCTION│  Close reduction
                               └──────────────┘
                ┌─────────────┴─────────────┐
                ▼                           ▼
        Late complications:            Good recovery
         Degenerative disease
         Narrowed pelvic canal
```

deformity may result in impairment of large bowel function (see p 78).

References

Bojarb MJ. Current techniques in small animal surgery. Philadelphia: Lea & Febiger, 1983.

Brinker WO et al. Handbook of small animal orthopedics and fracture treatment. Philadelphia: WB Saunders, 1983.

Denny HR. Pelvic fractures in the dog: a review of 123 cases. J small Anim Pract 1978; 19:151.

Robins GM, Dingwall JS, Sumner-Smith G. The plating of pelvic fractures in the dog. Vet Rec 1973; 93:550.

Slatter DH. Textbook of small animal surgery. Philadelphia: WB Saunders, 1985.

ACETABULAR FRACTURE

Joanne R. Cockshutt

A. A complete physical examination is essential as most acetabular fractures are the result of trauma, and concurrent injuries are likely. Assessment of neurologic function is mandatory (see p 80). Crepitation may be apparent on manipulation of the hip joint. Rectal examination may aid assessment of the pelvis, as well as the size of the pelvic canal.

B. Both ventrodorsal and lateral radiographic views of the pelvis are required. An oblique view may aid in assessment of the acetabulum. In large breed dogs, the hips should be examined for evidence of dysplasia, which may complicate postoperative return to function.

C. Upon confirmation, the acetabular fracture should be classified to assist in treatment selection. Fractures with little or no displacement of fragments and fractures of the caudal third of the acetabulum may be treated conservatively. Fractures through the weightbearing region of the acetabulum, fractures with marked instability or displacement, comminuted fractures, and those in which crepitus is elicited upon palpation should be managed surgically. Without treatment, degenerative joint disease is a likely sequela.

D. Conservative treatment consists of strict confinement with minimal exercise for 3 to 4 weeks. Good nursing care is mandatory to prevent decubitus ulcers and skin excoriation by urine. Laxatives and enemas may be required to prevent or treat constipation. A non-weightbearing sling may be used for 1 or 2 weeks in an active patient. Physiotherapy, consisting of passive joint manipulation and massage helps to maintain joint mobility and muscle tone. An exercise program can gradually be initiated after 1 month if the fracture is stable.

E. Open reduction and internal fixation is the treatment of choice for fractures that involve the cranial two-thirds of the acetabulum. A dorsal approach to the acetabulum provides the best exposure and aids in obtaining anatomic reduction. Plates and screws provide the best fixation in most cases, but pins, wire, and Kirschner-Ehmer external fixator may work well in some cases (Fig. 1 and 2).

Careful surgical closure is important in order to restore stability to the joint. A non-weightbearing sling may be advisable for 10 days postoperatively if fracture fixation is tenuous.

F. An excision arthroplasty can be performed in animals with concurrent damage to the femoral head or when reconstruction of the acetabulum cannot be accomplished. It is advisable to examine the acetabulum carefully prior to performing femoral head excision since fractures that appear comminuted radiographically may not involve the articular surface. Such fractures may be readily repairable. Excision arthroplasty should be considered a salvage procedure only and not used as first choice treatment.

G. Degenerative joint disease is the most common long-term complication associated with acetabular fractures. With adequate reduction and fixation the likelihood of osteoarthritis developing is greatly reduced. Ischiatic nerve injury can occur at the time of fracture, during surgery, or as a result of entrapment by callus during fracture healing. Femoral head luxation or subluxation may occur postoperatively if surgical closure is inadequate or if there is preexisting acetabular dysplasia.

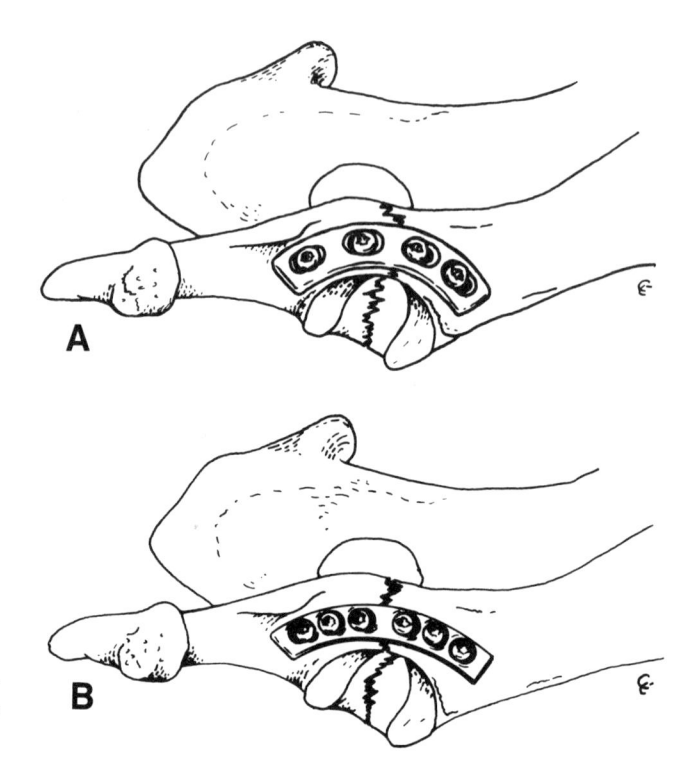

Figure 1 Acetabular fractures stabilized by (A) a four- or (B) six-hole plate.

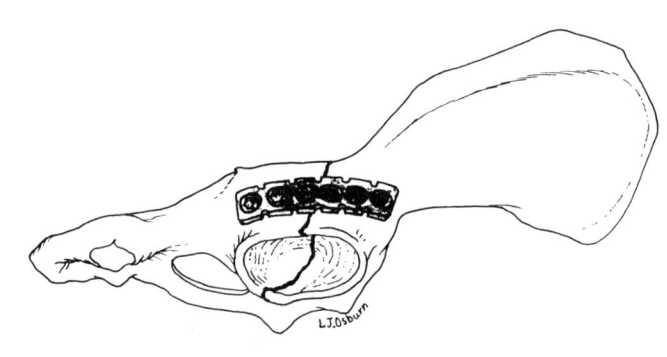

Figure 2 The same fracture is stabilized by means of a reconstruction plate. The size of plate and screws are determined by the breed of the animal.

ACETABULAR FRACTURE Suspected

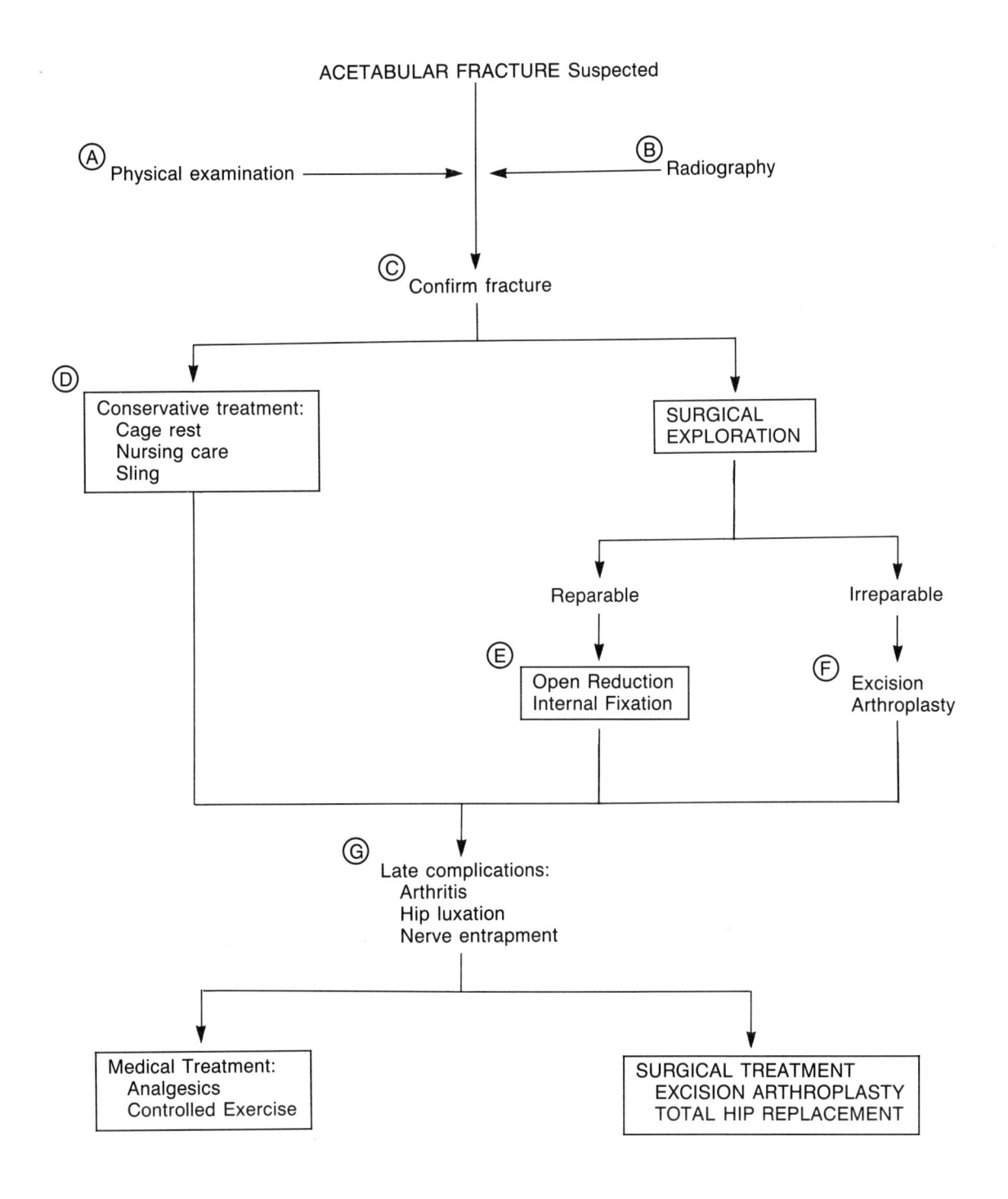

- Ⓐ Physical examination
- Ⓑ Radiography
- Ⓒ Confirm fracture
- Ⓓ Conservative treatment:
  - Cage rest
  - Nursing care
  - Sling
- SURGICAL EXPLORATION
  - Reparable → Ⓔ Open Reduction Internal Fixation
  - Irreparable → Ⓕ Excision Arthroplasty
- Ⓖ Late complications:
  - Arthritis
  - Hip luxation
  - Nerve entrapment
- Medical Treatment:
  - Analgesics
  - Controlled Exercise
- SURGICAL TREATMENT
  - EXCISION ARTHROPLASTY
  - TOTAL HIP REPLACEMENT

References

Bojrab MJ. Current techniques in small animal surgery. Philadelphia: Lea & Febiger, 1983.

Brinker WO et al. Handbook of small animal orthopedics and fracture treatment. Philadelphia: WB Saunders, 1983.

Gilmore DR. Traumatic intestinal injuries associated with pelvic fractures. JAAHA 1983; 19:667.

Husle DA et al. Management of acetabular fractures: long-term evaluation. Comp Cont Ed 1980; 2:189.

Ost PC, Kederly RE. Use of reconstruction plates for the repair of segmental ilial fractures involving acetabular comminution in four dogs. Vet Surg 1985; 13(3):259.

Slatter DH. Textbook of small animal surgery. Philadelphia: WB Saunders, 1985.

FRACTURES INVOLVING THE HIP JOINT

W. Dieter Prieur

A. Clinical signs are the same in all cases of trauma to the hip joint. The leg is carried with flexed hip and stifle. There is pain in the joint region and sometimes swelling. Crepitation and abnormal movement may also be present when the animal is examined under anesthesia.

B. Radiography should show the whole pelvis in ventrodorsal view. Sometimes special views are necessary. In the case of an acetabular fracture, look carefully for other fracture lines or sacroiliac separation.

C. Acetabular fractures may be in the central acetabulum, the cranial half (majority), or the caudal half; sometimes with protrusion of the femoral head into the pelvic cavity—protruso acetabula.

D. Conservative treatment should be avoided if possible. However it may be recommended in growing dogs in which there is no fragment displacement; especially in caudal acetabular fractures. The hip joint is a heavily loaded joint with forces working within the joint surface causes degenerative joint disease. Therefore, in order to achieve full joint function, precise fragment reduction and rigid fixation is essential (p 84). In central acetabular fractures only an attempt may be made to reduce the head from the pelvic canal when either conservative or operative treatment may prove to be extremely difficult. The trochanter major is pulled lateral with a pointed bone forceps, and with the index finger pressure from the rectum, the head is reduced.

E. Sometimes femoral head resection, especially in small dogs and cats, provides limited function. Total hip replacement in large or giant dogs is preferred.

F. Cases with additional fracture of the ischiatic crest are repaired by internal fixation. The fracture in the acetabular floor and the pubic bone cannot be repaired by operative techniques. The limb is supported in an Ehmer sling for about 1 month. The results are variable. In the proximal femur fracture, the following fracture types are seen:
  1. Physeal separation (in growing dogs only)
     fixation by Kirschner wires
     fixation by lag screws (if the animal is nearly skeletally mature)
  2. Femoral head fractures (treatment see p 106)
  3. Femoral neck fractures, lag-screw fixation (treatment see p 108)
  4. Multifragment fractures of the proximal femur (treatment see p 110)

The blood supply to the femoral head may be destroyed by the accident or additionally damaged during surgery, resulting in subsequent necrosis. Avascular necrosis of the head may also appear after successful fixation. In such cases, a resection of the femoral head is necessary. This is acceptable in small dogs. A total hip replacement is the solution in large breeds. Even following successful surgery, the original trauma to the cartilage may still result in degenerative joint disease.

References

Brown SG, Biggart JF. Plate fixation of iliac shaft fractures in the dog. JAVMA 1978; 167(6):462.

Denny HR. Pelvic fractures in the dog: a review of 123 cases. J small Anim Pract 1978; 19:151.

Henry WB. A method of bone plating for repairing iliac and acetabular fractures. Comp Cont Ed. 1985; 7:924.

FRACTURES INVOLVING THE HIP JOINT

- Ⓐ Clinical diagnosis
- Ⓑ Radiologic diagnosis
- Ⓒ Acetabular fractures
  - Central
  - Caudal
  - Cranial
  - Not operable
  - Operable
- Fractures of the proximal femur (see p 110)
- Ⓓ Conservative Treatment
- Ⓔ RESECTION OF FEMORAL HEAD / TOTAL HIP REPLACEMENT
- Ⓕ PRIMARY INTERNAL FIXATION
  - Necrosis of femoral head
- Satisfactory function
- Normal function
- Degenerative joint disease

PELVIC FRACTURE COMPLICATIONS

Allen G. Binnington

Complications are not a common occurrence, but do occasionally occur following pelvic trauma. Associated clinical signs may become evident shortly after trauma (2 to 4 weeks) or as long as a year or more following the incident. Often, at the time of initial treatment, evidence that warrants consideration of the possibility of future complication may be present. The initial traumatic incident may have been treated conservatively, surgically, or received no treatment at all.

A. The animal is usually presented with a history of previous trauma to the pelvic region. The owner may complain of the animal being constipated or passing small ribbon-like stools and possibly being anorexic and losing weight. Another presenting complaint may be of knuckling on a hindlimb, scuffing of the toes, or walking on the dorsum of the paw. A third owner complaint may be of decreased physical activity, abnormal gait, reluctance to climb stairs or jump into the car, or of a hindlimb lameness following exercise.

B. The physical examination should include digital examination of the rectum to assess pelvic canal size and rule out prostatic enlargement as a cause of tenesmus. A neurologic examination that concentrates on the lower spine and course of the ischiatic nerve in the pelvic region is necessary in cases of abnormal neurologic function. The possibility of degenerative joint disease in the coxofemoral joint is assessed through determining the range of motion of the joint, pain elicited on extension and flexion, muscle mass loss, and crepitus from the hip joint region.

C. Lateral and ventrodorsal radiographs are used to assess the following:
   1. The pelvic canal size and, if present, the degree of pelvic narrowing and colonic distention caused by fecal material.
   2. The presence of callous formation in a healing pelvic fracture, which could entrap the ischiatic nerve.
   3. The coxofemoral joint for evidence of degnerative joint disease.

D. Pelvic collapse or stenosis can be treated either medically or surgically, depending on the degree of collapse, the owner's willingness to treat medically, and the degree of secondary colonic changes. Medical therapy consists of enemas to break up the fecal mass and allow evacuation of the colon and rectum and the feeding of laxative dietary additives such as bran or purified phyphilline. The occasional enema may still be necessary to prevent fecal build-up. In cases in which severe collapse is present, owners are reluctant to use enemas, and colonic pathology is present, surgical correction is necessary. If a large portion of the colon is distended, a total or subtotal colectomy may be performed to eliminate the abnormal portion and/or alter fecal consistency to allow easier passage. A widening of the pelvic canal can be accomplished by a pubic osteotomy and insertion of a bone graft or metal plate or the performance of a partial hemipelvectomy.

E. If a high ischiatic deficit is present, surgical exploration of the ischiatic nerve on the affected side should be undertaken. If fibrous or bony entrapment is encountered, the nerve should be carefully freed.

F. Coxofemoral degenerative joint disease can be treated medically or surgically depending on the severity of the clinical signs and the response to medical therapy.

References

Alexander JW, Carb AV. Subtotal hemipelvectomy in the dog. J Vet Orthopaed 1979; 1(2):9.

Bright RM. Medical and surgical management of megacolon in the dog and cat. Chicago: ACVS Surg Forum, Gastrointest Surgery Notes, 1984.

Walker TL. Ischiatic nerve entrapment. JAVMA 1981; 178(12):1284.

PELVIC FRACTURE COMPLICATION

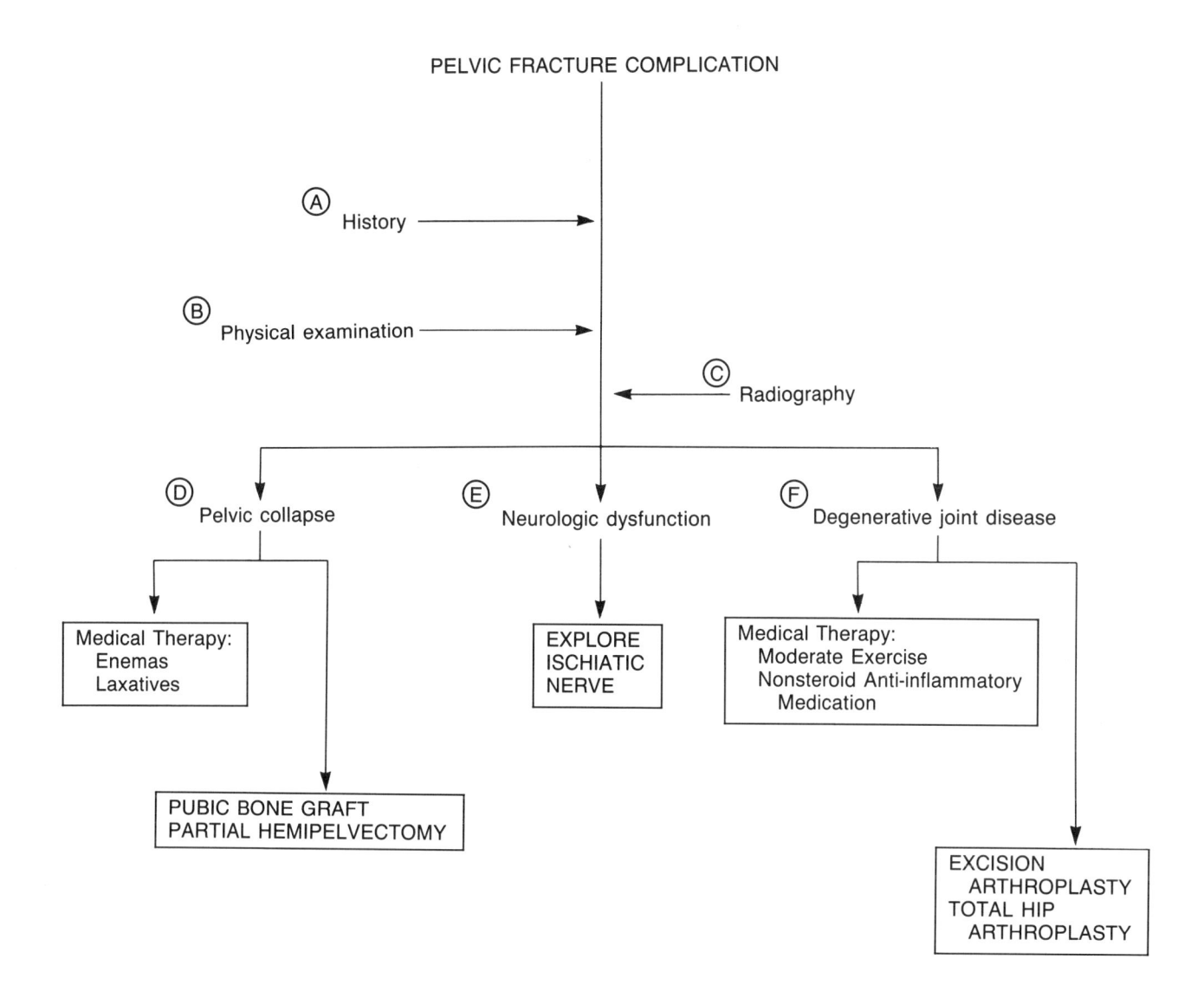

- (A) History
- (B) Physical examination
- (C) Radiography

- (D) Pelvic collapse
  - Medical Therapy:
    - Enemas
    - Laxatives
  - PUBIC BONE GRAFT
  - PARTIAL HEMIPELVECTOMY

- (E) Neurologic dysfunction
  - EXPLORE ISCHIATIC NERVE

- (F) Degenerative joint disease
  - Medical Therapy:
    - Moderate Exercise
    - Nonsteroid Anti-inflammatory Medication
  - EXCISION ARTHROPLASTY
  - TOTAL HIP ARTHROPLASTY

COXOFEMORAL LUXATION

Allen G. Binnington

A. The history may be one of an acute or chronic hind leg lameness. The onset may be related to a traumatic incident. In the chronic situation the use of the limb may have returned with the passage of time.

B. Examination to preclude neurologic dysfunction and eliminate other bone and joint problems is essential. The toes may be slightly rotated externally, a unilateral loss of pelvic muscle mass may be evident, and crepitus may be ellicited upon coxofemoral joint movement. The limb may appear to be longer or shorter than the contralateral limb depending upon the direction of dislocation. Abnormal location of the greater trochanter, in relation to the wing of the ileum and the tuber ischia, and failure of the examiner's thumb to be forced out of the space between the greater trochanter and tuber ischia upon external rotation of the hip, is diagnostic of a dislocation or fracture of the hip joint.

C. Ventrodorsal and lateral radiographs rule out the possibility of a greater trochanter fracture, proximal femoral shaft or neck fracture, acetabular fracture, or avulsion of a fragment of bone with the teres ligament from the fovea region of the femoral head. The dislocation can be classified as anterodorsal, posterior, ventral, or medial (Fig. 1) and the joint assessed for acetabular depth and changes caused by degenerative joint disease.

D. No treatment may be an appropriate approach in the cat with an anterodorsal luxation as they usually recover with the formation of a false acetabulum. Open reduction and internal stabilization is appropriate in the case of severe hip dysplasia; or an accompanying fracture of the femoral head, neck, or acetabulum; or chronic fibrosis of surrounding tissue. Open reduction also allows evaluation of acetabular and femoral head cartilage. In all other situations, closed reduction should be first attempted.

E. Closed reduction should be attempted under general anesthetic and is more easily accomplished if the luxation is converted to an anterodorsal position before attempting reduction by manual manipulation. Upon successful reduction, pressure is applied to the greater trochanter in a medial direction and the hip put through a full range-of-motion to expel blood clots and fibrin from the joint. Failure to achieve reduction may be due to the interposition of soft tissue between the head and acetabulum, organized debris, or hypertrophy of a remnant of the teres ligament filling the acetabulum. Chronic fibrosis of surrounding tissues may also prevent reduction.

F. Following reduction, the stability is assessed by manipulating the joint through a normal range-of-motion. If the joint reluxates easily, the cause may be inversion of the joint capsule or torn muscle into the acetabulum,

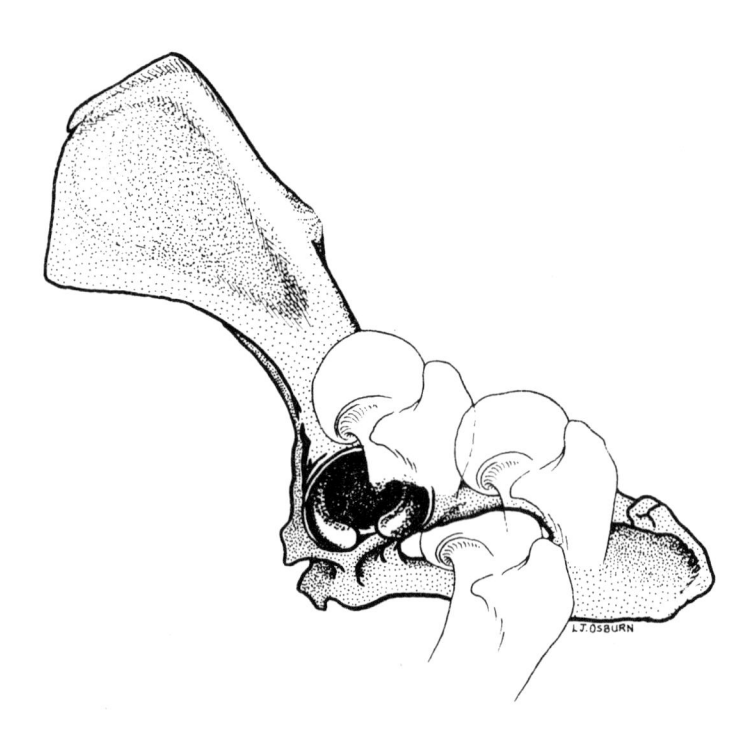

Figure 1 The various positions in which the dislocated femoral head may be found following luxation; the most common is the anterodorsal position.

COXOFEMORAL LUXATION Suspected

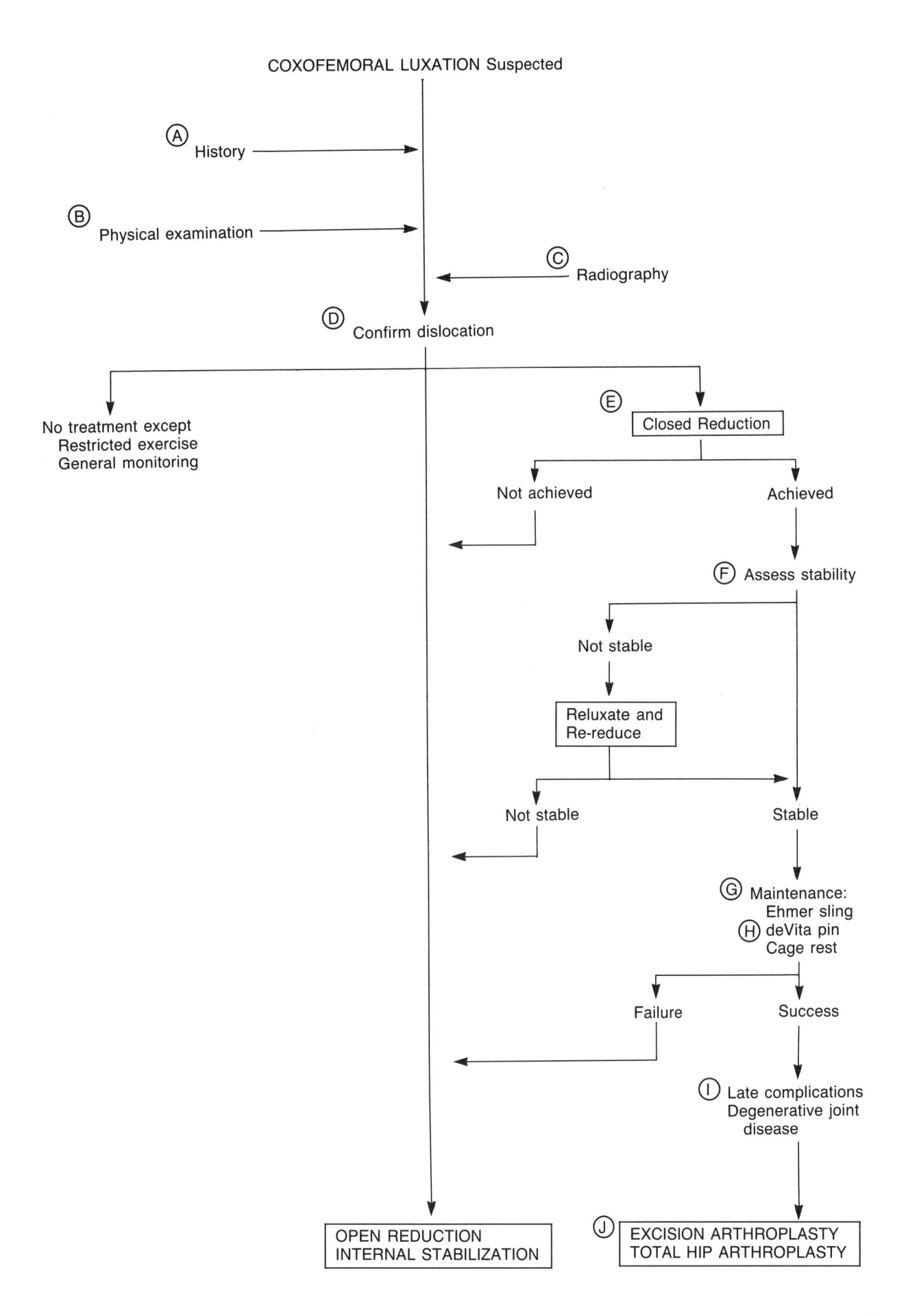

- Ⓐ History
- Ⓑ Physical examination
- Ⓒ Radiography
- Ⓓ Confirm dislocation
  - No treatment except Restricted exercise, General monitoring
  - Ⓔ **Closed Reduction**
    - Not achieved → OPEN REDUCTION / INTERNAL STABILIZATION
    - Achieved
      - Ⓕ Assess stability
        - Not stable → **Reluxate and Re-reduce**
          - Not stable → OPEN REDUCTION / INTERNAL STABILIZATION
          - Stable
        - Stable
          - Ⓖ Maintenance: Ehmer sling
          - Ⓗ deVita pin, Cage rest
            - Failure → OPEN REDUCTION / INTERNAL STABILIZATION
            - Success
              - Ⓘ Late complications, Degenerative joint disease
                - Ⓙ **EXCISION ARTHROPLASTY / TOTAL HIP ARTHROPLASTY**

too shallow an acetabulum, or extreme laxity of the surrounding tissues. In the case of inversion of tissue into the acetabulum, redislocation and further attempts at reduction should be performed. If stability is not achieved, open reduction is warranted.

G. An acute dislocation involving a hip, which radiographically has good joint conformation and feels solid upon reduction, may remain in place with a regimen of only strict cage rest for 5 to 7 days, followed by controlled exercise for a further 2 weeks. However, most reductions need some external support. This can be accomplished by the use of a figure-of-eight bandage (Ehmer sling) for 10 to 14 days, followed by a further 2 weeks of leash exercise, or the placement of a deVita pin for 14 to 28 days. A radiograph should be taken immediately following application of the maintaining device to assure a loss of reduction has not occurred during its placement.

H. Where failure to achieve closed reduction is due to acetabular filling, the craniolateral approach affords a less traumatic, although somewhat limited, exposure. A deVita pin or figure-of-eight bandage can be employed to maintain reduction following reduction, joint capsule imbrication, transacetabular pinning, placement of a toggle pin and a synthetic teres ligament. In cases of questionable joint conformation, chronic dislocation, or severe fibrosis, the dorsal approach of employing a trochanteric osteotomy affords greater exposure and less muscle resistance to reduction. Following reduction and joint capsule reconstruction, a trochanteric relocation to a more caudal and distal location is a method of choice (Fig. 2). A combination of toggle pin and trochanteric relocation have proved successful in cases of very shallow acetabulum.

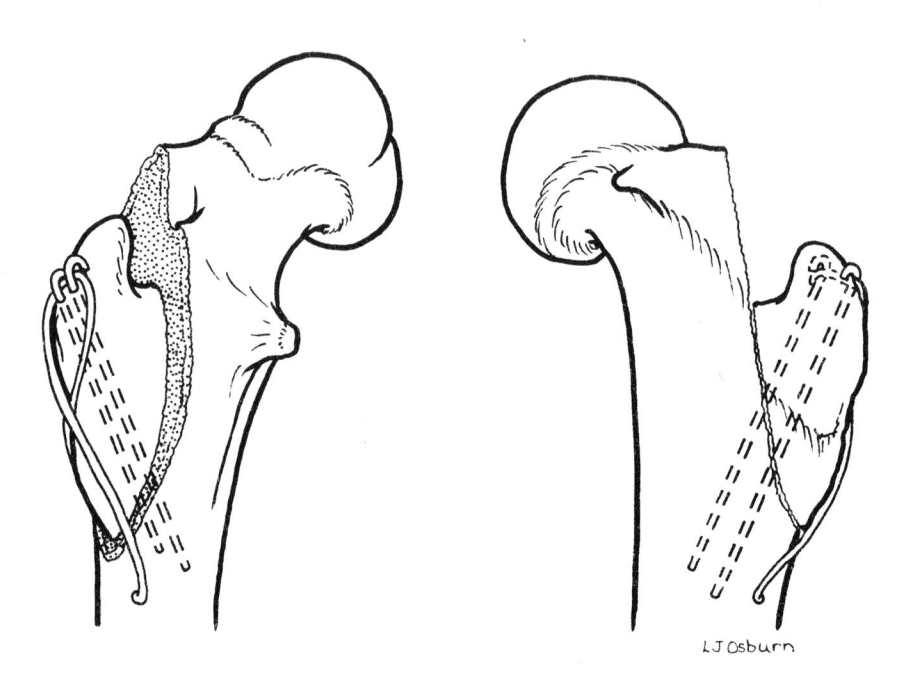

Figure 2 Lateral relocation of the trochanter major and fixation by a tension-band wire system.

I. Degenerative joint disease may develop months to years after successful repair of a dislocation because of joint damage that occurred during the dislocation or repair or subsequently through abnormal motion in the joint. Degenerative joint disease in this case is treated similar to any other form of degenerative joint disease.

J. Failing to achieve reduction during surgical treatment may result in irreparable damage to the acetabulum or femoral head or subsequent development of degenerative joint disease. Such a development may necessitate femoral head excision arthroplasty or total hip arthroplasty.

References

Alexander JW. Coxofemoral luxation in the dog. Comp Cont Ed 1982; 4(7):575.

Brinker WO, Piermattei DL, Flo GL. Handbook of small animal orthopedics and fracture treatment. Philadelphia: WB Saunders, 1983:267.

TRAUMATIC HIP LUXATION

W. Dieter Prieur

A. The majority of traumatic hip dislocations are caused by traffic accidents. Strong forces acting against the trunk when the leg is weightbearing cause the limb to move into the adducted position and the femoral head into increased anteversion. The long lever arm of the limb luxates the head from the acetabulum; also, there is increased abduction when the stifle is pressed to the ground and the pelvis rotated. Simultaneously, the femoral head slips into the craniodorsal position in about 80 percent of cases because of the traction of the cranial gluteal muscles.

B. The flat acetabulum and increased anteversion of the proximal femur in hip dysplasia predisposes to hip luxation. Such cases also are inclined to reluxate after reduction.

C. On physical examination the dog is found to carry the leg semiflexed and adducted. In extension the affected leg appears shorter than the opposite limb in caudodorsal luxations. There is an increased distance between trochanter major and tuber ischii, and it is impossible to rotate the femur internally. In the less common ventral luxations, the leg appears longer if extended perpendicular to the body axis.

D. Radiographic examination of the ventrodorsal view is sufficient. Only if there are additional fractures of the head or acetabulum is a lateral view sometimes necessary.

E. Two main groups have to be distinguished; they are fracture dislocation and simple luxations. In both groups the capsule is torn. Fracture dislocations of all types always require open reduction and internal fixation of the fragments. Simple luxations may be caudocranial (about 86 to 90 percent), caudoventral, ventral, or caudal. The last three are often the result of failed prolonged attempts at reduction. All cases of caudal luxation have to be operated upon as manipulating this type of dislocation can result in ischiatic nerve trauma.

F. Immediate reduction must be carried out in all cases suitable for such treatment. The joint cartilage is nourished by the synovial fluid combined with movement and weightbearing. The dislocation tears the capsule, and the synovial fluid escapes. Joint motion is impossible, resulting in a malnutrition of the hyaline cartilage. The longer the femoral head stays dislocated, the more likelihood of femoral head necrosis and degeneration. Formation of fibrous tissue within the luxated joint will, within a few days, make a closed reduction impossible. Reduction has to be done with a fully relaxed and anesthetized patient. If 3 to 5 attempts have failed, the hip must be operated upon. Too many attempts and too much force used to effect the reduction causes trauma to the femoral head and surrounding tissues and leads to muscle dystrophy, especially in young dogs. In most cases when closed reduction is impossible, there is interposition of soft tissue. If closed reduction is successful, the limb is fixed in inward rotation by an Ehmer sling for 10 days. In ventral luxations the Ehmer sling is contraindicated as it puts the leg in abduction, creating reluxation. The technique required is to hobble both rear legs together for about 6 days. If the femoral head reluxates after extending the limb or if the hip joint shows a widening of the joint space, there may be interposition of soft tissue and open reduction becomes necessary to avoid degenerative joint disease.

G. In the majority of cases, delay of treatment for more than 3 days postaccident makes closed reduction impossible because of filling of the acetabulum with fibrous tissue, causing loss of a functional hip joint. Open reduction provides a good chance for healing to take place without subsequent complications.

H. Failure to treat results in a pseudoarthrosis that, contrary to common belief, is without function. Most cases carry the leg completely resulting in muscle dystrophy and loss of function.

I. There are several methods described for open reduction and fixations of the joint. Those techniques that give the best final results are the ones that avoid too much damage to the joint and artificial or biological implants within the joint.

J. Degenerative joint disease and/or necrosis of the femoral head are complications that may follow closed and open reduction. Their incidence can be markedly decreased by early and correct reduction.

References

Alexander JW. Coxofemoral luxation in the dog. Comp Cont Ed 1982; 4(7):575.

Brinker WO, Piermattei DL, Flo GL. Handbook of small animal orthopedics and fracture treatment. Philadelphia: WB Saunders, 1983:267.

De Angelis M, Preta R. Surgical repair of coxo-femoral luxation in the dog. JAAHA 1973; 9:175.

Fry PD. Observations on the surgical treatment of hip dislocation in the dog and cat. J small Anim Pract 1974; 15:661.

Hauptman J. The hip joint. In: Slatter DH, ed. Textbook of small animal surgery. Philadelphia: WB Saunders, 1985:2161.

TRAUMATIC HIP LUXATION Suspected

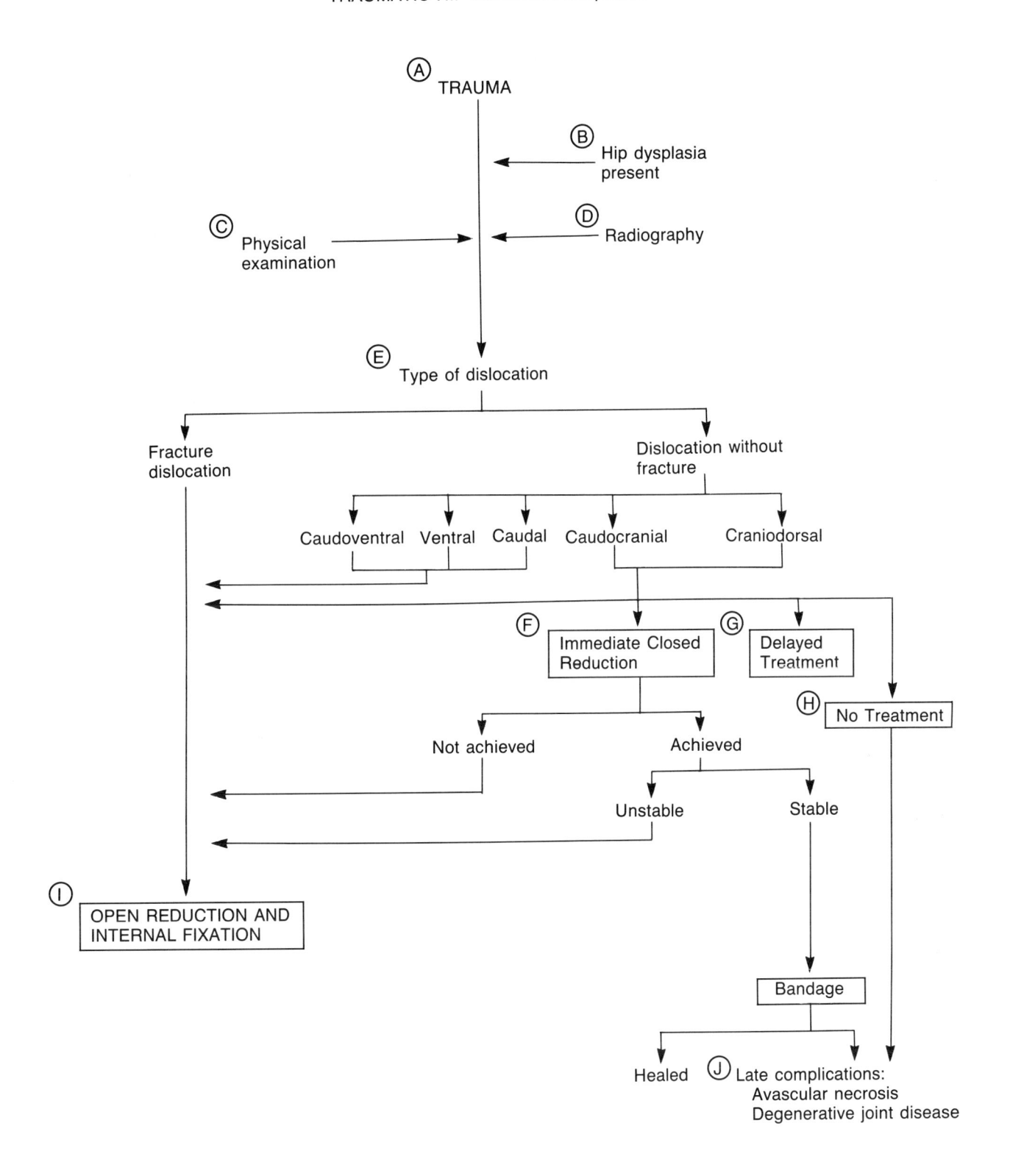

- **A** TRAUMA
- **B** Hip dysplasia present
- **C** Physical examination
- **D** Radiography
- **E** Type of dislocation
  - Fracture dislocation
  - Dislocation without fracture
    - Caudoventral
    - Ventral
    - Caudal
    - Caudocranial
    - Craniodorsal
- **F** Immediate Closed Reduction
  - Not achieved
  - Achieved
    - Unstable
    - Stable
- **G** Delayed Treatment
- **H** No Treatment
- **I** OPEN REDUCTION AND INTERNAL FIXATION
- Bandage
  - Healed
  - **J** Late complications:
    Avascular necrosis
    Degenerative joint disease

HIP DYSPLASIA

Joanne R. Cockshutt

Hip dysplasia (HD) occurs in all breeds, but is rare in dogs with adult body weights of less than 10 kg. The highest incidence is found in the working breeds. Dogs with disproportionately small pelvic muscle mass, caused by rapid skeletal development, are less likely to have normal hip joints.

A. Immature dogs frequently are presented with an acute onset of hind limb lameness evidenced by a decrease in activity, difficulty in rising, or a reluctance to climb stairs. Puppies may develop a waddling gait, or "bunny-hop" when running. The pain is prolonged, and a shifting foreleg lameness may result from increased weight transferral from the hips. The owner may report a change in personality if hip pain makes the dog irritable. Older animals may suffer from chronic degenerative joint disease (DJD) or develop acute lameness after heavy exercise. These animals usually exhibit bilateral lameness that worsens with intense or extended exercise. After prolonged rest, stiffness may be noted.

B. The dysplastic dog has a shortened stride, often with excessive lateral mobility of the greater trochanter (p 10). An audible clicking of the joint may occur with each stride in younger dogs. On palpation, most immature dogs have laxity of the hip joint, with subluxation of the femoral head and a positive Ortolani sign.* Mature dogs with chronic disease may have pain and crepitation in the hip joint concomitant with a reduced range-of-motion. There may be marked atrophy of the thigh muscles. In older dogs, particularly the German Shepherd, a careful neurologic assessment is essential to differentiate ataxia caused by myelopathy from the lameness of HD.

C. Radiographic confirmation of hip dysplasia is essential. A ventrodorsal view with fully extended hind limbs is standard. Sedation or general anesthesia is frequently necessary since conclusions drawn from improperly positioned radiographs are unreliable. Assessment should be made of the femoral head and acetabulum for congruity and evidence of degenerative changes. Femoral neck angles should be measured. There is often no correlation between the severity of radiographic changes and the clinical lameness of the dog.

D. The treatment of HD depends upon the age of the dog, the severity of clinical signs, the animal's general health, and its intended use. Many dogs with radiographic evidence of HD are not affected clinically and do not require treatment.

E. Euthanasia may be elected in the case of a dog used soley for working or breeding purposes. It may be an option in a dog with concurrent health problems, whose owner has financial restrictions.

F. The treatment chosen also depends upon the age of the dog, the severity of the dysplasia, and the presence or absence of arthritic change. Pectineal myectomy results in temporary symptomatic improvement in many dogs, although no effect on the development or progression of HD has been shown. Pelvic osteotomy should be reserved, in most instances, for dogs under 12 to 16 months of age with no evidence of secondary osteoarthritis. Results are best in dogs with mild or moderate HD in which femoral head luxation is not complete. Intertrochanteric varus osteotomy, like pelvic osteotomy, is reserved for immature dogs with minimal DJD. The congruency of the joint will be improved in those dogs with markedly abnormal femoral angles of anteversion and inclination. Pelvic osteotomy may be preferred if the acetabulum is shallow, as femoral neck angles are corrected by remodelling following acetabular redirection.

G. Restriction of exercise to a level which results in freedom from pain may be sufficient treatment for many dogs. Weight reduction is essential for obese animals and will benefit any animal with DJD. Analgesic and anti-inflammatory drugs may be indicated. Aspirin at 25 mg per kilogram is the first choice. Phenylbutazone at 10 mg per kilogram in divided doses may be more effective. Other nonsteroidal anti-inflammatory drugs (NSAID) may also be used. Intermittent medical treatment may be sufficient to minimize discomfort. Young dogs with HD often become sound at 12 to 14 months of age regardless of treatment or degree of HD. Clinical signs of lameness may not return, or DJD may cause lameness later in life. Accordingly, medical treatment of the immature dog can be discontinued after this acute phase.

H. Pectinectomy may result in symptomatic improvement in the mature dog with DJD, although pain may return months to years afterwards. Excision of the femoral head and neck is usually the preferred treatment for the non-working dog. If properly performed, the majority of dogs become pain free, although the range of motion of the hip is reduced. Larger dogs may have a quicker and better postoperative recovery of function if soft tissue such as biceps femoris muscle is interposed between the femur and acetabulum. Total hip replacement provides the best functional result in the mature dog with DJD of the hip. The surgery is technically demanding and for good results should be performed only by a specially trained surgeon.

I. There is a genetic predisposition in the development of HD. Many genes are involved, and environmental factors are superimposed upon the genetic predisposition. The use of only radiographically HD free dogs in breeding programs has consistently reduced the prevalence and severity of HD in the line. Therefore, neutering of affected dogs should be part of the protocol of any HD treatment.

* (In animals with hip joint laxity, femoral head subluxation occurs upon adduction of the affected limb. Abduction results in reduction of the joint and a palpable or audible click. The elicitation of a click by manipulation of the hip is a positive Ortolani sign.)

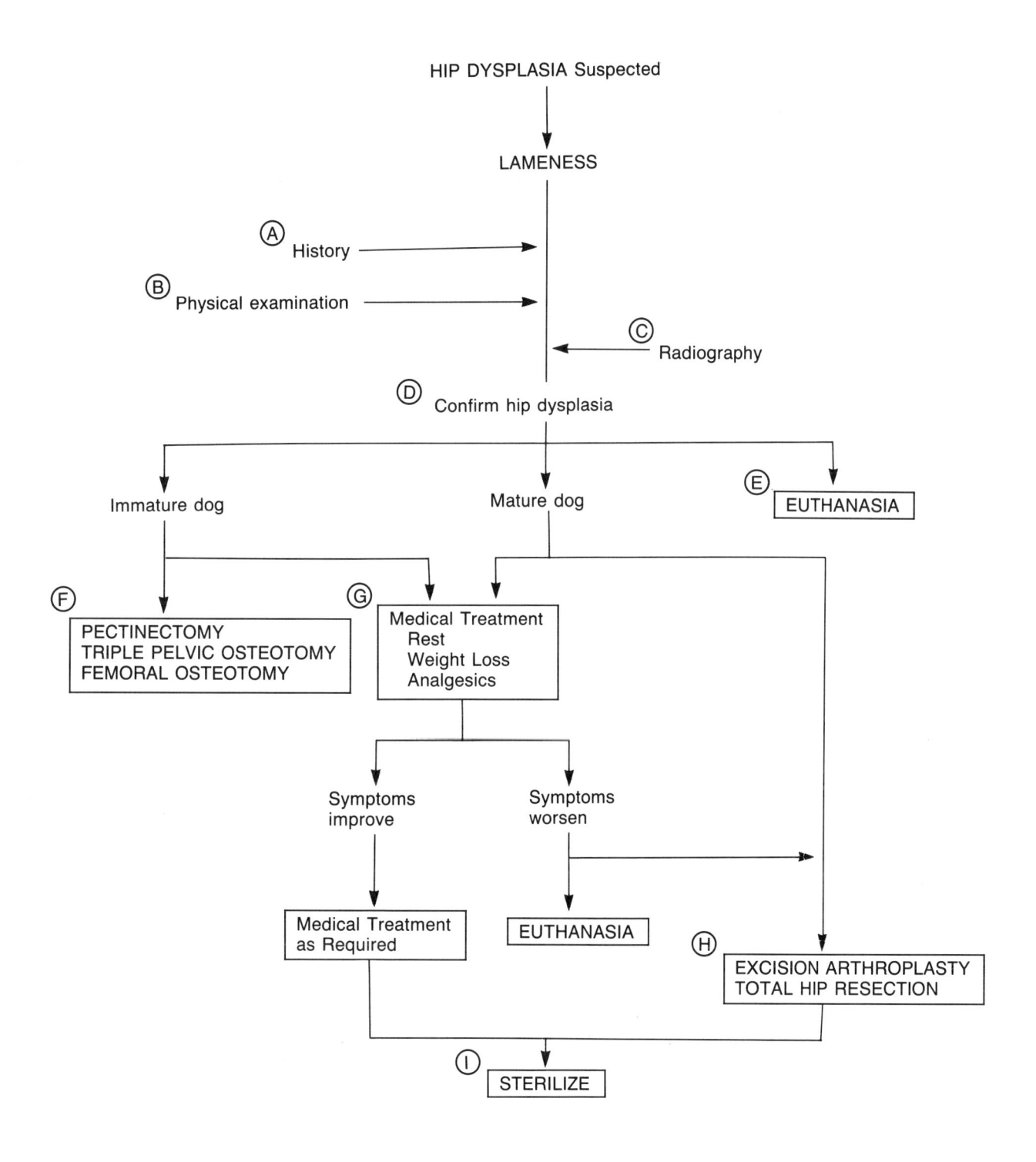

```
                    HIP DYSPLASIA Suspected
                              │
                              ▼
                         LAMENESS
                              ▲
           (A) History ───────┤
                              │
      (B) Physical examination ┤
                              │
                              ├──────── (C) Radiography
                              │
                         (D) Confirm hip dysplasia
              ┌───────────────┼───────────────┐
              ▼               ▼               ▼
         Immature dog    Mature dog      (E) EUTHANASIA
```

(F)
PECTINECTOMY
TRIPLE PELVIC OSTEOTOMY
FEMORAL OSTEOTOMY

(G) Medical Treatment — Rest, Weight Loss, Analgesics

- Symptoms improve → Medical Treatment as Required
- Symptoms worsen → EUTHANASIA

(H) EXCISION ARTHROPLASTY / TOTAL HIP RESECTION

(I) STERILIZE

References

Barr ARS, Denny HR, Gibbs C. Clinical hip dysplasia in growing dogs: the long-term results of conservative management. J small Anim Pract 1987; 28:243.

Bojrab MJ. Current techniques in small animal surgery. Philadelphia: Lea & Febiger, 1983.

Chalman JA. Coxofemoral joint laxity and the Ortolani sign. JAAHA 1985; 21:671.

Lippincott CL. Improvement of excision arthroplasty of the femoral head and neck utilizing a biceps femoris muscle sling. JAAHA 1981; 17:668.

Olmstead ML et al. A five-year study of 221 total hip replacements in the dog. JAVMA 1983; 183:191.

Schrader SC. Triple osteotomy of the pelvis as a treatment for canine hip dysplasia. JAVMA 1980; 178:39.

Slatter DH. Textbook of small animal surgery. Philadelphia: WB Saunders, 1985.

CANINE HIP DYSPLASIA

W. Dieter Prieur

Canine hip dysplasia (HD) is the unilateral or bilateral abnormal development of the hip joint in the dog during the first year of life. This condition is observed in all breeds of dogs, but mostly occurs in fast growing large breeds (including the Greyhound who for a long time was believed not to suffer from this disease). The etiology is multifactorial; heredity, exercise, feeding, growth rate, and other factors play a part. The incorrect development of the hip causes biomechanical overstressing, which results in degenerative joint disease (DJD) that can be seen histologically at about 5 to 7 months of age. The European classification of hip dysplasia includes the osteoarthritic changes. This is not correct as (1) there are other causes of degenerative joint disease besides hip dysplasia and (2) DJD is the result of, but not a sign of, hip dysplasia. The American classification has 7 degrees that describe the so-called questionable cases, but it is complicated and does not give clear information to the owner. For breeding purposes, a positive or negative diagnosis is of the most help. There is no proof that the degree of dysplasia has any relationship to subsequent stages and degree of development of the condition.

A. Most dogs of large breeds are examined routinely and radiographically for hip dysplasia before clinical signs appear. Dogs are presented with signs of hip pain and uncoordinated motion of the hind legs (see p 14) between 4 and 9 months or even later. After the onset of degenerative joint disease of the hip (see p 10) pain develops, and the owner may notice that the animal has difficulty in rising, poor exercise tolerance, rolling gait, and reluctance to climb stairs, varus deviation (increased adduction), and outward rotation of the femur. Pain can be evoked during examination by abducting, rotating, and overextending the hip. The pain is caused by the contracture of the periarticular muscles, induced to compensate for the loose hip, stretching of the joint capsule that will later thicken by fibrosis, and the venous stasis in the proximal femur. Lameness is caused by pain or joint instability.

B. Physical examination. Palpation and moving the joint in extreme position causes pain, as does pressure on the hip itself. Adducting the limb with cranial pressure against the trochanter or lifting the limb laterally can cause subluxation, and the following abduction causes a "popping" sound called the "Ortolani sign," but this is only possible in a relaxed dog with a severe joint laxity. Pain causes contraction of the periarticular muscles and inhibits the "Ortalani sign." A negative Ortolani sign does not prove the dog free of hip dysplasia.

C. Radiographs provide the diagnosis. Normally the dog is positioned in dorsal recumbancy for ventrodorsal view with extended legs. When examining a hip joint, one must always consider that the joint is not projected on the radiograph in a physiological position. This makes the estimation of subluxation and loose joint a matter for debate. As subluxation is related to muscle relation, the anesthetic may influence laxity. Different joint measurements develop due to the inadequacy of this radiologic technique, and they are not reliable.

D. The Canadian classification of degenerative joint disease is as follows:

   Grade I   Sclerosis of the cranial rim of the acetabulum.
   Grade II   Osteophyte formation at the cranial acetabular rim and femoral neck.
   Grade III Deformation of the femoral neck and acetabular rim.

E. In devising a treatment plan for the animal, the veterinarian should take into account the primary use of the dog. A dog with a recognized hip dysplasia will develop a severe degeneration joint disease of the hip within the next 2 years. If the owner wants a hunting dog, a trained police dog, or one to be used for a lot of running and walking, he should be advised against keeping the dog. If the dog is only a house dog, in most cases there is not a great problem. If necessary, hip osteotomy delays the development of DJD and improves the motion of the joint. If the dog is young and the dysplasia is not too severe, medical treatment in the form of analgesics overcomes the pain; otherwise, surgical treatment should be considered. A breeder should consider changing his breeding stock on account of the heredity element. Conservative or medical therapy consists of aspirin, butazolidin, oral corticosteroids for a short time in a low concentration, intra-articular crystalline corticosteroids

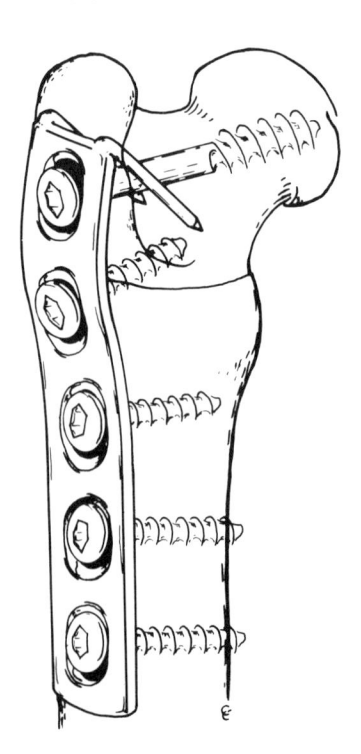

Figure 1 the appearance of the proximal femur following a varising osteotomy and fixation with a five-hole hook plate.

CANINE HIP DYSPLASIA

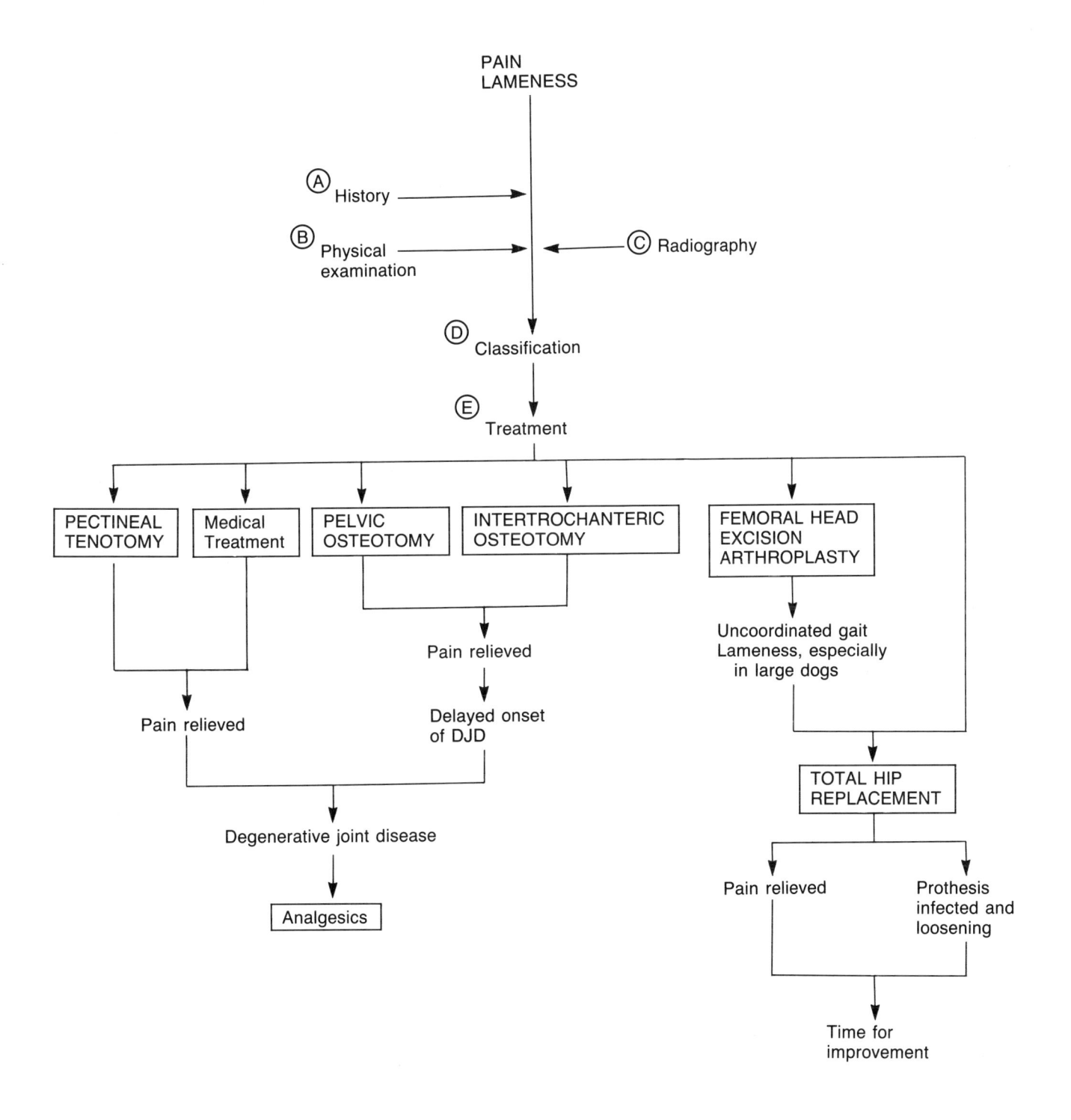

```
                    PAIN
                  LAMENESS
                     │
  Ⓐ History ────────▶│
                     │
  Ⓑ Physical ───────▶│◀─── Ⓒ Radiography
     examination     │
                     ▼
                  Ⓓ Classification
                     │
                     ▼
                  Ⓔ Treatment
```

| PECTINEAL TENOTOMY | Medical Treatment | PELVIC OSTEOTOMY | INTERTROCHANTERIC OSTEOTOMY | FEMORAL HEAD EXCISION ARTHROPLASTY |

- Pectineal Tenotomy / Medical Treatment → Pain relieved
- Pelvic Osteotomy / Intertrochanteric Osteotomy → Pain relieved → Delayed onset of DJD
- → Degenerative joint disease → Analgesics

- Femoral Head Excision Arthroplasty → Uncoordinated gait, Lameness, especially in large dogs → TOTAL HIP REPLACEMENT
  - → Pain relieved
  - → Prothesis infected and loosening
  - → Time for improvement

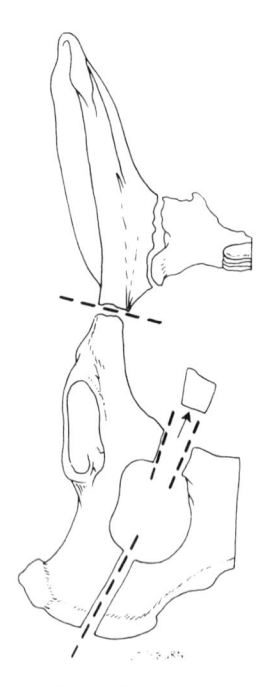

Figure 2 Sites for osteotomy of the pelvis, prior to rotation.

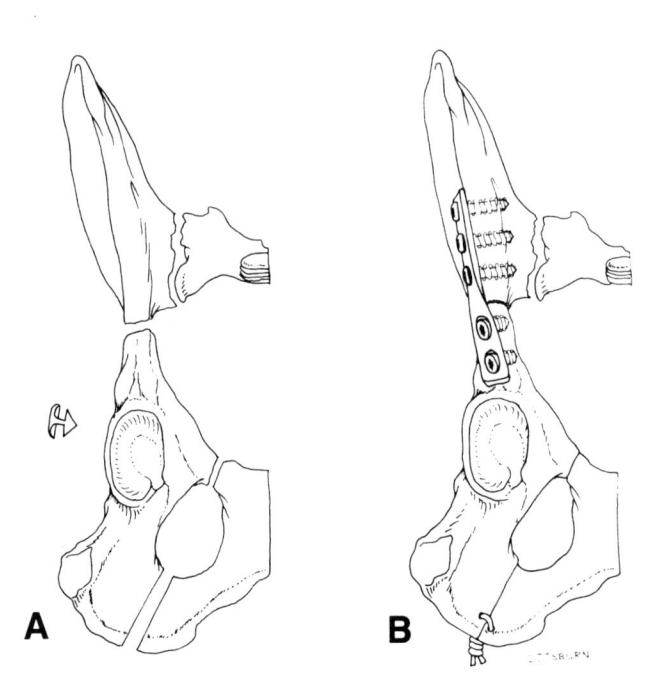

Figure 3 *A*, Rotation of the acetabular segment. *B*, Stabilization of the osteotomies by means of a five-hole plate on the ilial shaft and wiring of the tuber ischii. The pubic site is not stabilized.

should not be administered. Operative therapy may comprise of a pectineal myotomy or myotectomy, an intertrochanteric osteotomy (Fig. 1), a pelvic osteotomy (Figs. 2 and 3) or a total hip replacement. When degenerative joint disease is diagnosed, injections of special proteoglycans and antirheumatic drugs (NSAIDs) may be helpful.

References

Barr ARS, Denny HR, Gibbs C. Clinical hip dysplasia in growing dogs: the long-term results of conservative management. J small Anim Pract 1987; 28:243.

Hauptman J. The hip joint. In: Slatter DH, ed. Textbook of small animal surgery. Philadelphia: WB Saunders, 1985:2167.

Olmstead ML, Hohn RB, Turner TM. A five year study of 221 consecutive clinical total hip replacements in the dog. JAVMA 1983; 183:91.

Schrader SC. Triple osteotomy of the pelvis in the treatment of canine hip dysplasia. JAVMA 1971; 178:39.

SLIPPED CAPITAL EPIPHYSIS

W. Dieter Prieur

A. This trauma occurs in dogs between 4 and 10 months of age. It can occur with or without dislocation. If there is dislocation, the capsule is torn and the blood supply to the epiphysis may be destroyed. Slipped capital epiphysis may occur concomitant with avulsion of the trochanteric epiphysis.

B. In small dogs and cats, fixation by Kirschner wires may be attempted by an experienced surgeon, but excision arthroplasty may be the method of choice.

C. In medium-sized dogs and giant dogs, internal fixation preferably with Kirschner wires, should be performed. Avascular necrosis may still result within a year, requiring excision arthroplasty or total hip replacement. Lag-screw fixation is preferred if the growth plate is near to closure.

References

Lee R. Proximal femoral epiphyseal separation in the dog. J small Anim Pract 1976; 2:669.

Milton JL, Newman ME. Fractures of the femur: capital physeal fractures. In: Slatter DH, ed. Textbook of small animal surgery. Philadelphia: WB Saunders, 1985:2183.

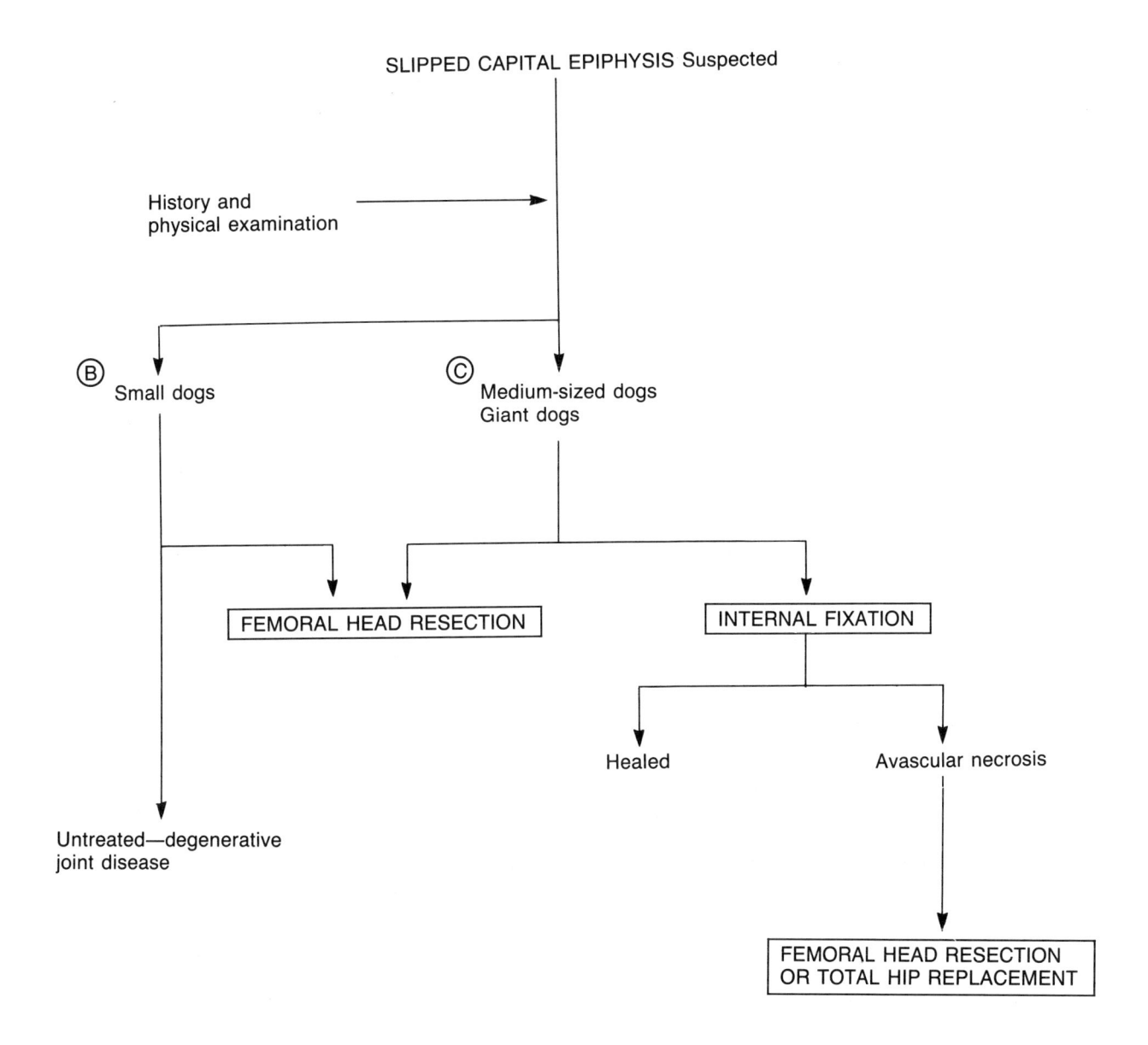

SLIPPED CAPITAL EPIPHYSIS Suspected

History and physical examination

Ⓑ Small dogs

Ⓒ Medium-sized dogs
Giant dogs

FEMORAL HEAD RESECTION

INTERNAL FIXATION

Healed

Avascular necrosis

Untreated—degenerative joint disease

FEMORAL HEAD RESECTION OR TOTAL HIP REPLACEMENT

AVASCULAR NECROSIS OF THE FEMORAL HEAD
(Legg-Calvé-Perthes Disease)

W. Dieter Prieur
Geoff Sumner-Smith

A. Avascular necrosis of the femoral head (also called Legg-Calvé-Perthes disease) normally occurs around the age of 7 months, but the range may be between 3 to 12 months in small and miniature breeds. It is believed to be caused by an interference with the blood supply to the femoral head and neck. The following causes have also been suggested:
   (1) thrombosis of the blood supply by trauma,
   (2) imbalance of sex hormones, and
   (3) genetic factors (the condition is seen more frequently in special blood lines).

B. Clinical signs include a gradual and increasing onset of hind limb lameness (uni- or bilateral) with intermittent carrying or use of the limb. The lameness is accompanied by muscle atrophy and contracture. Manipulation of the limb evokes acute pain.

C. In the beginning, the ischemia does not cause any clinical or radiologic signs. Both appear to be caused by decreased tissue resistance against joint loading, with trabecular fragmentation that results in deformation of the femoral head. Highly vascularized invading tissue partially replaces the cancellous bone and causes the typical radiologic appearance. Flattening and an uneven shape of the femoral head results in cartilage overloading and altered mechanism and congruity of the joint; this causes degenerative joint disease in which osteophyte formation is the main radiologic sign. In severe cases, the femoral neck fractures.

D. If the lameness and radiologic signs are not severe, the animal should be treated conservatively by means of light exercise and analgesics. Guard against the psychologic habit of carrying the limb. There is little pain on manipulation of the hip. In such cases, the opposite hind limb may be slung for a few hours each day. Inactivity of the joint tends to promote contracture of local muscles.

E. In severe cases, and following femoral neck fracture, perform excision arthroplasty, followed, once the soft tissues have healed, by local physiotherapy and general exercise in order to avoid the animal using only three legs out of habit; this ability is common to very small dogs.

References

Lee R. A study of radiographic and histological changes occurring in Legg-Calvé-Perthes disease (LCP) in the dog. J small Anim Pract 1970; 11:621.

Ljunggren GL. Legg-Perthes disease in the dog. Acta Orthop Scand (Suppl) 1967; 95:7.

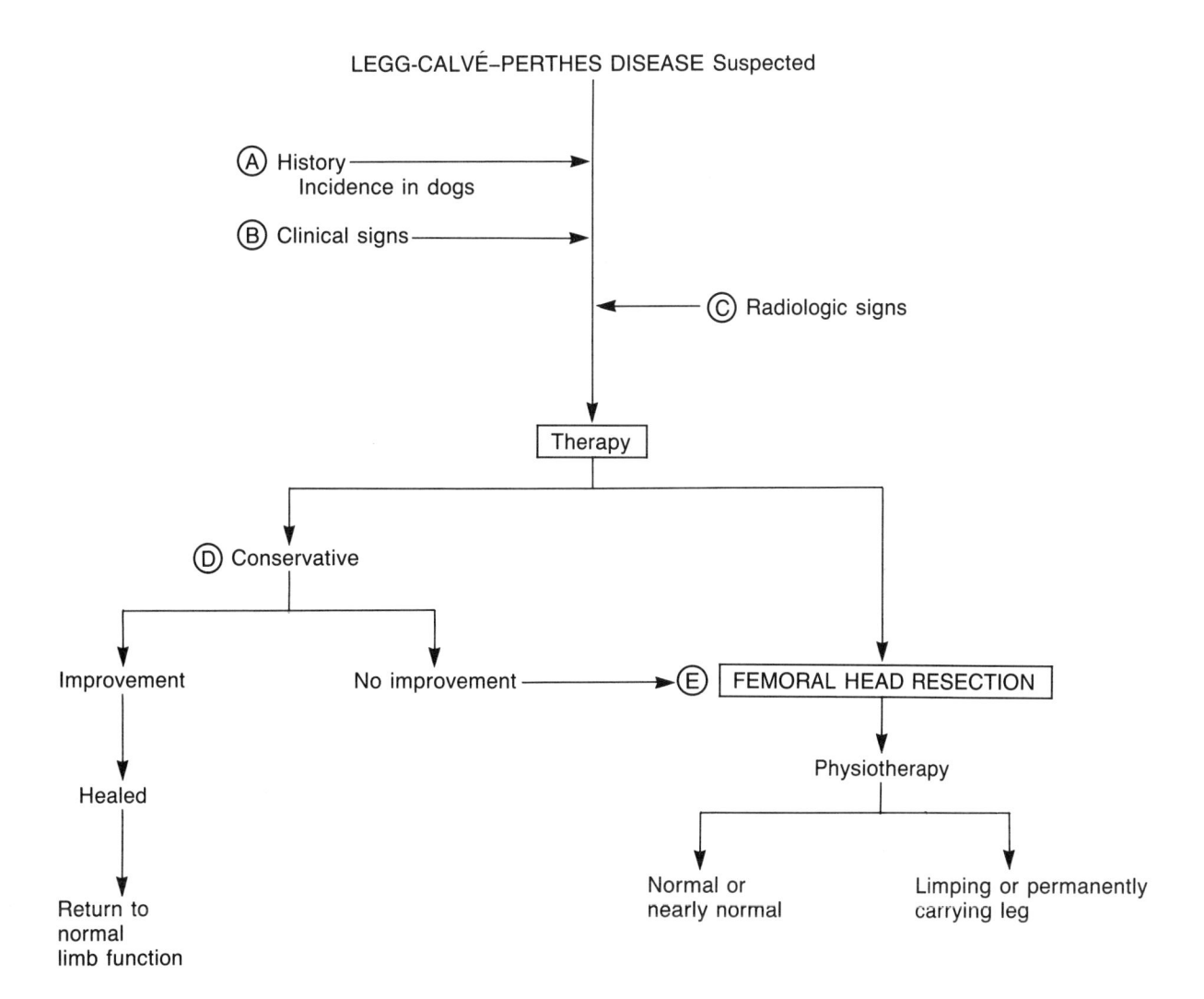

LEGG-CALVÉ–PERTHES DISEASE Suspected

- (A) History — Incidence in dogs
- (B) Clinical signs
- (C) Radiologic signs

↓

Therapy

- (D) Conservative
  - Improvement → Healed → Return to normal limb function
  - No improvement → (E) **FEMORAL HEAD RESECTION**
- FEMORAL HEAD RESECTION → Physiotherapy
  - Normal or nearly normal
  - Limping or permanently carrying leg

SEPSIS IN TOTAL HIP REPLACEMENT

Geoff Sumner-Smith

Occasionally postoperative sepsis occurs following total hip replacement. This situation is less common when cementless implants are used.

A. If an animal is presented with acute lameness and obvious distress following total hip replacement, sepsis should be suspected. The presence of a draining sinus confirms the suspicion, and the early stage identification of infection is most important because secondary infection that tracks from the skin surface may obscure the primary infectious organism, which invariably gains entrance at the time of the original operation.

B. Any hip joint aspirates and samples taken from the sinus tract should be cultured to establish the cause of the organism, to determine whether the prosthesis has loosened, and to observe the condition of the bone surrounding the implant. Sinograms may also aid in identifying the extent of the sinus tracts.

C. Acute sepsis following total hip replacement is usually seen within the first 2 or 3 postoperative weeks; in fact, the animal may have never regained reasonable use of the limb. Unfortunately, there may be considerable spread of deep infection via fascial planes before sinuses to the exterior are formed. Any sinus tract should be assumed to communicate with the hip joint area itself. Although aggressive medical treatment may limit the spread of infection, total debridement of the sinus tract is mandatory. If the implant is found to be firmly imbedded and not showing signs of loosening, a long-term course of antibiotics should be commenced; initially this is given intravenously for 10 to 14 days and then continued by oral administration. Immobilization of the hip is not recommended, although it would be beneficial to the wound healing; in dogs, the danger of total fibrosis and a subsequently useless appendage is high. Monitoring of the blood picture, particularly the sedimentation rate, gives the surgeon an idea as to the resolution of the sepsis. If infection cannot then be controlled, the implant should be removed. If infection cannot be controlled, the hip should be allowed to develop into a pseudarthrosis, such as occurs following excision arthroplasty. Positive physiotherapy is essential if the joint is not to fibrose and become useless. Should the organism then prove susceptible to treatment and once the infection is totally controlled, a revision may be carried out, preferably with a cementless prosthesis.

D. Chronic sepsis may be sequel to acute infection or may develop many months after the insertion of a total hip prosthesis. In the latter case considerable bone destruction is likely to have occurred and removal of the implant and cement is recommended. Once infection is controlled, this may be followed either by revision to produce a result similar to an excision arthroplasty, or by the insertion of a new implant. If the animal is suffering from a chronic draining sinus without generalized sepsis, febrile episodes, or bone resorption, treatment with long-term antibiotics or other forms of chemotherapy is a reasonable approach.

References

Denny HA. A guide to canine orthopaedic surgery. Blackwell Scientific (Oxford), 1986:153.

Harris WH. Revision surgery for failed, nonseptic total hip arthroplasty. Clin Orthop Rel Res 1982; 170:8.

Hunter G, Dandy D. The natural history of the patient with an infected total hip replacement. J Bone Joint Surg 1977; 59-B:293.

Olmstead ML, et al. Technique for canine total hip replacement. Vet Surg 1981; 10:44.

Olmstead ML, et al. A five-year study of 221 consecutive clinical total hip replacements in the dog. JAVMA 1983; 193:91.

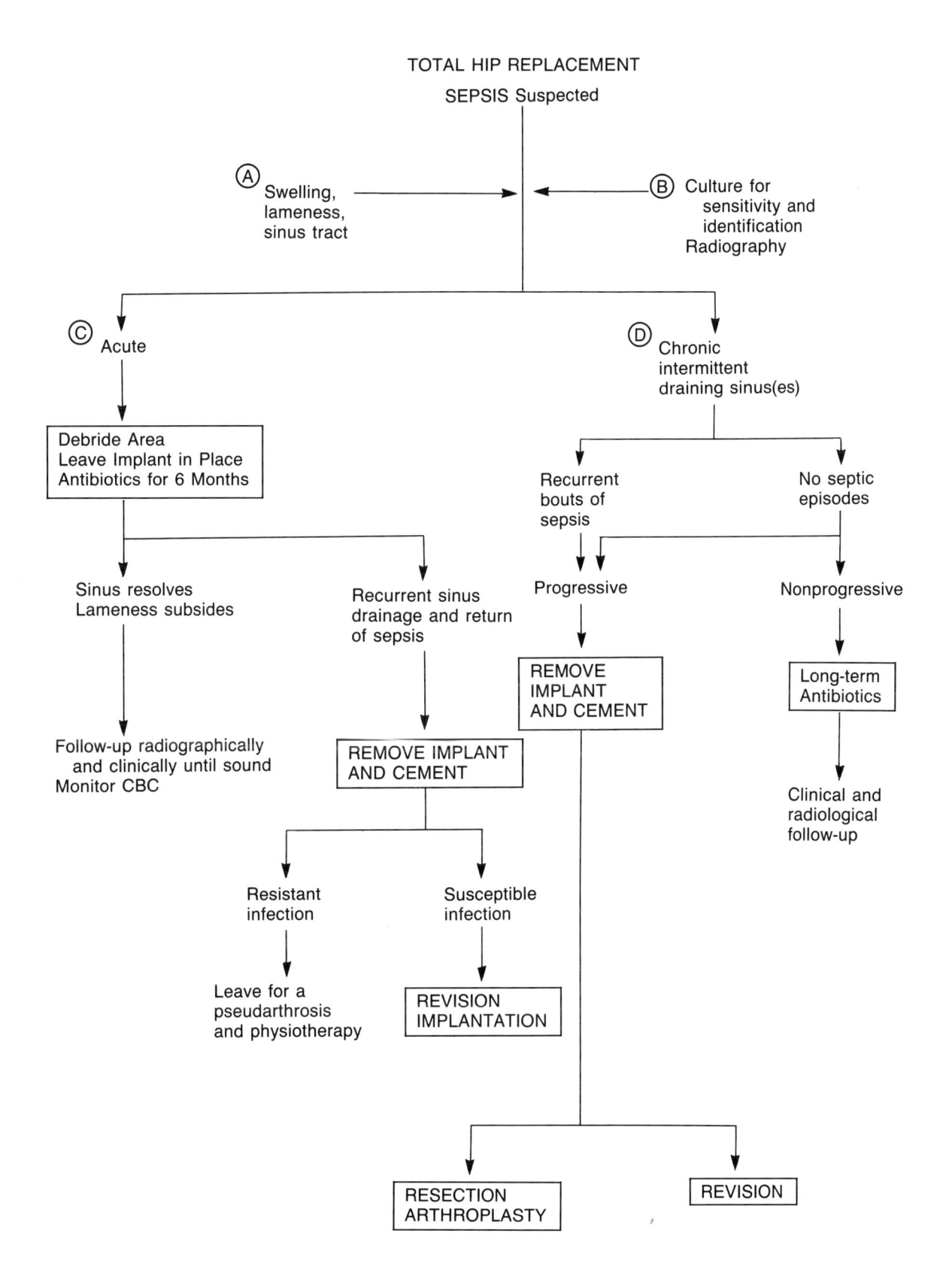

TOTAL HIP REPLACEMENT
SEPSIS Suspected

- Ⓐ Swelling, lameness, sinus tract
- Ⓑ Culture for sensitivity and identification Radiography

Ⓒ **Acute**
→ Debride Area / Leave Implant in Place / Antibiotics for 6 Months
- Sinus resolves / Lameness subsides → Follow-up radiographically and clinically until sound / Monitor CBC
- Recurrent sinus drainage and return of sepsis → **REMOVE IMPLANT AND CEMENT**
  - Resistant infection → Leave for a pseudarthrosis and physiotherapy
  - Susceptible infection → **REVISION IMPLANTATION**

Ⓓ **Chronic intermittent draining sinus(es)**
- Recurrent bouts of sepsis
  - Progressive → **REMOVE IMPLANT AND CEMENT** → **RESECTION ARTHROPLASTY** or **REVISION**
- No septic episodes
  - Nonprogressive → Long-term Antibiotics → Clinical and radiological follow-up

105

FEMORAL HEAD AND NECK FRACTURE

W. Dieter Prieur

A. The clinical signs are similar to those presented with other hip injuries, i.e., hip dislocation, acetabular fracture. Therefore, the diagnosis must be confirmed by radiography.

B. Radiographs must be taken with the patient in the ventrodorsal position. Lateral radiographs are of little value.

C. Many different types of femoral head and neck fractures should be considered. A slipped capital epiphysis is more likely to occur in growing animals (see p 100). These are (1) normally Salter I fractures, (2) seldom Salter II fractures with a small piece of the epiphysis, and (3) seldom Salter III fractures with additional fractures of the epiphysis.

D. Fracture of the femoral head in adult animals may present in the following ways: (1) avulsion fracture of the ligamentus teres insertion are normally combined with hip dislocation; (2) horizontal fracture; often three fragment fractures, combining and avulsion fracture of the ligamentus teres insertion and dislocation; and (3) vertical fractures; also involving the neck, combined with dislocation. Multifragment fractures occur infrequently.

E. Femoral neck fractures may be intra- or extracapsular with often two, but seldom three or more fragments.

F. The chief aim, if at all possible, is to reconstruct the femoral head and neck. The treatment modality depends on the severity of the fracture, the size of the animal, and the experience of the veterinary surgeon. Treatment of an avulsion fracture of the insertion of the teres ligament varies with the size of the animal. In a miniature dog or cat weighing 5 kg, surgical removal of the avulsed piece of bone with fixation of the dislocation is the treatment of choice. In a medium-sized dog weighing 5 to 15 kg, a small piece of bone requires surgical removal; larger pieces may possibly be stabilized by an experienced veterinary surgeon. In a large dog weighing 15 kg or more, if the piece is very small, surgical removal is required; otherwise fixation may be attempted.

G. In a miniature dog or cat weighing up to 5 kg, the best mode of treatment for two-fragment femoral head fracture is excision arthroplasty; if the fragment is very small, surgical removal may be attempted. In the medium-sized dog weighing 5 to 15 kg with horizontal fractures, if the piece is large, rigid internal fixation must be attempted with lag-screw fixation. Smaller fragments that cannot be adequately fixed should be removed. In vertical fractures (in mose cases the neck is involved), stabilization by lag screws is required. If fixation is not possible, excision arthroplasty is the other choice. In the large dog weighing 15 kg or more, if possible, the fragment should be fixed by internal fixation as excision arthroplasty is not suitable for large and heavy dogs. Total hip replacement is an alternative choice. When there are three or more fragment fractures of the head and neck, in miniature and medium-sized dogs, excision arthroplasty is the easiest method. If the femoral head fracture is combined with an avulsion of the teres ligament, the fracture is fixed, and the avulsed bony insertion of the teres ligament is removed.

H. In all cases, the main complication is subsequent avascular necrosis of the head and neck with radiographic loss of density, demineralization, and nonunion. The neck may disappear, partially or completely in 3 to 6 weeks, but necrosis may appear up to 12 months later in cases that previously appeared to have healed. Treatment requires excision arthroplasty in cats and small and medium-sized dogs, or total hip replacement, or as a final choice, excision arthroplasty in large dogs. Degenerative joint disease may appear up to 2 years after surgery. For treatment see *Degenerative Joint Disease* (p 16).

References

Brinker WO, Hohn RB, Prieur WD. Manual of internal fixation in small animals. Heidelberg: Springer-Verlag, 1984.

Hulse DA. Femoral head and neck fractures. In: Bojrab MJ, ed. Current techniques in small animal surgery. Philadelphia: Lea & Febiger, 1983; 636.

Milton JL, Newman ME. Fractures of the femur: capital epiphyseal fractures. In: Slatter DH, ed. Textbook of small animal surgery. Philadelphia: WB Saunders, 1985:2183.

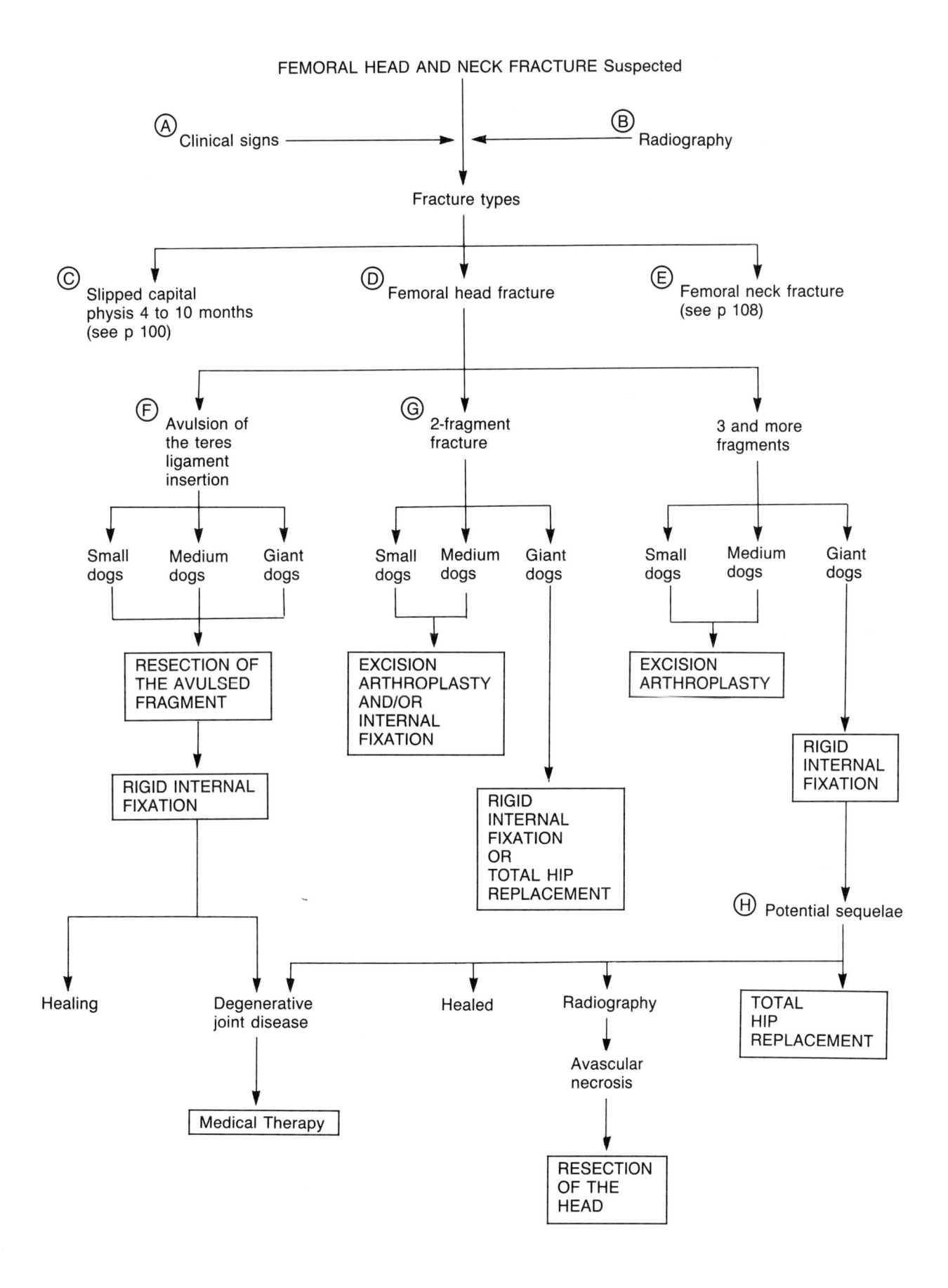

FEMORAL HEAD AND NECK FRACTURE Suspected

- Ⓐ Clinical signs
- Ⓑ Radiography

→ Fracture types

- Ⓒ Slipped capital physis 4 to 10 months (see p 100)
- Ⓓ Femoral head fracture
- Ⓔ Femoral neck fracture (see p 108)

Femoral head fracture

- Ⓕ Avulsion of the teres ligament insertion
  - Small dogs / Medium dogs / Giant dogs → **RESECTION OF THE AVULSED FRAGMENT** → **RIGID INTERNAL FIXATION** → Healing / Degenerative joint disease → **Medical Therapy**

- Ⓖ 2-fragment fracture
  - Small dogs / Medium dogs → **EXCISION ARTHROPLASTY AND/OR INTERNAL FIXATION**
  - Giant dogs → **RIGID INTERNAL FIXATION OR TOTAL HIP REPLACEMENT**

- 3 and more fragments
  - Small dogs / Medium dogs → **EXCISION ARTHROPLASTY**
  - Giant dogs → **RIGID INTERNAL FIXATION**

Ⓗ Potential sequelae:
- Healed
- Radiography → Avascular necrosis → **RESECTION OF THE HEAD**
- **TOTAL HIP REPLACEMENT**

107

FEMORAL NECK FRACTURES

W. Dieter Prieur

A. Two-fragment fractures may be intra- or extracapsular. To date there are no reports to indicate differences between the healing patterns of the two types.

B. Complicated femoral neck fractures with three or more fragments are very infrequent, and often the femoral head and the greater trochanter are involved. In young dogs, the femoral neck fracture is often combined with avulsion of the epiphysis.

C. In miniature breeds, only a very skilled veterinary surgeon is able to achieve rigid internal fixation by a lag screw; however, in many cases, avascular necrosis of the femoral head may destroy a good initial result within 12 months. Excision arthroplasty is the treatment of choice, but only if the animal is clinically unsound.

D. In medium- and large-size breeds, internal fixation by lag-screw fixation must be attempted. Fixation by Kirschner wires is too weak, and interfragmentary movement promotes avascular necrosis (Fig. 1).

E. In large breeds, total hip replacement is preferred as excision arthroplasty impedes the locomotion of these dogs (Fig. 2).

References

Brinker WO, Piermattei DL, Flo GL. Handbook of small animal orthopedics and fracture treatment. Philadelphia: WB Saunders, 1983:76.

Hulse DA. Femoral head and neck fractures. In: Bojrab MJ, ed. Current techniques in small animal surgery. Philadelphia: Lea & Febiger, 1983:636.

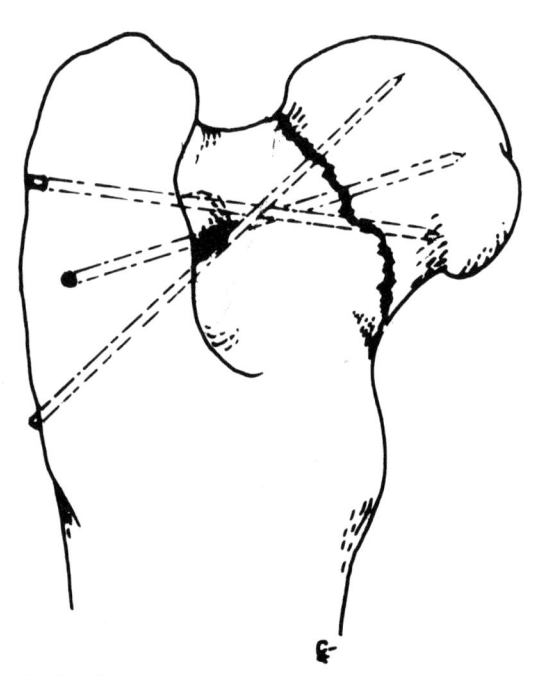

Figure 1 Stabilization of a femoral neck fracture by three Kirchner wires normally only used in small- to medium-sized dogs.

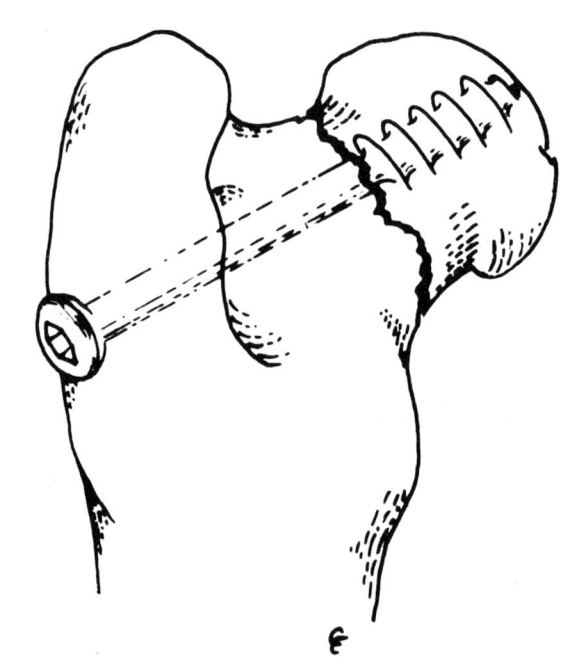

Figure 2 The same fracture is stabilized by means of a cancellous lag screw. This method is preferable, if sufficient purchase may be obtained on the femoral head to permit compression.

FEMORAL NECK FRACTURE Suspected

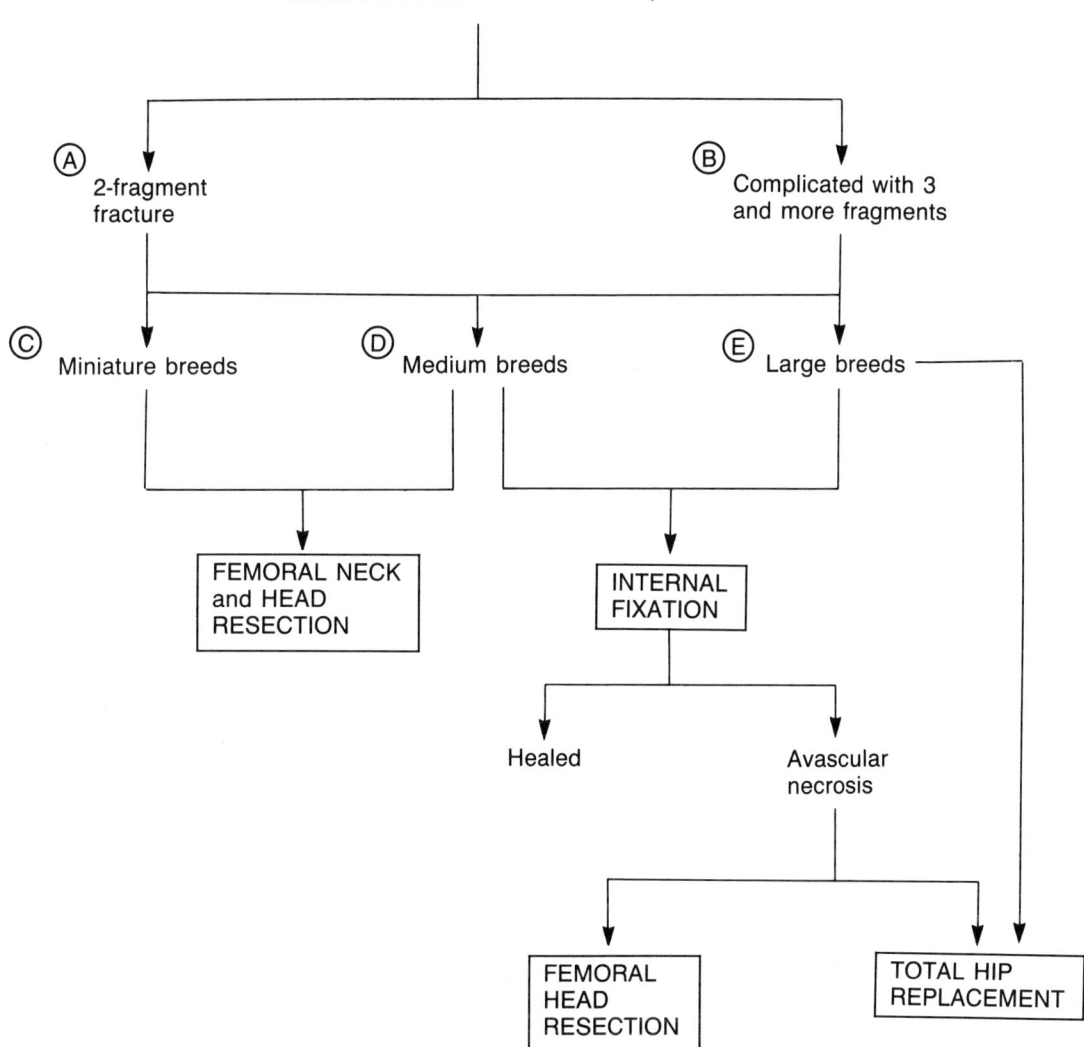

- (A) 2-fragment fracture
- (B) Complicated with 3 and more fragments

- (C) Miniature breeds
- (D) Medium breeds
- (E) Large breeds

FEMORAL NECK and HEAD RESECTION

INTERNAL FIXATION
- Healed
- Avascular necrosis

FEMORAL HEAD RESECTION

TOTAL HIP REPLACEMENT

PROXIMAL FEMUR FRACTURE

W. Dieter Prieur

A. Physical examination reveals fractures that are often compound or have severe associated contusion of the soft tissue. The integrity of the ischiatic nerve must be determined. This is often difficult in the first 48 hours.

B. Radiographs in both mediolateral and anteroposterior projections should be taken in order to check for femoral neck fractures, as well as for acetabular and other pelvic fractures and hip luxations.

C. Fracture of the trochanter major is most commonly seen in the young animal with avulsion of the apophysis. Fixation by tension band wiring is preferred. Screw fixation destroys the physis in the growing dog; furthermore, there is the tendency for a screw to bend on account of the tension of the gluteal muscles.

D. Subtrochanteric or intertrochanteric fractures are often combined with femoral neck fractures. Therefore the radiographs must be carefully studied. Fixation is best performed with screws and plates. If there are short fragments, the double hookplate should be used (Fig. 1, p 96).

References

Brinker WO, Hohn RB, Prieur WD. Manual of internal fixation in small animals. Heidelberg: Springer-Verlag, 1984.

Milton JL, Newman ME. Fractures of the femur. In: Slatter DH, ed. Textbook of small animal surgery. Philadelphia: WB Saunders, 1985.

PROXIMAL FEMUR FRACTURE Suspected

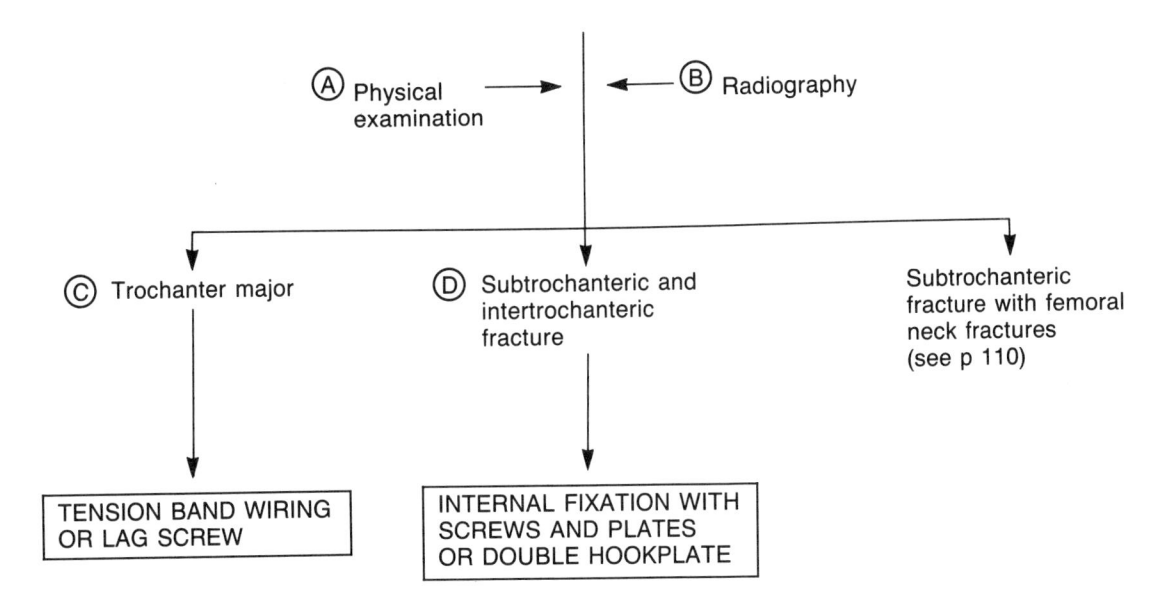

- (A) Physical examination → ← (B) Radiography

- (C) Trochanter major
  - **TENSION BAND WIRING OR LAG SCREW**

- (D) Subtrochanteric and intertrochanteric fracture
  - **INTERNAL FIXATION WITH SCREWS AND PLATES OR DOUBLE HOOKPLATE**

- Subtrochanteric fracture with femoral neck fractures (see p 110)

FEMORAL SHAFT FRACTURE

W. Dieter Prieur

A. Femoral fractures result from high energy trauma. Therefore, they are often comminuted, with severe soft tissue damage. Always check the thorax, abdomen, and pelvis for additional trauma. Lung and cardiac contusions are often missed and cause death during or after surgery. With femoral fractures, especially if comminuted, a radiograph of the thorax is mandatory. Surgery must be delayed if lung contusions are present. Check for ischiatic nerve integrity. This is essential for successful treatment and outcome.

B. Radiographs must be taken in both lateral and anteroposterior positions and must be carefully examined for additional fissures.

C. Open fractures are treated as follows:
   Grade I - after cleaning the skin and removing necrotic or contused skin, the fracture is treated in the same way as the closed.
   Grade II - after correct cleaning of the wound, the bone is fixed and the wound left open and treated routinely.
   Grade III - treatment as for Grade II, or in severely infected cases, the main fragments are fixed by external fixator in order to maintain bone length and treat the soft tissue and infection first, delaying internal fixation until the soft tissue has healed sufficiently.

D. Because of the shape of the limb, there is no reliable conservative treatment for femoral shaft fractures by casts and splints. The thick muscle layer and the impossibility to include the pelvis in the cast makes such techniques inadequate. The Schröder-Thomas splint may cause additional interfragmentary motion, especially in proximal midshaft fractures, and causes nonunion. The fixed and extended stifle joint causes contracture of the quadriceps group of muscles. If it is not possible to treat the fracture operatively, 6 weeks of cage rest allows fracture healing, but subsequent limb function is questionable.

E. Operative treatment with rigid internal fixation by lag screws, plates, and external fixator achieves, when applied correctly, the best results in all fracture types. Rigid fixation is neither achieved by medullary pins nor Küntscher nail alone. The use of cerclage wires in special fracture types is possible, but can create problems. All open fractures must be treated by rigid fixation in cases with severe soft tissue damage. External fixation of the main fragments is achieved until the soft tissue is in good condition. If necessary the fracture can be rigidly fixed at a second operation.

F. Transverse and short oblique fractures are best treated by compression plating, especially if additional fissures are visible on the radiograph. This technique permits function of the traumatized limb soon after surgery. Other types of fixation are: external fixation with Kirschner-Ehmer apparatus or medullary nailing with Steinmann pins and Küntscher nails. Medullary nailing has the tendency to create rotational instability and additional fragments if fissures break during implant insertion, or when the animal begins to bear weight.

G. Long oblique or butterfly fractures are best treated by lag-screw compression with additional stabilization with a neutralization plate (Fig. 1) or less securely by an external fixator. Fixation with cerclage wire is possible if the surgeon has proper experience with this technique. Otherwise, the fixation breaks down and often creates additional fragments or nonunion. All too commonly, wire that is too thin is employed, and this either stretches or breaks.

H. Comminuted fractures can be fixed by a plate or external fixator. The most rigid plate suitable for the size of the bone must be selected; otherwise, the implant may become loose, bend, or break. Larger fragments are first fixed with lag screws. If the external fixator is used, the fixation must be rigid for the whole period of healing (3 to 4 months).

I. Nonunions occur mainly following medullary fixation or by loosening of plates and pins of the external fixator. All external fixators have the potential danger of being caught on surrounding objects, and the transfixing pins can impede muscle function.

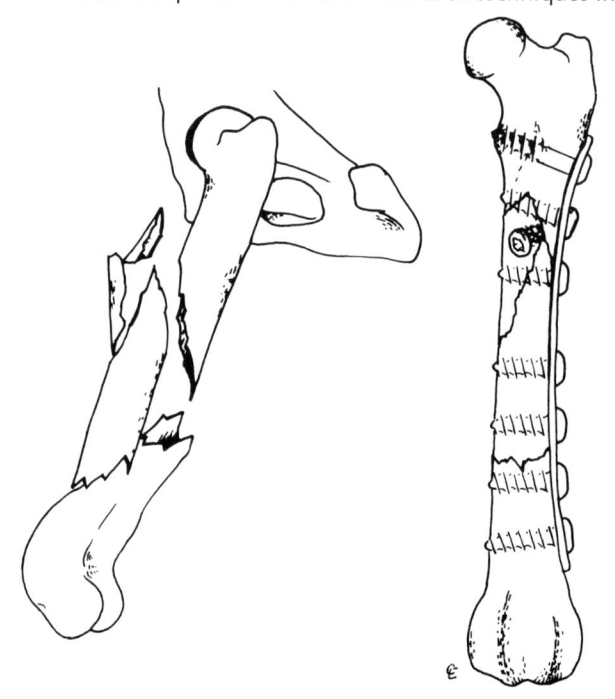

Figure 1 A multiple fracture of the femoral shaft stabilized by intrafragmentary lag-screw compression and a plate placed partly in neutralization and partly in compression according to the particular fracture.

References

Brinker WO, Hohn RB, Prieur WD. Manual of internal fixation in small animals. Heidelberg: Springer-Verlag, 1984:174.

Milton JL, Newman ME. Fractures of the femur. In: Slatter DH, ed. Textbook of small animal surgery. Philadelphia: WB Saunders, 1985:2186.

FEMORAL SHAFT FRACTURE Suspected

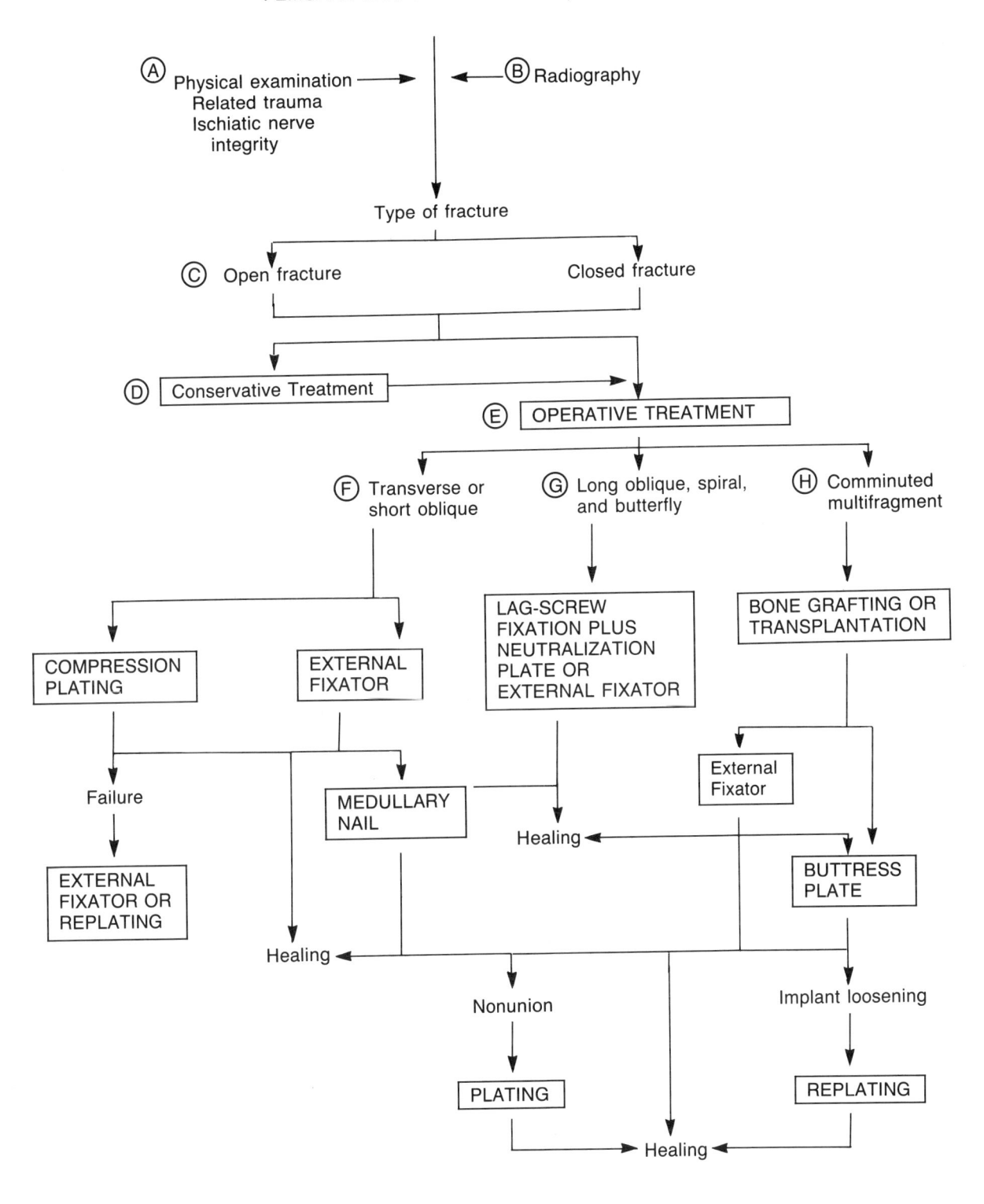

- **A** Physical examination
  - Related trauma
  - Ischiatic nerve integrity
- **B** Radiography

Type of fracture

- **C** Open fracture
- Closed fracture

- **D** Conservative Treatment
- **E** OPERATIVE TREATMENT
  - **F** Transverse or short oblique
    - COMPRESSION PLATING
      - Failure → EXTERNAL FIXATOR OR REPLATING
    - EXTERNAL FIXATOR
      - MEDULLARY NAIL → Healing
      - Nonunion → PLATING → Healing
  - **G** Long oblique, spiral, and butterfly
    - LAG-SCREW FIXATION PLUS NEUTRALIZATION PLATE OR EXTERNAL FIXATOR → Healing
  - **H** Comminuted multifragment
    - BONE GRAFTING OR TRANSPLANTATION
      - External Fixator
      - BUTTRESS PLATE
        - Implant loosening → REPLATING → Healing

113

DISTAL FEMUR FRACTURE

W. Dieter Prieur

A. Fracture types differ in growing and in adult animals. In the immature animal, the presence of a growth plate must be borne in mind.

B. Lateral and anteroposterior radiographs are essential to determine the site of the fracture, fracture type, and the number of fragments.

C. Normally, in growing animals, the fracture line runs fully or partially through the distal femoral growth plate, as this is the weakest part.

D. Avulsion of the long distal extensor tendon of origin may result in a fragmentation of the lateral femoral condyle. The clinical signs are pain, joint effusion, joint laxity, and lameness. To avoid degenerative joint disease, surgery is essential. In recent cases, the avulsed piece is fixed to the femur. In cases of longer duration, the hypertrophied bony fragment must be removed, and the tendon is fixed to the soft tissue adjacent to the tibia.

E. Most cases may be classified as Salter I or Salter II fractures with differing caudal displacement of the epiphysis by the tension of the gastrocnemias muscle. Treatment may be accomplished by cross pinning.

F. Salter III fractures require lag-screw fixation and pinning.

G. In adult dogs, distal femoral fractures can be supracondylar, condylar, and intercondylar. They may be simple or comminuted and may be complicated by damage to the joint capsule and rupture of stifle joint ligaments. The epiphyseal fragments are fixed to one another by lag screws of appropriate size. Kirschner wires used for fixation have to be inserted obliquely as cross pins, otherwise they tend to migrate into the joint. In simple fractures, fixation of the epiphysis to the shaft can be carried out by medullary pinning with an additional external fixator. Multifragment condylar fractures must be reduced and stabilized by plating.

References

Brinker WO, Hohn RB, Prieur WD. Manual of internal fixation of fractures in small animals. Heidelberg: Springer-Verlag, 1984.

Milton JL, Newman ME. Fractures of the femur. In: Slatter DH, ed. Textbook of small animal surgery. Philadelphia: WB Saunders, 1985:2189.

Sumner-Smith G, Dingwall JS. A technique for repaired fractures of the distal femoral epiphysis in the dog and cat. JAAHA 1973; 9(2):171.

DISTAL FEMORAL FRACTURE Suspected

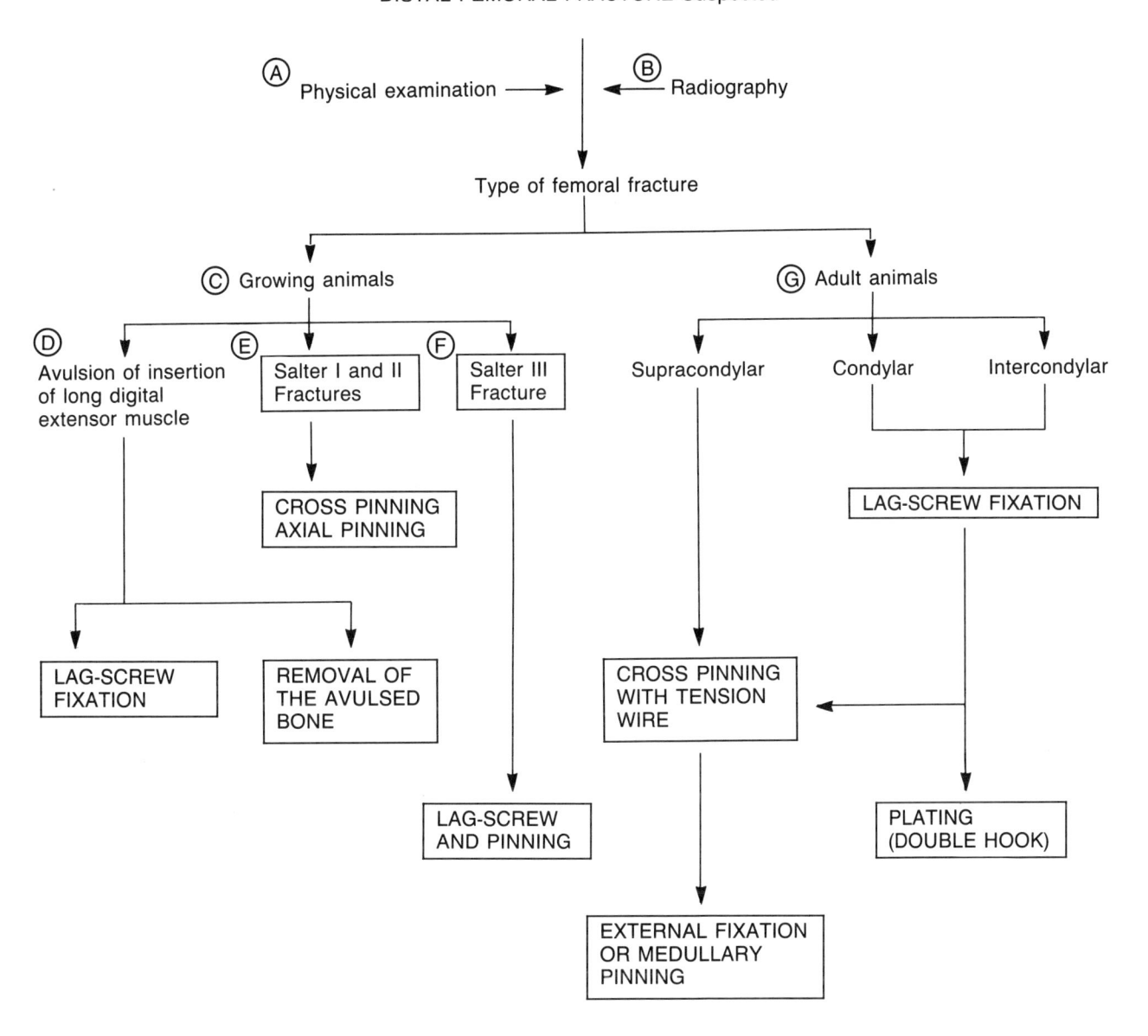

- (A) Physical examination → ← (B) Radiography
- Type of femoral fracture
  - (C) Growing animals
    - (D) Avulsion of insertion of long digital extensor muscle
      - LAG-SCREW FIXATION
      - REMOVAL OF THE AVULSED BONE
    - (E) Salter I and II Fractures
      - CROSS PINNING AXIAL PINNING
    - (F) Salter III Fracture
      - LAG-SCREW AND PINNING
  - (G) Adult animals
    - Supracondylar
      - CROSS PINNING WITH TENSION WIRE
        - EXTERNAL FIXATION OR MEDULLARY PINNING
    - Condylar / Intercondylar
      - LAG-SCREW FIXATION
        - CROSS PINNING WITH TENSION WIRE
        - PLATING (DOUBLE HOOK)

FRACTURE OF THE PATELLA AND RUPTURE OF THE PATELLA LIGAMENT

Geoff Sumner-Smith

Although neither fracture of the patella nor rupture of the patella ligament are particularly common injuries, when they do occur, they can be crippling and need appropriate attention.

A. Unless the stifle joint is flexed, it is occasionally possible for a fissure fracture at the patella to be missed. Radiographs in both the A-P and lateral position are necessary in order to determine the severity of the fracture.

B. As with all injuries to the stifle area, careful digital palpation, either under sedation or under a general anesthetic, of the whole stifle joint is essential in order to determine whether there is concurrent instability caused by damage to other supporting structures.

C. If the articular surface is intact and displacement of the fragment is minimal, the limb may be restrained in a conforming bandage for 3 to 6 weeks and re-radiographed before removal of the support.

D. If the animal is unable to extend the stifle and if the articular surface is disrupted, open reduction with internal fixation is essential.

E. A simple transverse fracture may be repaired with one or two Kirschner wires and a tension band wire. Fissure fractures of the patella may be treated by tension band wires alone. These pass through the quadriceps tendon and the straight ligament of the patella. It should be noted that equatorial wires are not recommended for any fracture of the patella because when the stifle joint is flexed the cranial surface of the patella gapes open (Figs. 1A and B).

F. Comminuted fractures of the patella can be extremely challenging. Some may be fixed with Kirschner wires in conjunction with two tension band wires, but it may be necessary to remove fragments of the patella if the particular element does not have any articular surface. Very comminuted fractures, particularly in small dogs, may well require total patellectomy.

G. Partial rupture of the straight ligament of the patella may be handled by a conforming bandage that keeps the stifle in extension. The bandage should also involve the hock so as to minimize the action of the stay apparatus.

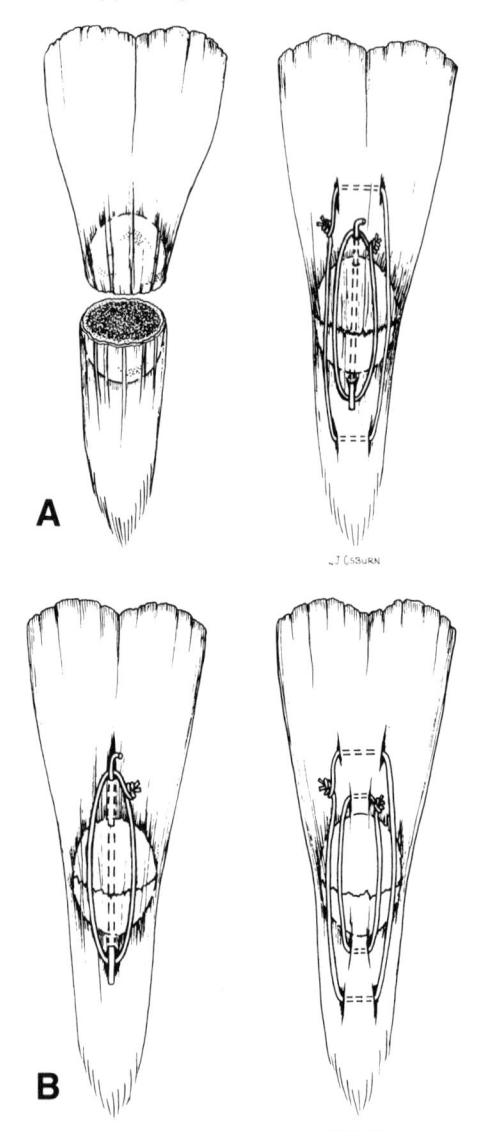

Figure 1 Transverse patella fracture repaired by A, Transfixing pin and tension wire and B, Double tension wire. Note: The tension wires are never placed as equatorial cerclage wires.

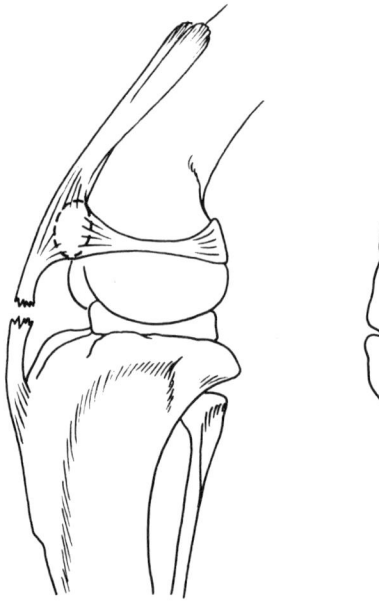

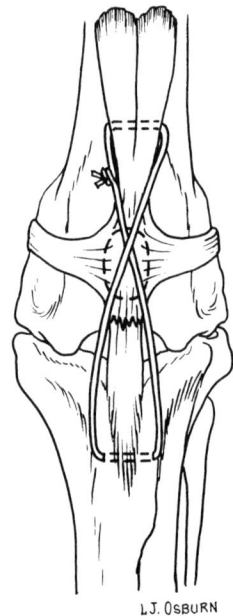

Figure 2 Rupture of the straight patella ligament repaired by a superimposed tension wire that passes under the quadriceps tendon and through a hole drilled in the tibial crest.

FRACTURE OF THE PATELLA Suspected

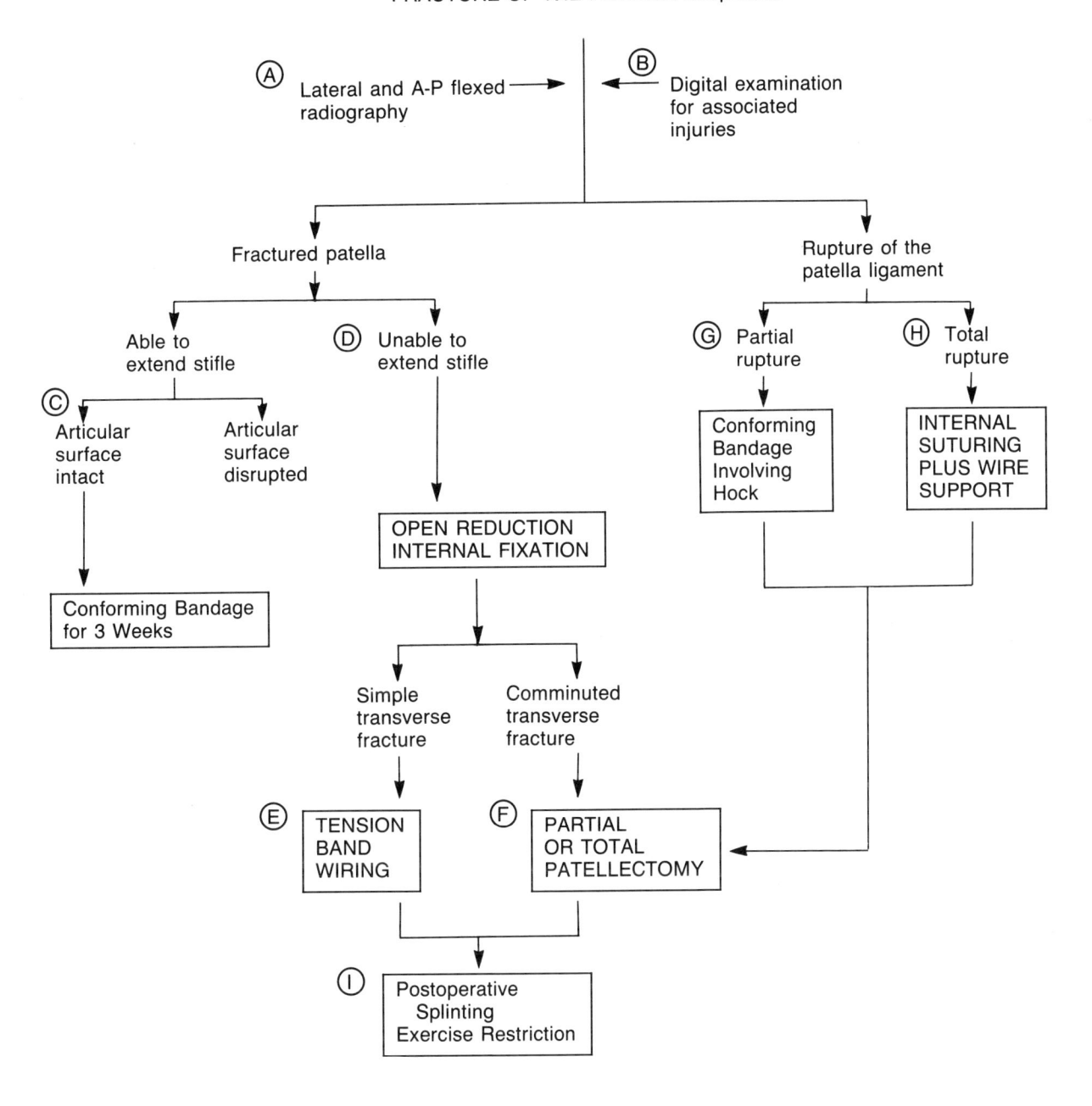

```
                    (A) Lateral and A-P flexed  ──→  ←── (B) Digital examination
                        radiography                        for associated injuries

        ┌───────────────────────────────────────┴─────────────────────────────────┐
        ▼                                                                         ▼
   Fractured patella                                                    Rupture of the
        │                                                               patella ligament
   ┌────┴────┐                                                    ┌──────────┴──────────┐
   ▼         ▼                                                    ▼                     ▼
Able to   (D) Unable to                                   (G) Partial           (H) Total
extend    extend stifle                                       rupture              rupture
stifle        │                                                 │                     │
   │          │                                                 ▼                     ▼
(C)│          │                                           Conforming            INTERNAL
 ┌─┴──┐       │                                           Bandage               SUTURING
 ▼    ▼       │                                           Involving             PLUS WIRE
Articular Articular                                       Hock                  SUPPORT
surface   surface
intact    disrupted
   │          ▼
   ▼       OPEN REDUCTION
Conforming INTERNAL FIXATION
Bandage       │
for 3 Weeks   │
          ┌───┴────┐
          ▼        ▼
        Simple  Comminuted
        transverse transverse
        fracture  fracture
          │        │
          ▼        ▼
     (E) TENSION  (F) PARTIAL
         BAND         OR TOTAL
         WIRING       PATELLECTOMY
              │    │
              └─┬──┘
                ▼
          (I) Postoperative
              Splinting
              Exercise Restriction
```

H. Total rupture of the straight ligament of the patella is a crippling injury. The tendon should be repaired by a Bunnell suture supported by a figure-of-eight wire, which is inserted in the quadriceps tendon, passed through and crossed over the patella ligament distal to the patella, and then transversed through a hole that has been drilled in the proximal tibial crest (Fig. 2).

I. Most injuries to the patella and the patella straight ligament should be supported in a splint over the early healing period (1 to 2 weeks). Activity should be restricted to short walks on a leash, and it must be appreciated that some or all of the implants may need to be removed at a later date.

References

Brinker WO, Piermattei DL, Flo GL. Handbook of small animal orthopedics and fracture treatment. Philadelphia: WB Saunders, 1983.

Hulse DA, Shires PK. The stifle joint. In: Slatter DH, ed. Textbook of small animal surgery. Philadelphia: WB Saunders, 1985:2231.

Stoll SG. In: Brinker WO, Hohn RB, Prieur WD, eds. Manual of internal fixation of small animals. Heidelberg: Springer-Verlag, 1984:176.

CHRONIC SWELLING OF THE STIFLE JOINT

Geoff Sumner-Smith

A number of conditions may cause swelling of the stifle joint; the swelling may originate from distension of the joint capsule or fusion of the surrounding tissue.

A. The owner may be able to report the history of an acute onset of lameness, although more often the dog arrives home carrying a limp. Alternatively, the owner may report that the joint swells from time to time and then the effusion subsides. A general examination of the animal should be carried out in order to determine whether the condition is part of an overall malaise. The local temperature of the swelling has a distinct effect upon the treatment chosen.

B. The initial investigation should commence with a general blood picture examination and aspiration of the swollen area. The appearance of the aspirated material determines the next step in the diagnosis. At the same time, routine radiographs of the joint should be taken, and these should include not only AP and lateral but also the skyline view. Such conditions as degenerative joint disease, loose bodies, osteochondrosis, patella luxation, and stifle malalignment are identifiable radiographically. An arthrogram, particularly a double contrast study, may well aid in diagnosing the degree of synovial membrane and any defects in the cartilage components. Even if the aspirate does not give a clear indication of major changes, it should still be sent for culture, sensitivity, cell count, and personal examination. The sedimentation rate of the blood gives an indication as to whether or not there is an underlying infection, as does the differential leucocyte count. A synovial biopsy may be helpful, but in the routine practice, suitable needles are rarely available.

C. If swelling of the stifle is cool and chronic, one may suspect an underlying biomechanical abnormality, which should be diagnosed by radiography. However, if nothing abnormal is seen on the plates, the diagnosis should follow from an examination of the previously collected aspirate. If the swelling subsides following rest, a gradual controlled exercise program should be instituted; but if it does not do so, then a surgical approach should be taken. If the radiographs demonstrate an underlying abnormality of either the bone or the joint cartilage, the underlying condition should then be treated (p 122).

D. Heat around the stifle joint denotes an inflammatory response, and the character of the aspirate determines the treatment to be followed. If it is purely inflammatory and not infectious, a synovial biopsy is necessary in order to determine the preferred treatment. Septic groinitis is extraordinarily painful and requires aspiration and irrigation of the joint. Antibiotics should be used vigorously, but irrigation of the joint with antibiotics is counterindicated after a primary flushing.

References

Allan G. Radiographic signs of joint disease. In: Thrall DE, ed. Textbook of veterinary diagnostic radiology. Philadelphia: WB Saunders, 1986:121.

Denny HD. A guide to canine orthopaedic surgery. Oxford: Blackwell Scientific Publications, 1980.

Harris AM. Bacterial sensitivity to antibiotics. In: Yoxal AT, Hird JFR, eds. Pharmaceutical basis of small animal medicine. Oxford: Blackwell Scientific Publications: 1979:40.

CHRONIC SWELLING OF THE STIFLE JOINT

- **Ⓐ** History
  Lameness
  Temperature

- **Ⓑ** ASPIRATION
  Sedimentation rate

Ⓒ Cold → Radiographs

No abnormality → ASPIRATE
- Swelling subsides → Exercise
- Swelling persists → Arthrography / Arthroscopy / ARTHROTOMY

Abnormality of bone or joint function
- Treat underlying condition(s) (p 122)

Ⓓ Hot → ASPIRATE

Inflammatory
- SYNOVIAL BIOPSY → ARTHROTOMY / Medication / SYNOVECTOMY

Bacterial
- ASPIRATION / ARTHROTOMY / Antibiotics

STIFLE LIGAMENT INJURY

Geoff Sumner-Smith

A. The accurate clinical assessment as to which ligament(s) are injured is imperative in order that appropriate therapy may be instituted. The history, if available, may be helpful; usually, but not always, collateral ligaments are injured by direct violence and cruciate ligaments by indirect violence, such as sudden arrest or turning. Breed predisposition should be taken into account.

B. Physical examination should be performed in order to localize instability and pain. Place the joint into valgus and varus, and elicit the drawer sign. Rotatory instability usually indicates that more than one structure has ruptured.

C. If the animal remains lame after 4 to 5 days the examination should be repeated and surgical intervention recommended.

D. If the lameness disappears the animal should be kept on restrictive exercise for 2 to 3 weeks. Partial ruptures of ligaments may repair but are more likely to remain divided; hence, joint instability remains with the consequent development of degenerative joint disease. Following stifle ligament injury the joint capsule invariably suffers some degree of trauma; during healing it thickens and reduces the joint laxity. Nonoperative management of stifle injuries should probably be confined to patients who have associated life-threatening medical conditions.

E. Persistent instability and lameness require that the damage be defined. Although physical examination is usually sufficient, on occasion the total damage is only assessible on exploration of the joint.

F. Pain and apprehension invariably make deep sedation, or general anesthesia, essential for proper assessment of stifle joint injury; the animal's resistance makes good relaxation of the limb impossible. Some practice is required to properly assess the instability; both the eyes and the fingers play important parts in the examination. In examining for collateral ligament instability an attempt to "break open" the joint is made on the side under examination. Pressure with the thumbs on the opposite side of the joint fixes the pivot point and increases the leverage.

G. The drawer test is employed to test the cruciate ligament instability; it should be applied in both extended and flexed positions. Rotatory instability is seen sometimes in partial ruptures and in chronic cases. The drawer sign to test for cruciate ligament rupture can be confusing to the inexperienced. It must be appreciated that there is some laxity in the normal joint; this laxity requires that the joint return to the normal position before the joint is assessed. Brinker, Pierrmattei, and Flo list the following sequences for the cranial drawer sign: (1) tibial reduced position, (2) cranial drawer position, and (3) reduced position. Similarly, the caudal drawer sign sequence is ordered as follows: (1) tibial caudal drawer position, (2) reduced position, and (3) caudal drawer position. A large number of techniques have been described for repair of stifle joint injuries involving the use of either the animal's own tissue (e.g., fascia, tendon) or synthetic prostheses. The surgeon should use the technique and material with which he/she has the most familiarity and success.

References

Brinker WO, Pierrmattei DL, Flo GF. Handbook of small animal orthopedics and fracture treatment. Philadelphia: WB Saunders, 1983:315, 321.

Flo GF. Modification of the lateral retinacular implication technique for stabilizing cruciate ligament injuries. JAAHA 1975; 11:570.

Pond MJ, Campbell JR. The canine stifle joint. I. Rupture of the anterior cruciate ligament. An assessment of conservative and surgical management. J small Anim Pract 1972; 13:1.

INSTABILITY OF THE STIFLE JOINT

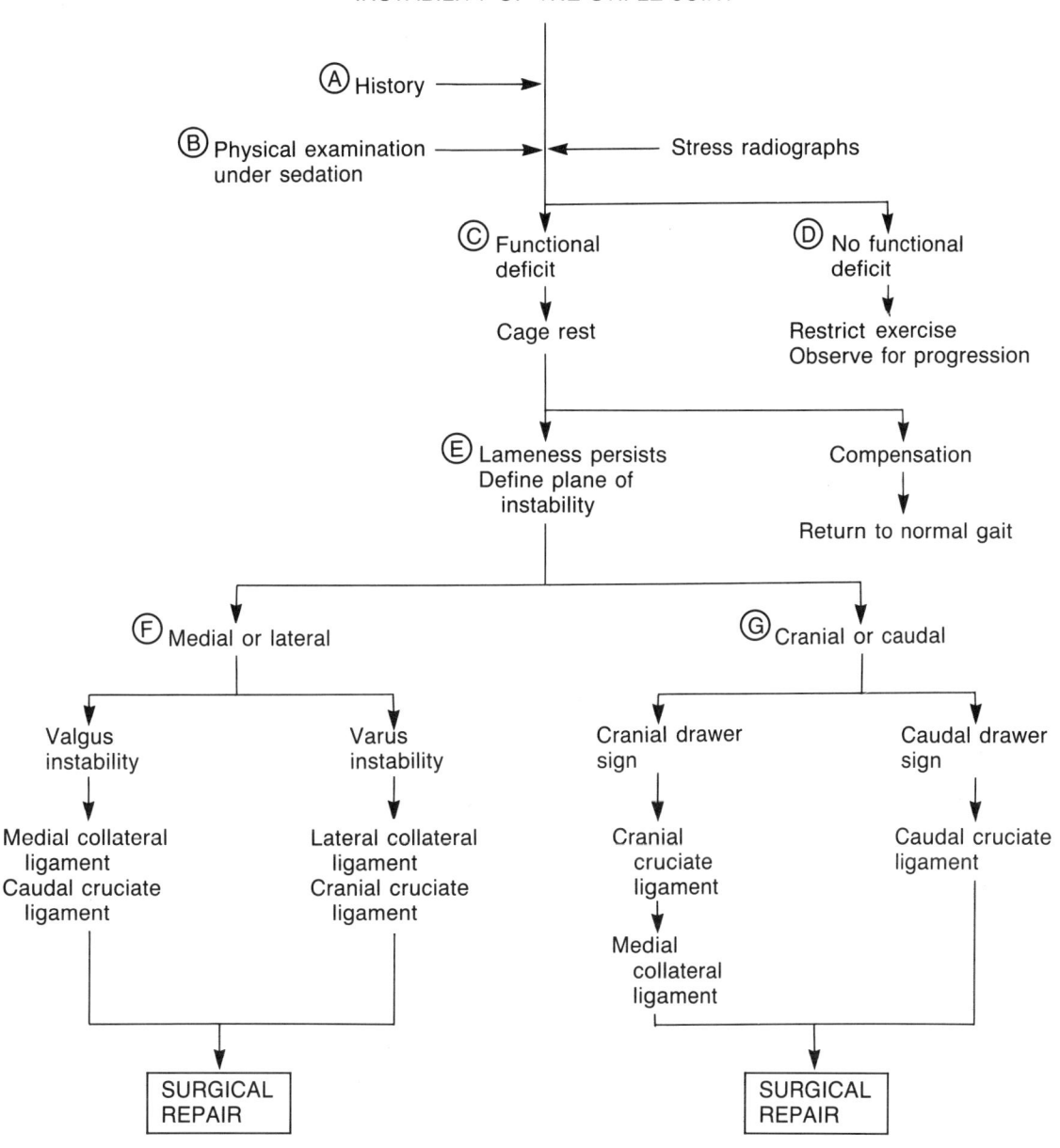

- Ⓐ History
- Ⓑ Physical examination under sedation
- Stress radiographs

- Ⓒ Functional deficit
  - Cage rest
    - Ⓔ Lameness persists. Define plane of instability
      - Ⓕ Medial or lateral
        - Valgus instability
          - Medial collateral ligament
          - Caudal cruciate ligament
        - Varus instability
          - Lateral collateral ligament
          - Cranial cruciate ligament
        - **SURGICAL REPAIR**
      - Ⓖ Cranial or caudal
        - Cranial drawer sign
          - Cranial cruciate ligament
          - Medial collateral ligament
        - Caudal drawer sign
          - Caudal cruciate ligament
        - **SURGICAL REPAIR**

- Ⓓ No functional deficit
  - Restrict exercise
  - Observe for progression
    - Compensation
    - Return to normal gait

MENISCAL INJURY

Geoff Sumner-Smith

A. During weight bearing, a clicking of the joint may be seen and heard. This may be substantiated by a positive tibial compression test, although the latter is not always present, and results in a limited range of motion of the stifle joint. A displaced horn may impair movement.

B. Although, in larger dogs, arthroscopy is both possible and helpful, the instrumentation is rarely available except in referral institutes. An exploratory arthrotomy is strongly recommended, at which time corrective surgery may also be carried out.

C. Resect bucket-handle tears. These tears may be slightly displaced, causing partial locking of the joint, or totally separated and displaced into the posterior pouch. In all cases they lose their attachment to the annular segment and never reunite. They should be removed.

D. If the meniscus is only partially separated from the capsule, reattachment may be attempted employing nonabsorbable horizontal mattress sutures. In large dogs, this technique may succeed, but in the smaller individual meniscectomy is advised.

E. Remove the separated portion in cases that display limited cleavage (i.e., small tags or flaps). In such cases of partial meniscectomy, retain as much of the annular ligament as possible. The future stability of the joint is enhanced if the periphery remains intact. Some rejuvenation of the resected portion may take place by the growth of fibrocartilage, which aids in joint stability.

F. Extensive tearing and destruction of one or both menisci require either subtotal or total meniscectomy. Residual instability of the joint often ensues, with the consequent development of degenerative joint disease.

G. In order to prevent fibrosis of the joint capsule and surrounding tissue, such as seen in "fracture disease", early postoperative ambulation is essential. Encourage positive movement of the joint as well as passive flexion and extension.

References

Brinker WO, Pierrmattei DL, Flo G. Handbook of small animal orthopedic surgery and fracture treatment. Philadelphia: WB Saunders, 1983:319.

Halse DA, Shires PK. The stifle joint. In: Slatter DH, ed. Textbook of small animal surgery. Philadelphia: WB Saunders, 1985:2208.

Suspected MENISCAL INJURY

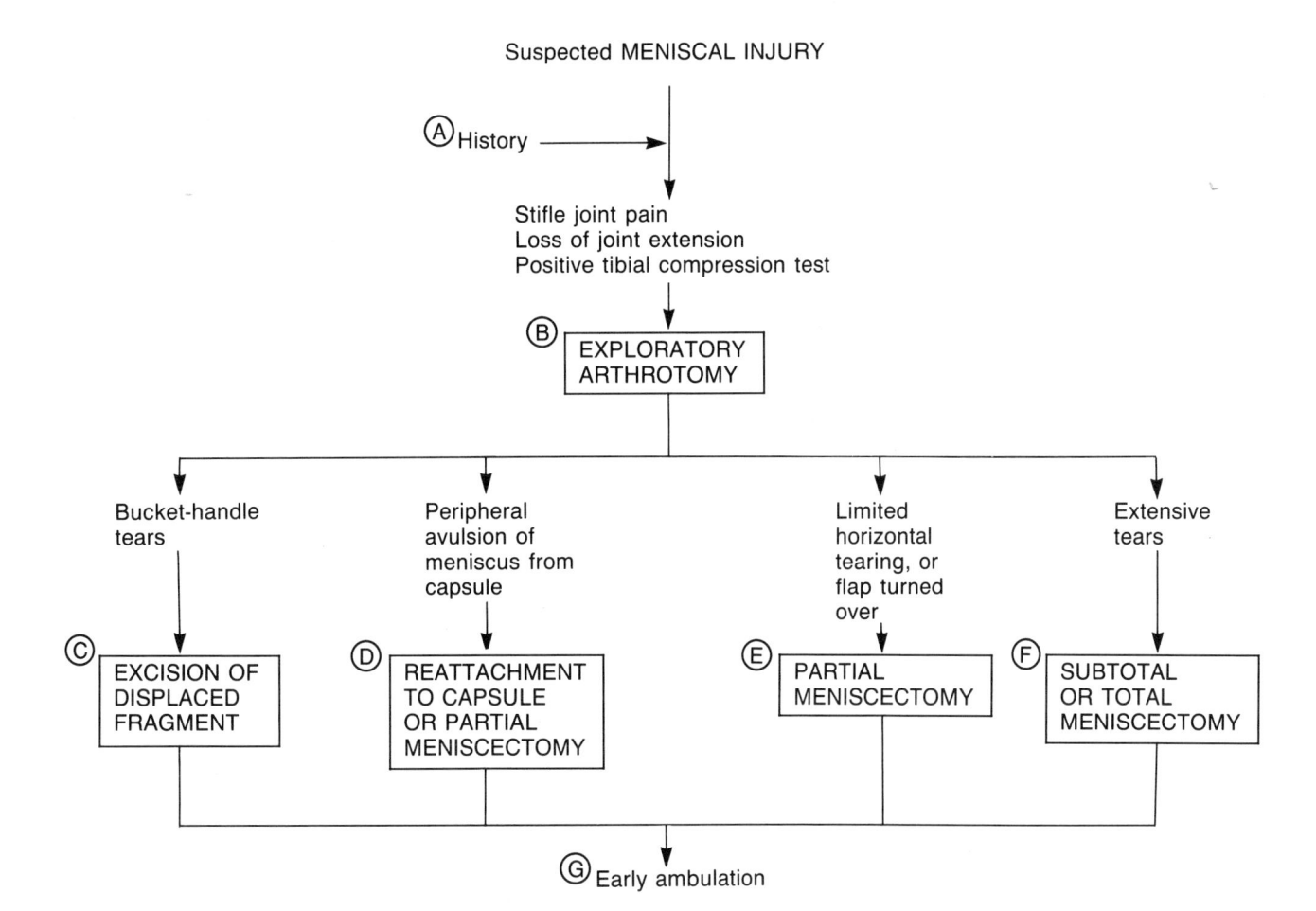

Ⓐ History

Stifle joint pain
Loss of joint extension
Positive tibial compression test

Ⓑ **EXPLORATORY ARTHROTOMY**

- Bucket-handle tears → Ⓒ **EXCISION OF DISPLACED FRAGMENT**
- Peripheral avulsion of meniscus from capsule → Ⓓ **REATTACHMENT TO CAPSULE OR PARTIAL MENISCECTOMY**
- Limited horizontal tearing, or flap turned over → Ⓔ **PARTIAL MENISCECTOMY**
- Extensive tears → Ⓕ **SUBTOTAL OR TOTAL MENISCECTOMY**

Ⓖ Early ambulation

PATELLA LUXATION

Geoff Sumner-Smith

A. A clear distinction should be made between luxations that are inherent and those that are acquired as a result of trauma. The former may require corrective surgery of the joint elements, whereas the latter requires reparative intervention.

B. Physical examination elucidates whether there is malformation of the joint or whether, as in congenital cases, there is malalignment of the limb with consequent valgus or varus deformity. In more severe cases rotational deformity is also present.

C. Congenital medial luxation (CML) is commonly seen in toy breeds and the incidence of CML as compared to congenital lateral luxation (CLL) is approximately 3:1. In older or larger animals there may be an associated traumatic rupture of the cranial cruciate ligament, which precipitates the signs of lameness. The Singleton Classification (Table 1) of CML aids in deciding upon the surgical technique to be employed.

D. Usually CLL is seen only in toy or miniature breeds and may not be evident until part way through the animal's life. In these cases luxation is only Grade I to Grade II in severity, and the changes are opposite to those seen in CML.

E. Traumatic medial luxation (TML) may exist on its own or in association with more severe injuries to the stifle joint. Early repair of the traumatized tissue, followed by early ambulation, is essential if full use of the joint is to be returned.

F. CLL is seen commonly in animals with hip dysplasia with associated coxa valga. Displacement of the quadriceps mechanism occurs along with genu valgum.

G. Surgical treatment of CML is dependent upon the severity of the condition (Fig. 1). Mild Grade I situations may be left alone if locking of the joint and limb carriage is rare and intermittent; otherwise, perform surgery to prevent erosion of the condylar cartilage and subsequent degenerative joint disease. The techniques listed in Table 2 may be employed singly or in association, depending upon the surgeon's assessment of what is required. Grade IV luxations (Fig. 2) rarely respond well to surgical correction; if unilateral, the animal usually ambulates well on the three remaining legs. Invariably, however, the opposite stifle joint is affected to some degree and likely requires corrective surgery. As all cases of congenital patella luxation are hereditary, offer advice to the owner as to the breeding program for an animal or a whole kennel.

References

Brinker WO, Pierrmattei DL, Flo G. Small animal orthopedics and fracture treatment. Philadelphia: WB Saunders, 1983:290.

Olmstead MR. Lateral luxation of the patella. In: Bojrab MJ, ed. Pathophysiology in small animal surgery. Philadelphia: Lea & Febiger, 1981:638.

Singleton WB. The surgical correction of stifle joint deformities in the dog. J small Anim Pract 1969; 10:59.

TABLE 1 Singleton Classification

Grade I
Intermittent patellar luxation causes the limb to be carried occasionally.
The patella easily luxates manually at full extension of the stifle joint, but returns to the trochlea when released. No crepitation is apparent.
The medial or, very occasionally, lateral deviation of the tibial crest (with lateral luxation of the patella) is only minimal with very slight rotation of the tibia. Flexion and extension of the stifle is in a straight line with no abduction of the hock.

Grade II
There is frequent patellar luxation, which in some cases becomes more or less permanent. The limb is usually carried, although a little weight bearing may occur with the stifle remaining slightly flexed.
It is often possible to reduce the luxation by manual lateral rotation of the tibia, especially under anesthesia, but the patella reluxates with ease when manual tension of the joint is released.
The tibia is rotated up to 30°; a slight deviation of the tibial crest may exist.
The hock is slightly abducted when the patella is resting medially.
If the condition is bilateral, more weight is thrown onto the forelimbs.
Many Grade II cases live with the condition reasonably well for many years, but the constant luxation of the patella over the medial lip of the trochlea causes erosion of both the articulating surface of the patella and the proximal area of the medial lip. This results in crepitation, which becomes apparent when the patella is luxated manually, and calls for a quite different surgical approach.

Grade III
The patella is permanently dislocated when the tibia is rotated and the tibial crest is deviated between 30° and 60° from the anterior-posterior plane. Although the luxation is not intermittent, many cases use the limb with the stifle held in a semi-flexed position.
Flexion and extension of the joint causes abduction and adduction of the hock.
The trochlea is very shallow or even flattened.

Grade IV
The tibia is rotated and the tibial crest may show further medial deviation. Consequently, it lies 60° to 90° from the anterior-posterior plane.
The patella is permanently luxated.
The patella lies just above the medial condyle and a "space" can be palpated between the patellar ligament and the distal end of femur.
The limb is carried or the animal moves in a crouched position with the limb partly flexed.
The trochlea is absent or even convex.

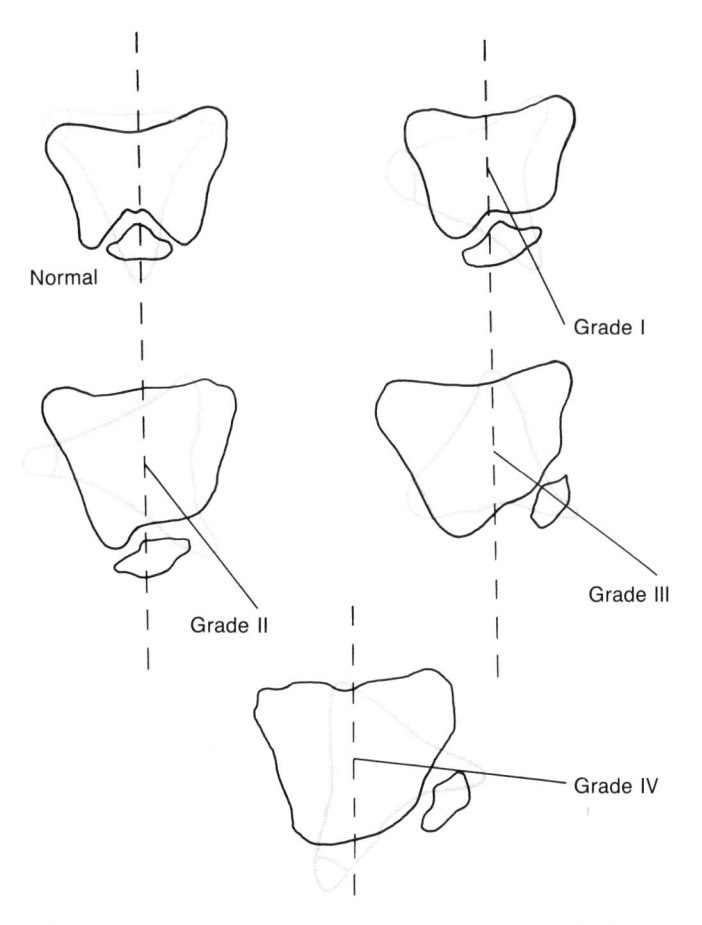

Figure 1 Diagrams illustrating the relationship between distal end of femur and proximal end of tibia in the normal joint and Grade I–IV deformities. (From Singleton WB. The surgical correction of stifle joint deformities in the dog. J small Anim Pract 1969; 10:59.

TABLE 2 Surgical Correction for Congenital Medial Luxation and Congenital Lateral Luxation

CML	CLL

Grade I
  Medial retinacular release
  Lateral retinacular overlap
  Tibial antirotational suture
	Grade I
	  Medial retinacular overlap
	  Medial antirotational suture

Grade II
  Tibial tubercle transposition
  Medial desmotomy
  Medial retinacular release
  Lateral retinacular overlap
  Trochleoplasty, if patella unstable
	Grade II
	  Lateral desmotomy
	  Medial tibial tubercle transposition
	  Medial retinacular overlap
	  Trochleoplasty
	  Medial antirotational sutures

Grade III
  Tibial tubercle transposition
  Medial desmotomy
  Trochleoplasty
  Lateral retinacular overlap
  Lateral antirotational sutures
	Grade III
	  As Grade II

Grade IV
  As Grade III
  Quadriceps release
  Femoral and tibial osteotomy	

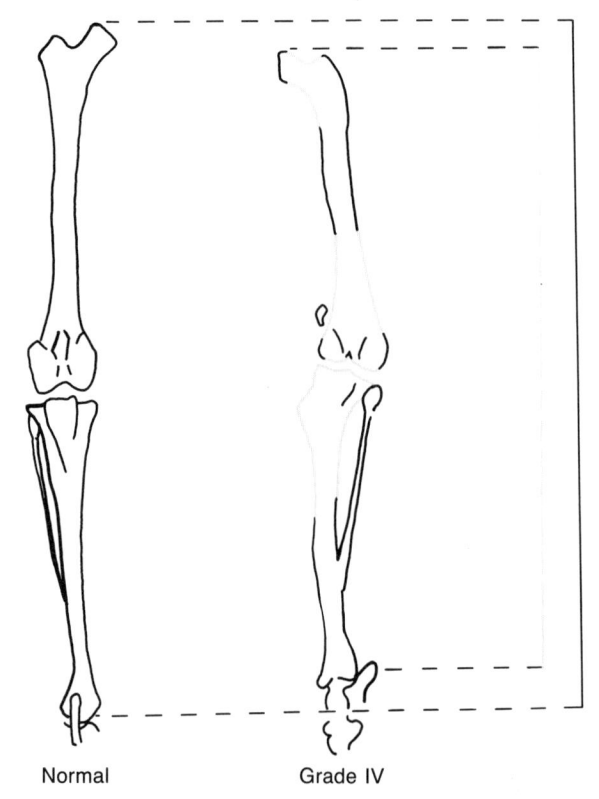

Figure 2 Illustrating the changes in the limb associated with Grade IV deformity. (From Singleton WB. The surgical correction of stifle joint deformities in the dog. J small Anim Pract 1969; 10:59.

PATELLA LUXATION

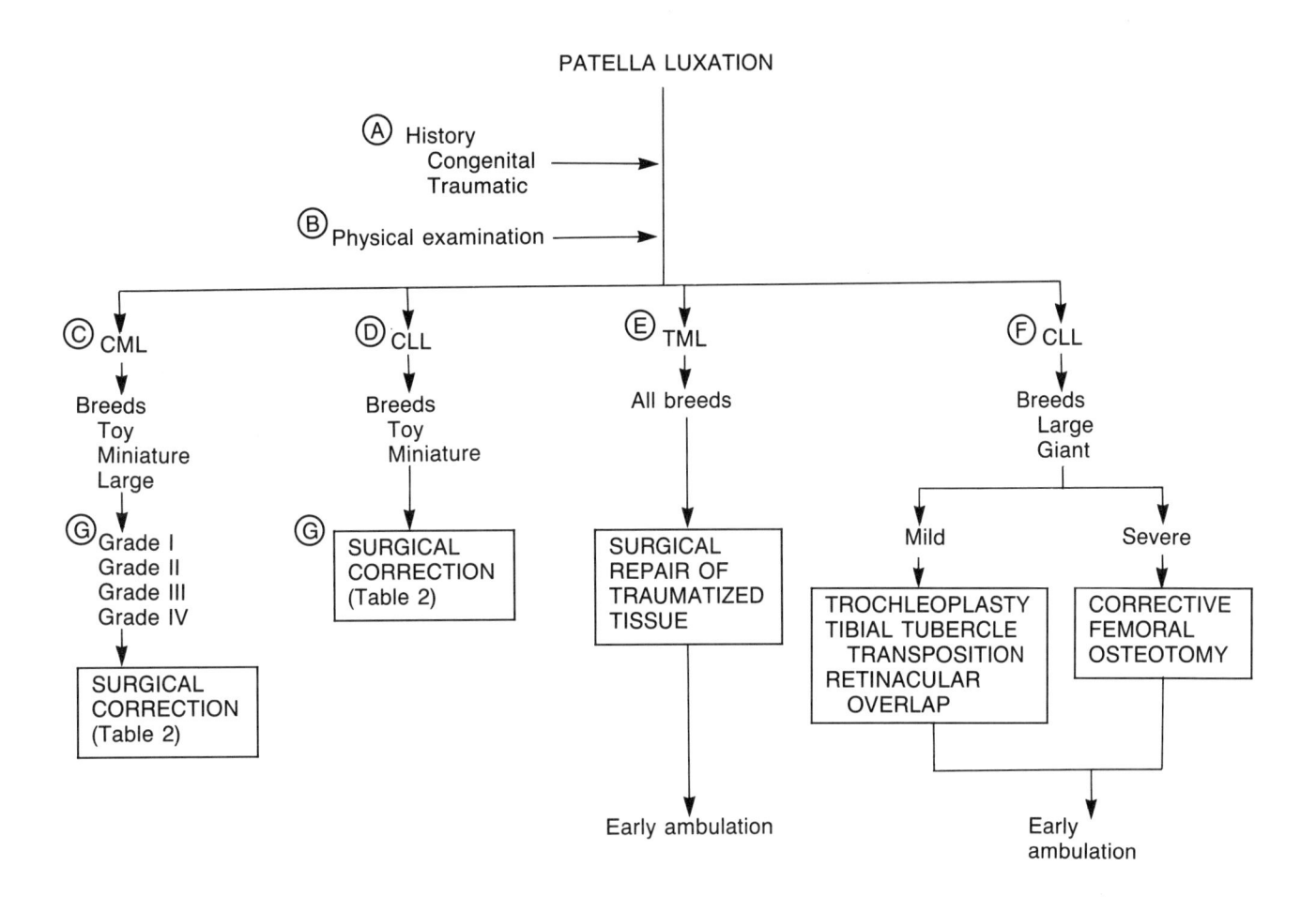

- (A) History
  - Congenital
  - Traumatic
- (B) Physical examination

- (C) CML
  - Breeds
    - Toy
    - Miniature
    - Large
  - (G) Grade I
    - Grade II
    - Grade III
    - Grade IV
  - **SURGICAL CORRECTION** (Table 2)

- (D) CLL
  - Breeds
    - Toy
    - Miniature
  - (G) **SURGICAL CORRECTION** (Table 2)

- (E) TML
  - All breeds
  - **SURGICAL REPAIR OF TRAUMATIZED TISSUE**
  - Early ambulation

- (F) CLL
  - Breeds
    - Large
    - Giant
  - Mild → **TROCHLEOPLASTY TIBIAL TUBERCLE TRANSPOSITION RETINACULAR OVERLAP**
  - Severe → **CORRECTIVE FEMORAL OSTEOTOMY**
  - Early ambulation

TIBIAL PLATEAU FRACTURE

Geoff Sumner-Smith

A. Slightly depressed fractures of the tibial plateau may give an impression of joint instability; consequently, both lateral and AP radiographs are mandatory. If the initial results are equivocal, the lateral radiograph may need to be repeated in both the flexed and stressed positions; similarly minor fractures of the tibial plateau may only be demonstrated in an oblique view. Ligamentous damage is often seen in association with minimally displaced fractures, and the injury may lead to a misleading diagnosis if palpation is not combined with radiography. When these fractures are minimally displaced, a conforming bandage is suitable, but when there is a major displacement, it should be dealt with by means of proper internal fixation (see G). Fracture of the fibula, which may be concomitant with fracture(s) of the lateral condyle, should be treated as a separate fracture.

B. Under sedation, or a general anesthetic, the stifle joint should be palpated to ascertain ligamentous injury (p 120). If the fracture is only minor but does not receive attention, there is the danger of long-term instability, malwear, and erosion.

C. The primary objective is to return the joint to normal function. The stifle joint is notorious for developing the sequela of "fracture disease," which, on account of retinacular fibrosis, results in a marked decrease of joint motion. Consequently, treatment is aimed at returning the joint to normal function as quickly as possible. Therefore, if the fracture is not displaced, the stifle joint should be supported by a conforming bandage, with the hock additionally flexed to prevent weight-bearing, for 4 weeks. The lack of weight-bearing does not prevent the animal from moving the stifle joint and consequently the development of "fracture disease" is minimized.

D. Displaced fractures of the proximal tibia can be extremely crippling to the stifle joint unless they are treated judiciously and with great care. Commonly these fractures are associated with a hemarthrosis, which adds considerable pain to that of the initial injury. The joint should be aspirated 24 hours after injury and placed in a conforming bandage until surgery is deemed advisable.

E. Small isolated fractures of the plateau, which do not involve the articular surface of the joint and in which fragment depression is less than 5 mm, may be treated in the same manner as in C. If the depression is greater than 5 mm, the joint is likely to be unstable and internal fixation necessary. (Although the figure of 5 mm has been given, it should be borne in mind that these measurements are relative to the size of the patient; 5 mm is a large amount for a toy dog, but a minimal amount for a giant dog.)

F. Severely depressed fractures of the tibial plateau require elevation and internal fixation by means of screws or Kirschner wires. In the elderly patient the depression is likely to be quite severe as there is no underlying cancellous bone, and it may be necessary to support the area with an additional bone graft taken from the ilial wing. In order to maintain good joint motion, early function is desirable, and it may be necessary to bandage the opposite hind limb once the clinician is satisified that the damaged limb is able to support the animal's weight without severe consequences.

G. When the joint surface is severely involved in the original fracture and condyles are involved, or if the whole of the proximal tibia has collapsed as may be seen following gunshot wounds, elaborate internal fixation is necesary. Complications of "fracture disease" with subsequent degenerative joint disease, stifle instability, and tendon contracture are minimized by careful anatomic reduction of the fragments. Sometimes the fragments are so small that they may not be stabilized by the internal fixation device and consequently have to be supported on massive cancellous bone grafts being held in position by fine Kirschner wires. In the elderly patient this is not possible, but bone cement may be used as a bed onto which the cortical bone is mounted and stabilized by wires. Great care should be taken to ensure that the cement does not protrude into the interphase between the cortical fragments. Invariably a buttress plate and associated screws is a method of choice of dealing with this type of injury (Fig. 1).

References

Brinker WO, Hohn RB, Prieur WD. Manual of internal fixation in small animals. Heidelberg: Springer-Verlag 1984:181.

Gofton N. Fractures of the tibia and fibula. In: Slatter DH, ed. Textbook of small animal surgery. Philadelphia: WB Saunders, 1985:2235.

Leger L, Sumner-Smith G, Gofton N, Prieur WD. A.O. hookplate fixation of metaphyseal fractures and corrective wedge osteotomies. J small Anim Pract 1982; 23:209.

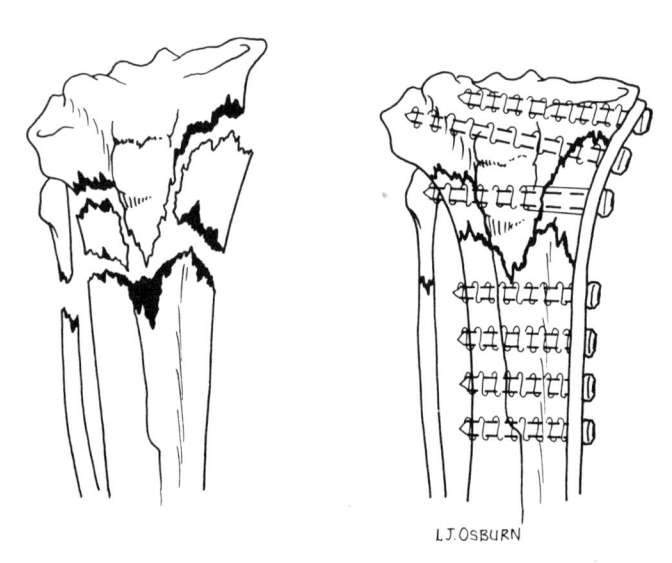

Figure 1 Multiple fracture of the proximal tibia supported with a buttress plate. Autogenous grafting is recommended if a defect exists.

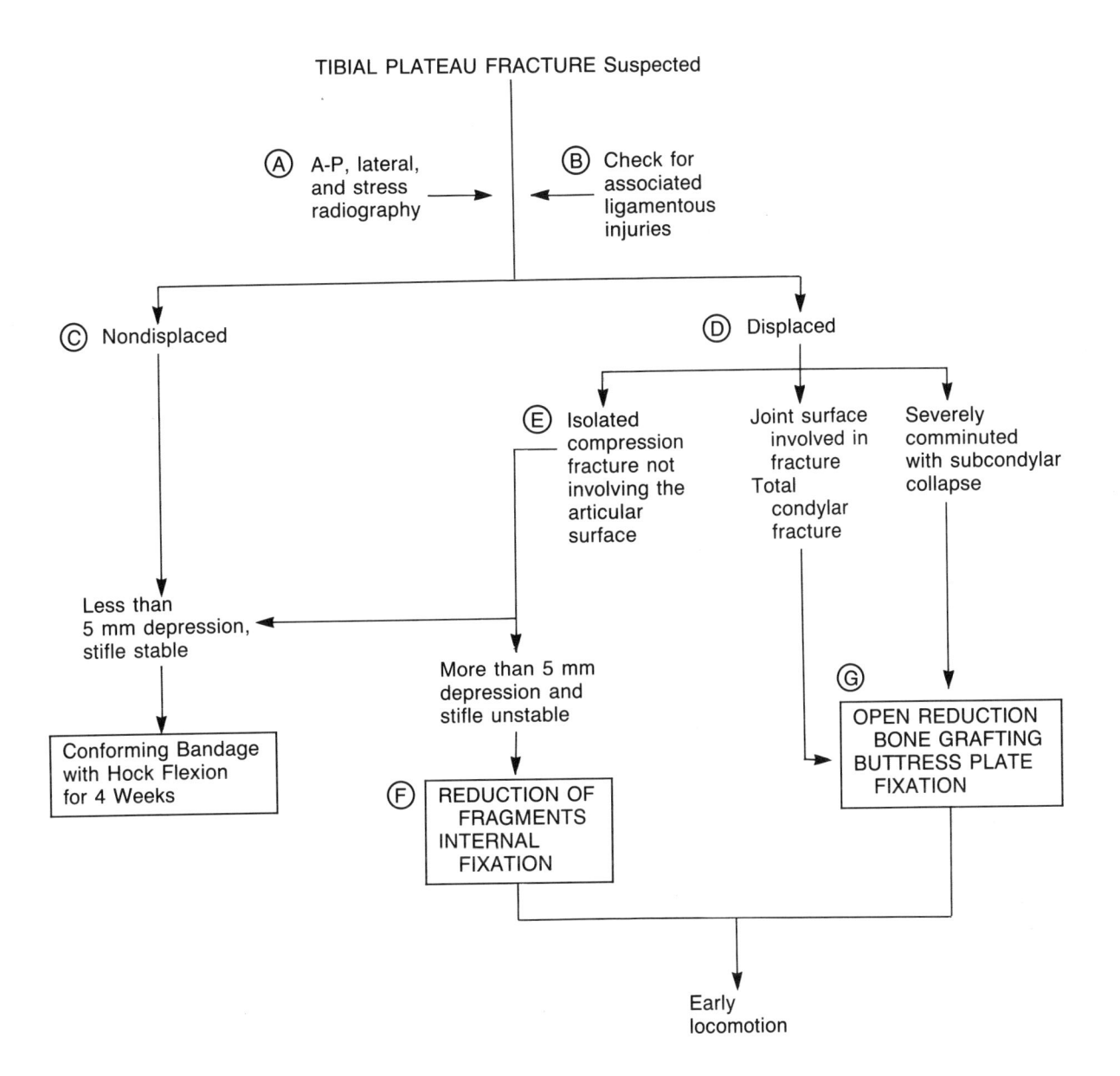

TIBIAL PLATEAU FRACTURE Suspected

- **A** A-P, lateral, and stress radiography
- **B** Check for associated ligamentous injuries

C Nondisplaced
Less than 5 mm depression, stifle stable
→ **Conforming Bandage with Hock Flexion for 4 Weeks**

D Displaced

- **E** Isolated compression fracture not involving the articular surface
  - Less than 5 mm depression, stifle stable → Conforming Bandage with Hock Flexion for 4 Weeks
  - More than 5 mm depression and stifle unstable → **F REDUCTION OF FRAGMENTS INTERNAL FIXATION**
- Joint surface involved in fracture / Total condylar fracture → **G OPEN REDUCTION BONE GRAFTING BUTTRESS PLATE FIXATION**
- Severely comminuted with subcondylar collapse → **G OPEN REDUCTION BONE GRAFTING BUTTRESS PLATE FIXATION**

→ Early locomotion

PROXIMAL TIBIAL GROWTH PLATE FRACTURE IN YOUNG ANIMALS

Geoff Sumner-Smith

The proximal tibia possesses two centers of ossification (p 202), one for the tibial plateau and the other for the tibial crest.

A. Avulsion of the tibial tuberosity occurs in athletic animals and is the result of sudden, violent exercise and contraction of the quadriceps. In young sight-hounds, the condition commonly occurs bilaterally.

B. If the patient is lightweight and the displacement is minimal, excellent healing occurs if exercise is restricted for 6 weeks and movement of the stifle joint is restricted in a conforming bandage, which may be stiffened by inclusion of a splint on the cranial aspect.

C. In athletic breeds or if the fragment is displaced a distance of more than its own mass, open reduction is mandatory. Although screws and pins are commonly employed (Fig. 1), frequently the tuberosity, which is still very soft in young animals, fragments and displaces. The stay-suture method is preferred (Fig. 2). This technique acts as a tension band; consequently, active motion of the stifle assists in compressing the fracture surfaces together. Nevertheless, the animal should be restricted to leash activity until the fracture is radiographically healed.

D. When both the tibial tuberosity and the plateau are involved in the fracture, they usually separate from the metaphysis as one unit (Salter II). The shaft of the tibia displaces caudally on account of traction of the stronger flexor muscles.

E. If it remains stable following reduction, the fracture may be treated conservatively; bandaging and restricted exercise may be sufficient.

F. Internal fixation by cross-pins, or in large animals by means of a screw, is the preferred method of treatment. Exercise should be severely restricted for 2 weeks, following which leash exercise is permitted until the fracture has healed radiographically.

Figure 1 Tibial growth plate fractures shown from the lateral and medial aspects, stabilized by: *A*, large screws; *B*, cross-pins.

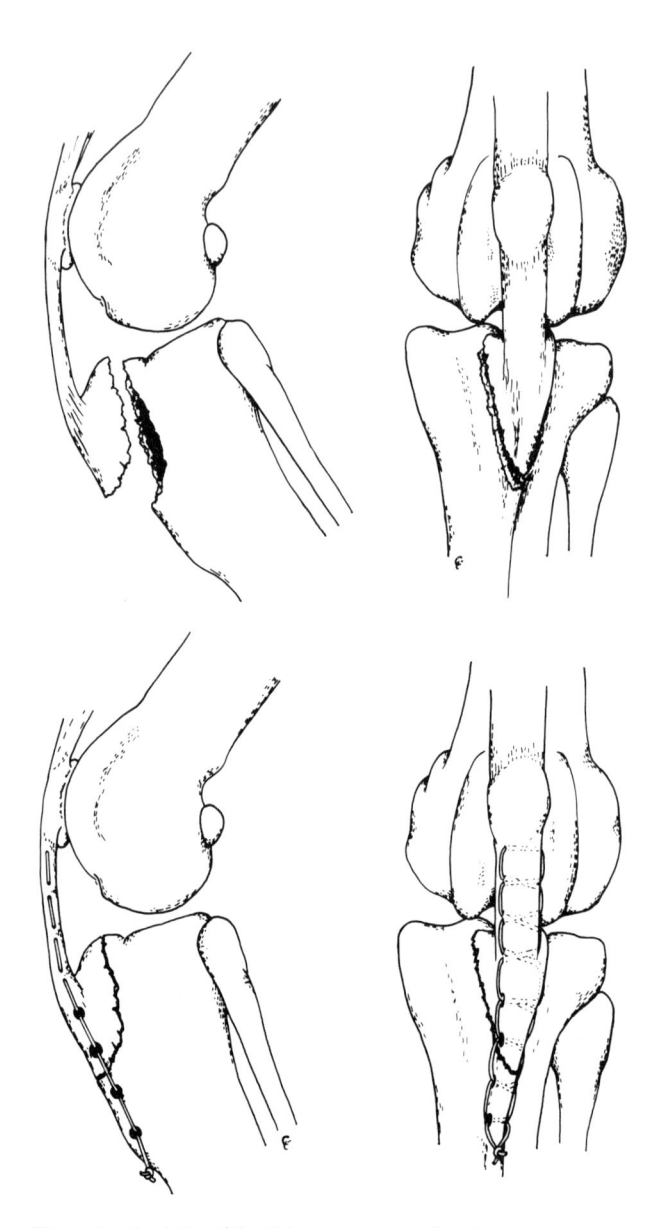

Figure 2 Avulsion of the tibial tubercle stabilized by a tension suture.

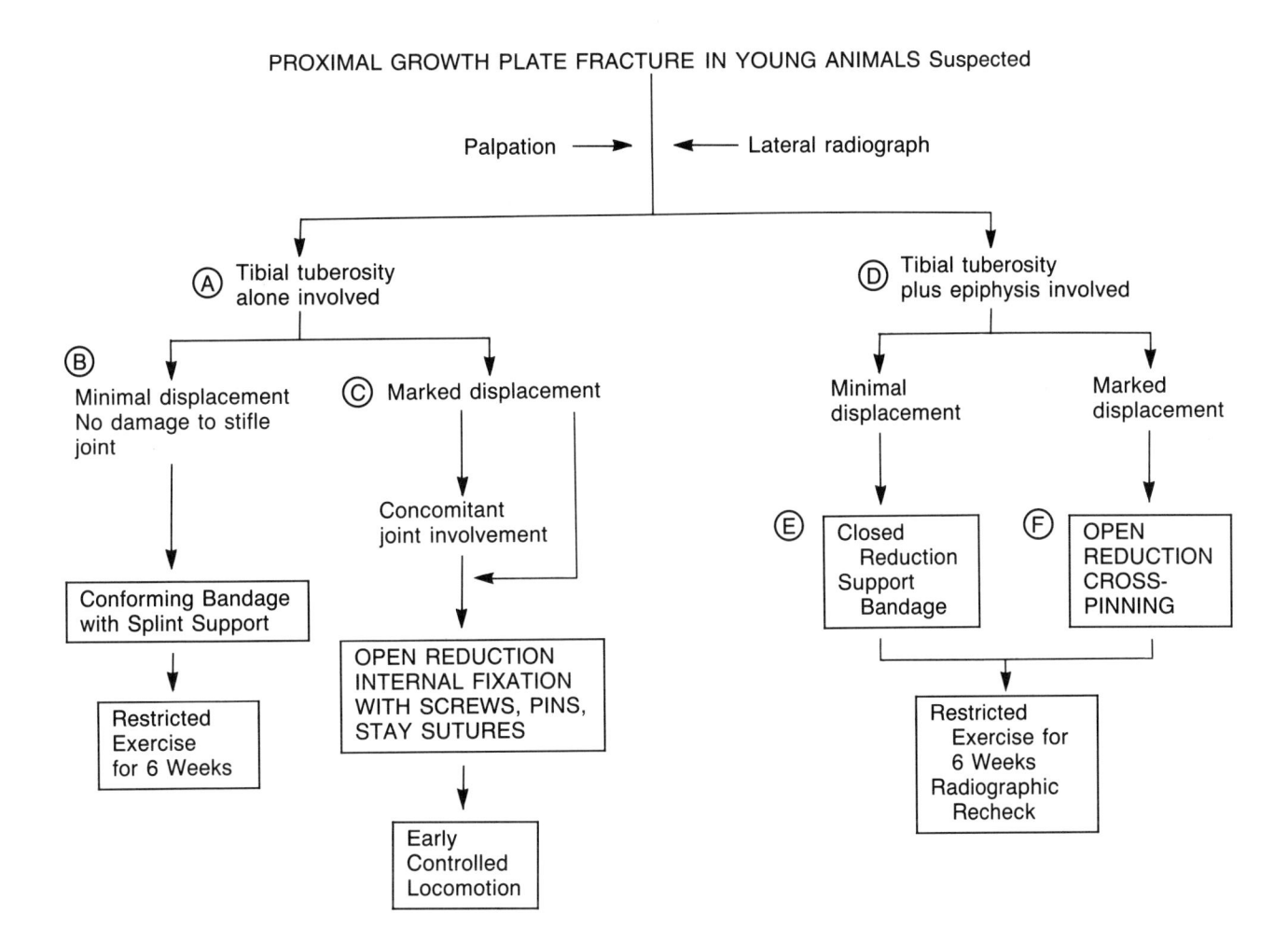

PROXIMAL GROWTH PLATE FRACTURE IN YOUNG ANIMALS Suspected

Palpation → ← Lateral radiograph

Ⓐ Tibial tuberosity alone involved

Ⓑ Minimal displacement No damage to stifle joint
→ Conforming Bandage with Splint Support
→ Restricted Exercise for 6 Weeks

Ⓒ Marked displacement
→ Concomitant joint involvement
→ OPEN REDUCTION INTERNAL FIXATION WITH SCREWS, PINS, STAY SUTURES
→ Early Controlled Locomotion

Ⓓ Tibial tuberosity plus epiphysis involved

Ⓔ Minimal displacement
→ Closed Reduction Support Bandage

Ⓕ Marked displacement
→ OPEN REDUCTION CROSS-PINNING

→ Restricted Exercise for 6 Weeks Radiographic Recheck

References

Dingwall JS, Sumner-Smith G. A technique for repair of avulsion of the tibial tuberosity in dogs. J small Anim Pract 1971; 12:665.

Sumner-Smith G. Observations on epiphyseal fusion in the canine appendicular skeleton. J small Anim Pract 1966; 7:303.

Withrow SJ. Treatment of fractures of the tibial tuberosity in the dog. JAVMA 1976; 168:122.

TIBIAL SHAFT FRACTURE

Geoff Sumner-Smith

Tibial shaft fractures vary considerably in their complexity and hence in the method of treatment required.

A. Simple midshaft fractures respond well to casting, provided good reduction is obtainable. Care must be exercised to ensure that the reduction is properly aligned, and that there is minimal rotation at the fracture site. Dogs are able to compensate for a rotation of up to 5 degrees by rotating the hip in the appropriate direction. Frequently small dogs, less than 6 kg in weight, do not respond well to casting of this fracture; the limb tends to rotate within the cast, resulting in either malunion or nonunion.

B. Radiographic rechecks, at intervals of 3 weeks, are recommended, whether be the fracture is treated by internal or external fixation.

C. Enclosing the stifle joint in a cast often produces unsatisfactory results; the proximal portion surrounding the femur develops the Wellington Boot effect, which produces a lever-arm that pivots at the fracture site. Consequently, frequent examination of the cast is advised. Because of these possible complications, use of a half (gutter) cast is recommended, especially for the occasional orthopaedist. The cast is secured to the limb by bandages and tape to prevent loosening and to facilitate inspection.

D. Although a simple closed fracture might, on its own, be treated by casting, this seriously impairs the animal's ambulation, and internal fixation is therefore strongly advised.

E. Multiple fractures of the tibia should be treated by internal fixation with a plate; grafting may be necessary if there is severe loss of devitalized bone (Fig. 1). Intramedullary pinning is not advised in such cases, as the fragments tend to collapse when threaded in Shish-Kebab fashion on the pin. However, transverse fractures and some oblique fractures respond well to intramedullary pinning, especially when this is supported by hemicerclage wiring.

F. Once hemorrhage has been controlled, cleaning and debridement of the wound should commence. If the wound is treated some hours post-injury, recognition of vitalised tissue may be difficult. This may be overcome by the intravenous injection of disulpheine blue—only the tissue receiving the blood supply turns blue. Irrigation of the wound should be thorough, but not traumatic to the tissue. The wound should be left open and dressed; it may be subsequently closed once infection has been controlled and healthy granulation tissue is present. A course of appropriate antibiotic therapy is routinely recommended. Some fractures may be treated by stabilization with a cast.

G. More severe fractures should *not* be stabilized by means of a cast as frequent attention to the wound is necessary. These fractures respond well to stabilization with the external fixator, which permits maintenance of normal length of the bone and prevents rotation.

H. If stability is insufficient, these fractures may subsequently be treated by plating and attendant bone graft. Closure of the wound may be primary or secondary, according to the nature of the fracture.

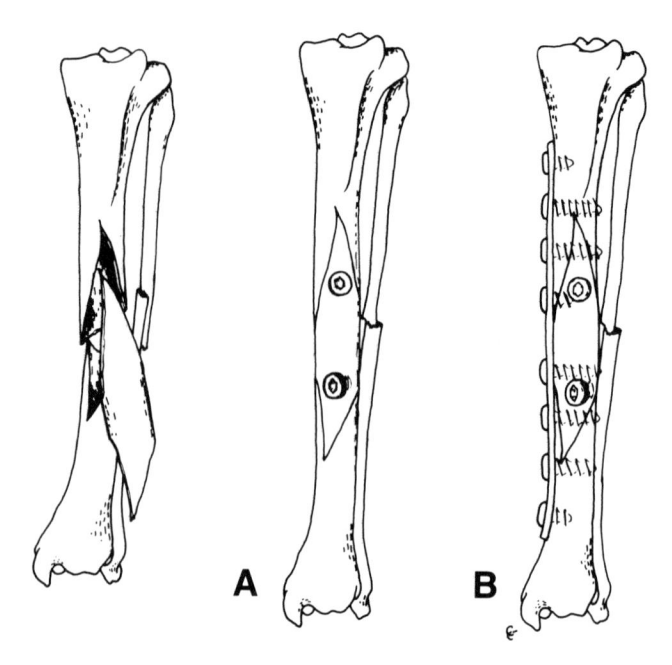

Figure 1 Multiple fracture of the tibial shaft; *A*, the butterfly fragment is first stabilized with large screws, which are then protected by a neutralization plate, *B*.

References

Brinker WO, Hohn RB, Prieur WD. Manual of internal fixation in small animals. Heidelberg: Springer-Verlag, 1984.

Brinker WO, Piermattei DL, Flo GL. Handbook of small animal orthopedics and fracture treatment. Philadelphia: WB Saunders, 1983.

Gofton N. Fracture of the tibia and fibula. In: Slatter DH, ed. Textbook of small animal surgery. Philadelphia: WB Saunders, 1985:2235.

TIBIAL SHAFT FRACTURE Suspected

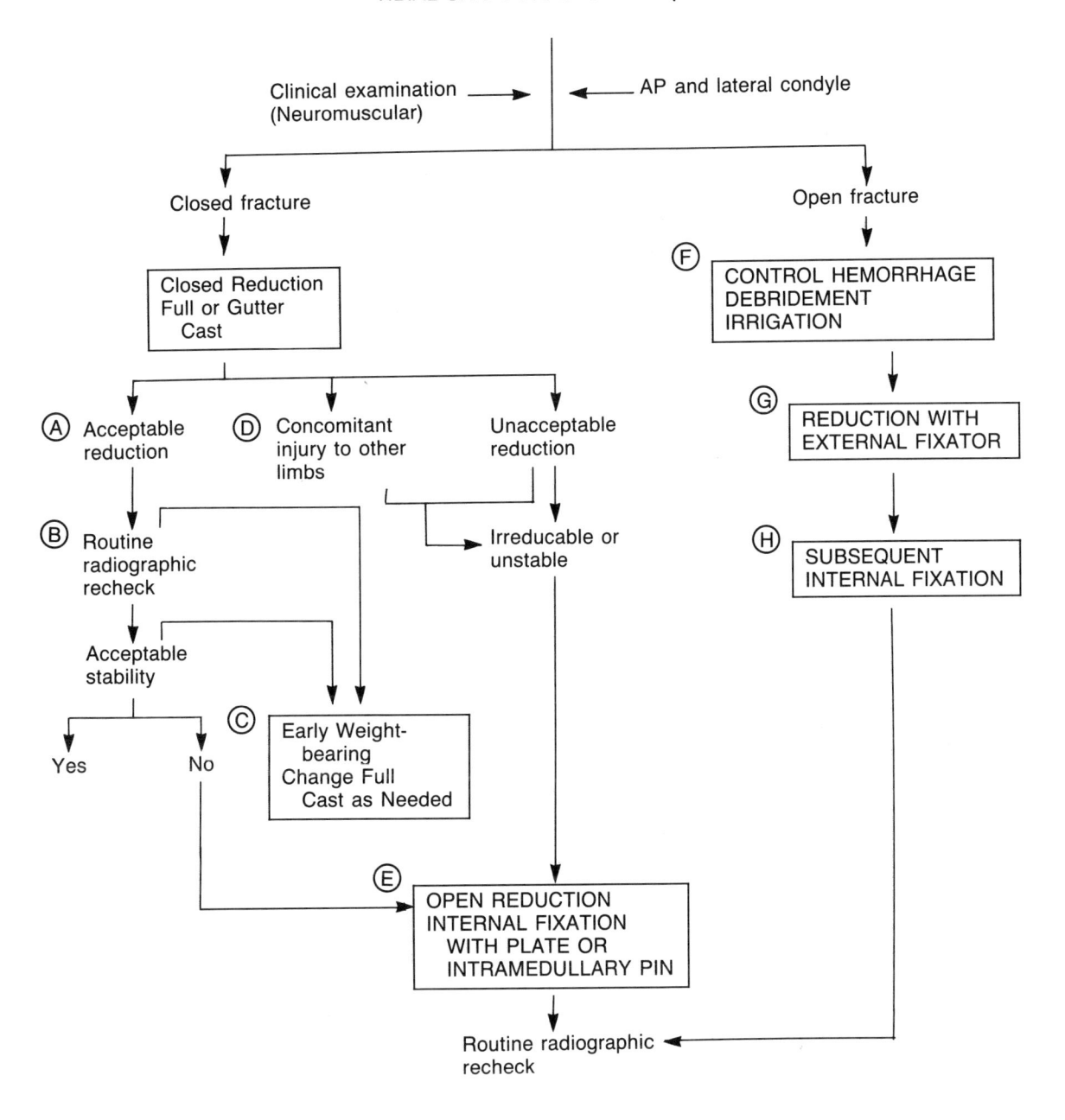

```
                    Clinical examination ──→  ←── AP and lateral condyle
                       (Neuromuscular)
                              │
                ┌─────────────┴─────────────┐
                ▼                           ▼
          Closed fracture              Open fracture
                │                           │
                ▼                      Ⓕ CONTROL HEMORRHAGE
         Closed Reduction                 DEBRIDEMENT
         Full or Gutter                   IRRIGATION
              Cast                           │
                │                            ▼
    ┌───────────┼───────────┐          Ⓖ REDUCTION WITH
    ▼           ▼           ▼             EXTERNAL FIXATOR
 Ⓐ Acceptable Ⓓ Concomitant Unacceptable       │
   reduction   injury to    reduction           ▼
               other limbs      │          Ⓗ SUBSEQUENT
    │                           ▼             INTERNAL FIXATION
    ▼                    Irreducable or
 Ⓑ Routine               unstable
   radiographic
   recheck
    │
    ▼
 Acceptable
  stability
    │
  ┌─┴─┐
  ▼   ▼
 Yes  No     Ⓒ Early Weight-
                bearing
                Change Full
                Cast as Needed

           Ⓔ OPEN REDUCTION
             INTERNAL FIXATION
             WITH PLATE OR
             INTRAMEDULLARY PIN
                    │
                    ▼
             Routine radiographic ←──
             recheck
```

NOMENCLATURE OF THE TARSAL JOINTS

Jon F. Dee

Articulatio tarsi (tarsal joint) refers to the collective joints that include the tarsocrural, intertarsal, and tarsometatarsal joints (Fig. 1).

A. Tarsocrural joint: the joint between the tibia and fibula and the talus.

B. Intertarsal joints: any of the joints between the tarsal bones, including those from side to side as well as proximodistally. Four of these have been given specific names.
   1. Talocalcaneal joint: the joint between the talus and calcaneus.
   2. Talocalcaneocentral joint: the joint between the talus and the central tarsal bone. Calcaneus is included in the name because the joint cavity also extends between the talus and the calcaneus.
   3. Calcaneoquartal joint: the joint between the central tarsal bone and the distal tarsal bones.
   4. Centrodistal joint: the joint between the central tarsal bone and the distal tarsal bones.

C. Tarsometatarsal joints: the joints between the distal tarsal bones and the metatarsal bones.

References

Dee JF. Injuries to the distal tibia and tarsus. Proc AAHA 1984:359.

Miller MF, Christensen GC, Evans HE. Anatomy of the dog. Philadelphia: WB Saunders, 1964.

Shively MJ. Personal communications. Nomina Anatomica Veterinaria Jan 1979.

Shively MJ. Tarsal nomenclature. Presented at the sixth annual meeting. Vet Orth Soc 1978.

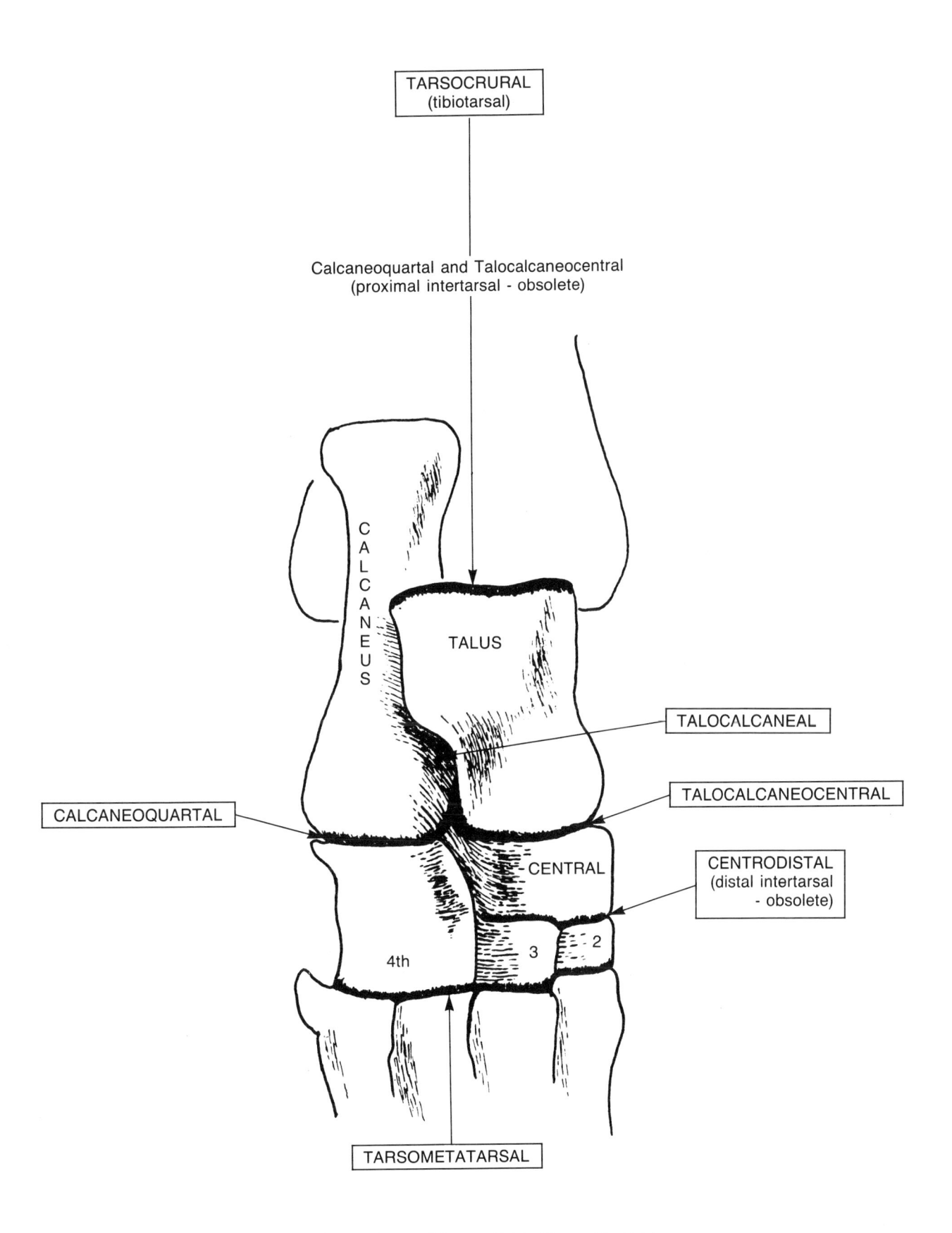

Figure 1 Nomenclature of the tarsal joints: The ventrical joints are the intertarsal joints.

MALLEOLAR SHEARING INJURY

Jon F. Dee

A. Early examination of malleolar shearing injuries consists of assessing the amount of tarsocrural tilt throughout the normal range of motion. Deep joint cultures are obtained, followed by thorough debridement and joint lavage.

B. Take radiographs in order to more accurately assess the extent of the bony damage.

C. Double ligament replacement which utilizes three bone screws and two figure-of-eight braided polyester sutures have been shown to be superior to single ligament replacement techniques which utilize two screws and a single figure-of-eight synthetic suture. The three screws are placed approximately at the origin and insertions of the destroyed medial or lateral ligamentous complex (Fig. 1). Protect the repair for approximately 1 month with a transarticular, external skeletal fixator during which time the wound is dressed daily and allowed to heal by second intention. After removal of the external fixator, the limb is supported with decreasing amounts of coaption (splints to soft roll dressings) for 4 to 6 weeks.

References

Aron DN. Prosthetic ligament replacement for severe tarsocrural joint instability. JAAHA 1987; 23:41.

Bjorling DE, Toombs JP. Transarticular application of the Kirschner Ehmer splint. Vet Surg 1982; 11:34.

Brinker WO, Piermattei DL, Flo GL. Handbook of small animal orthopedics and fracture treatment. Philadelphia: WB Saunders, 1983:336.

Dee JF. Injuries to the distal tibia and tarsus. Proc AAHA 1984:359.

Miller MF, Christensen GC, Evans HE. Anatomy of the dog. Philadelphia: WB Saunders, 1964:265.

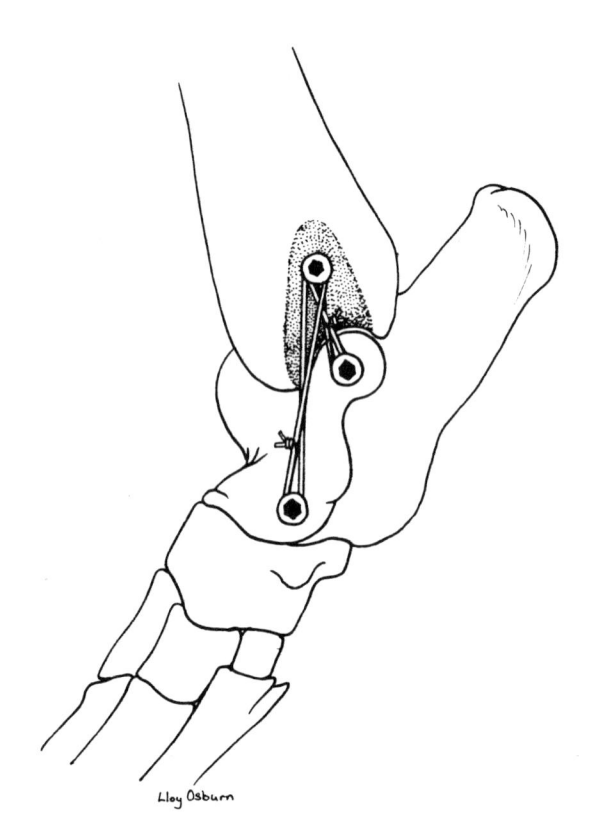

Figure 1 Prosthetic ligaments wound around bone screws inserted at the attachment of destroyed ligaments.

MALLEOLAR SHEARING INJURY Suspected

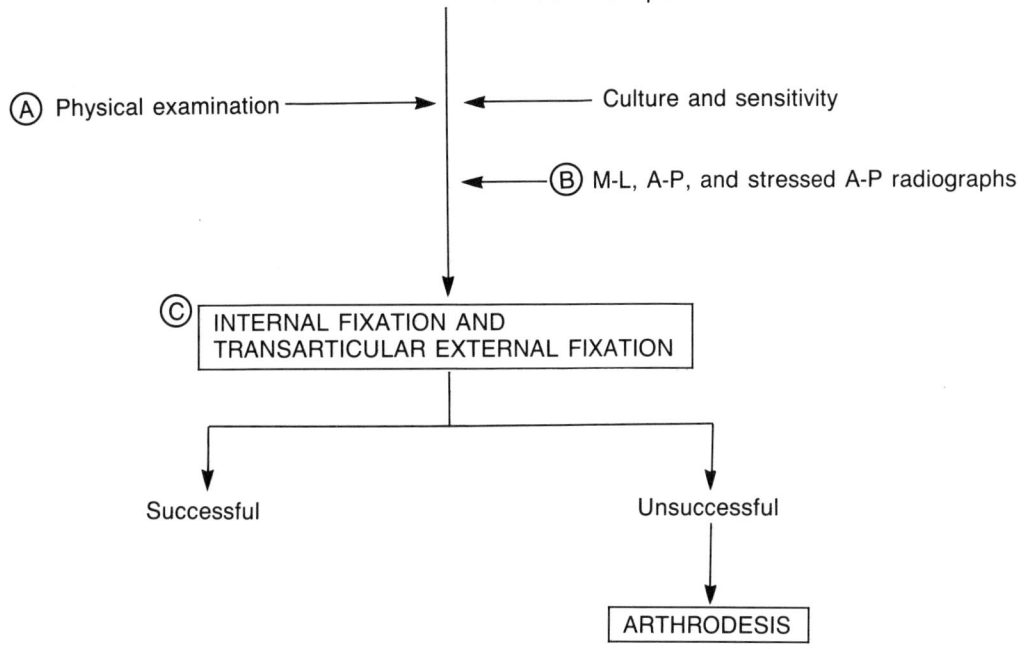

Ⓐ Physical examination ⟶ ⟵ Culture and sensitivity

Ⓑ M-L, A-P, and stressed A-P radiographs

Ⓒ **INTERNAL FIXATION AND TRANSARTICULAR EXTERNAL FIXATION**

Successful | Unsuccessful ⟶ **ARTHRODESIS**

MALLEOLAR FRACTURE

Jon F. Dee

A. Stress the tarsocrural joint medially and laterally throughout its normal range of motion in order to assist in the diagnosis of subtle lesions.

B. In addition to the customary views, anteroposterior views that are stressed both medially and laterally during extension and flexion are sometimes necessary.

C. The short components of the collateral ligaments of the tarsus may avulse independently of the long components. Very small fragments must be excised and the remaining soft tissues sutured. On occasion an anteroposterior transosseous tunnel may be utilized to pass a small gauge orthopaedic wire in order to "capture" an avulsed fragment too small for pinning (Fig. 1). Larger fragments may be repaired with a pin and a figure-of-eight tension band wire.

D. Larger avulsions that involve the short and long components of the collateral ligaments are routinely repaired with pin(s) and figure-of-eight tension band wire fixation. There is little application for Rush pins or "malleolar" screws (Fig. 2).

References

Dee JF, Dee LG, Earley TD. Fractures of carpus, tarsus, metacarpus and phalanges. In: Brinker WO, Hohn RB, Prieur WD, eds. Manual of internal fixation in small animals. Heidelberg: Springer-Verlag, 1983:190.

Earley TD, Dee JF. Trauma to the carpus, tarsus and phalanges of dogs and cats. Vet Clin North Am 1980; 10:717.

Earley TD, Piermattei DL, Dee JF, Weigel JP. Canine carpus and tarsus short course. Proceedings. Knoxville, TN: University of Tennessee, 1981:1.

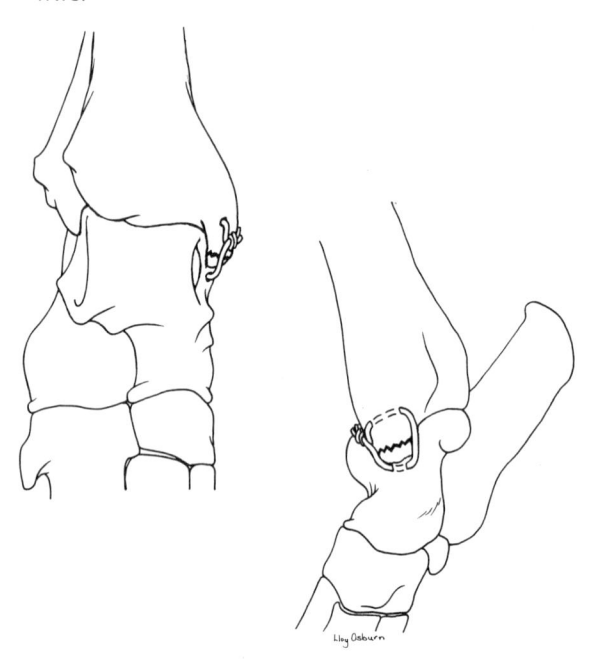

Figure 1 "Small fragment" fracture of the tibial malleolus stabilized by means of a wire suture.

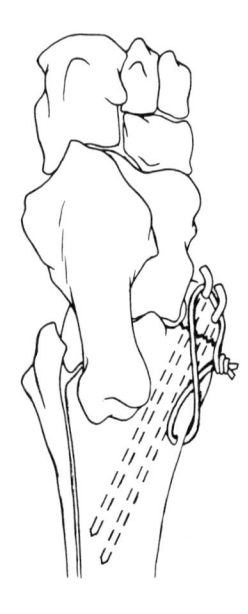

Figure 2 Tension-band wire fixation. Whenever possible, two pins should be employed.

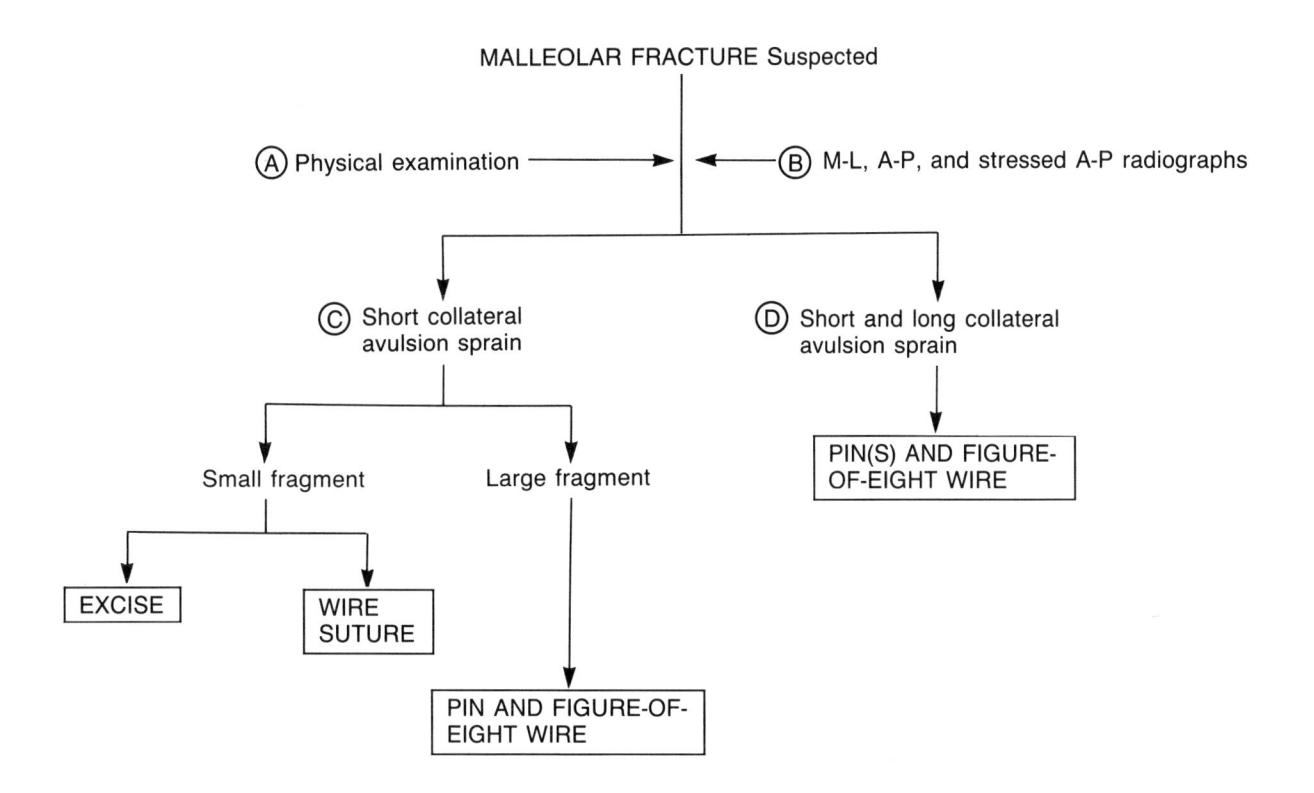

MALLEOLAR FRACTURE Suspected

- (A) Physical examination
- (B) M-L, A-P, and stressed A-P radiographs

- (C) Short collateral avulsion sprain
  - Small fragment
    - EXCISE
    - WIRE SUTURE
  - Large fragment
    - PIN AND FIGURE-OF-EIGHT WIRE
- (D) Short and long collateral avulsion sprain
  - PIN(S) AND FIGURE-OF-EIGHT WIRE

PROXIMAL INTERTARSAL SUBLUXATION

Jon F. Dee

A. Proximal intertarsal joint subluxations may involve either the dorsal or the plantar joint surfaces (Fig. 1A). The diagnosis of both is made by physical examination and verified or documented by appropriate radiograph.

B. The plantar ligaments are much thicker and stronger than those on the dorsal side of the hock (Fig. 1B). Plantar subluxations are often associated with avulsions of the plantar ligament from the base of the calcaneus, which can occur during excessive dorsiflexion.

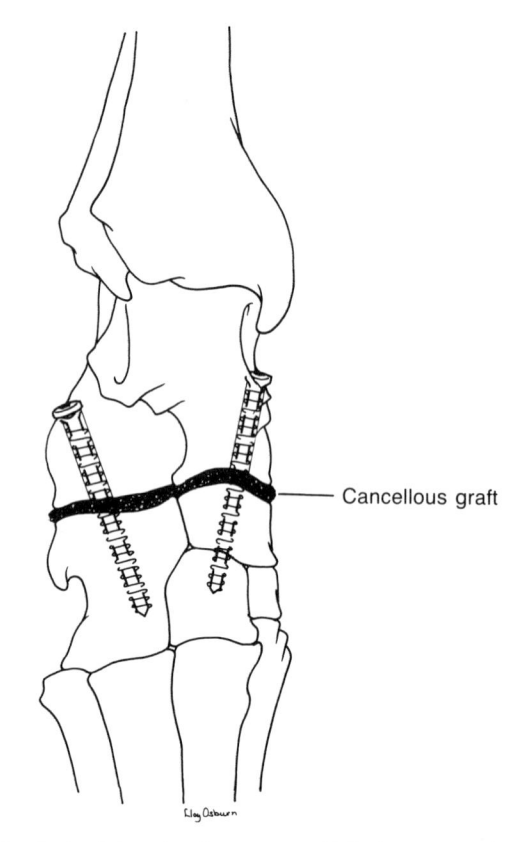

Figure 2 Arthrodesis of the talocalcaneocentral joint by means of lag screws.

C. Most repairs consist of primary arthrodesis of the calcaneoquartal joint by pin and figure-of-eight tension band wire (Fig. 1C). More severe instabilities require arthrodesis of the talocalcaneocentral joint as well.

D. A dorsal subluxation is an uncommon hyperextension injury and generally does not have associated bony fragments. This is a self-compressing injury that becomes more stable with weight-bearing and less stable during the swing phase of the gait. In contrast, a plantar proximal intertarsal subluxation becomes less stable during weight-bearing because the lesion is on the tension side of the tarsus.

E. Treat by coaptation in position of function for 6 to 8 weeks.

F. If coaptation is unsuccessful, arthrodesis is performed. Most have either a predominantly medial or lateral component. These are managed by arthrodesis of the talocalcaneocentral or the calcaneoquartal joints respectively, which utilizes a "lagged" cortical bone screw across the appropriate joint. A further 6 to 8 weeks of coaptation is recommended (Fig. 2).

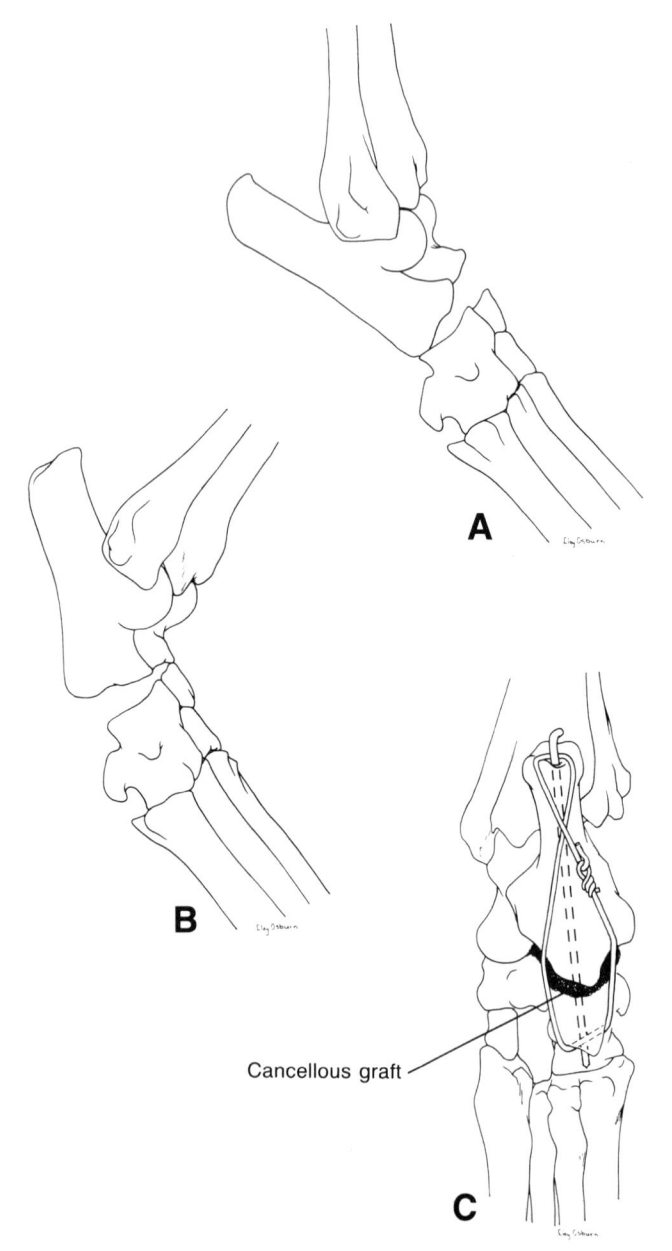

Figure 1 *A*, dorsal intertarsal subluxation. *B*, plantar intertarsal subluxation. *C*, arthrodesis by means of a figure-of-eight tension band wire and incorporated graft (posterior view).

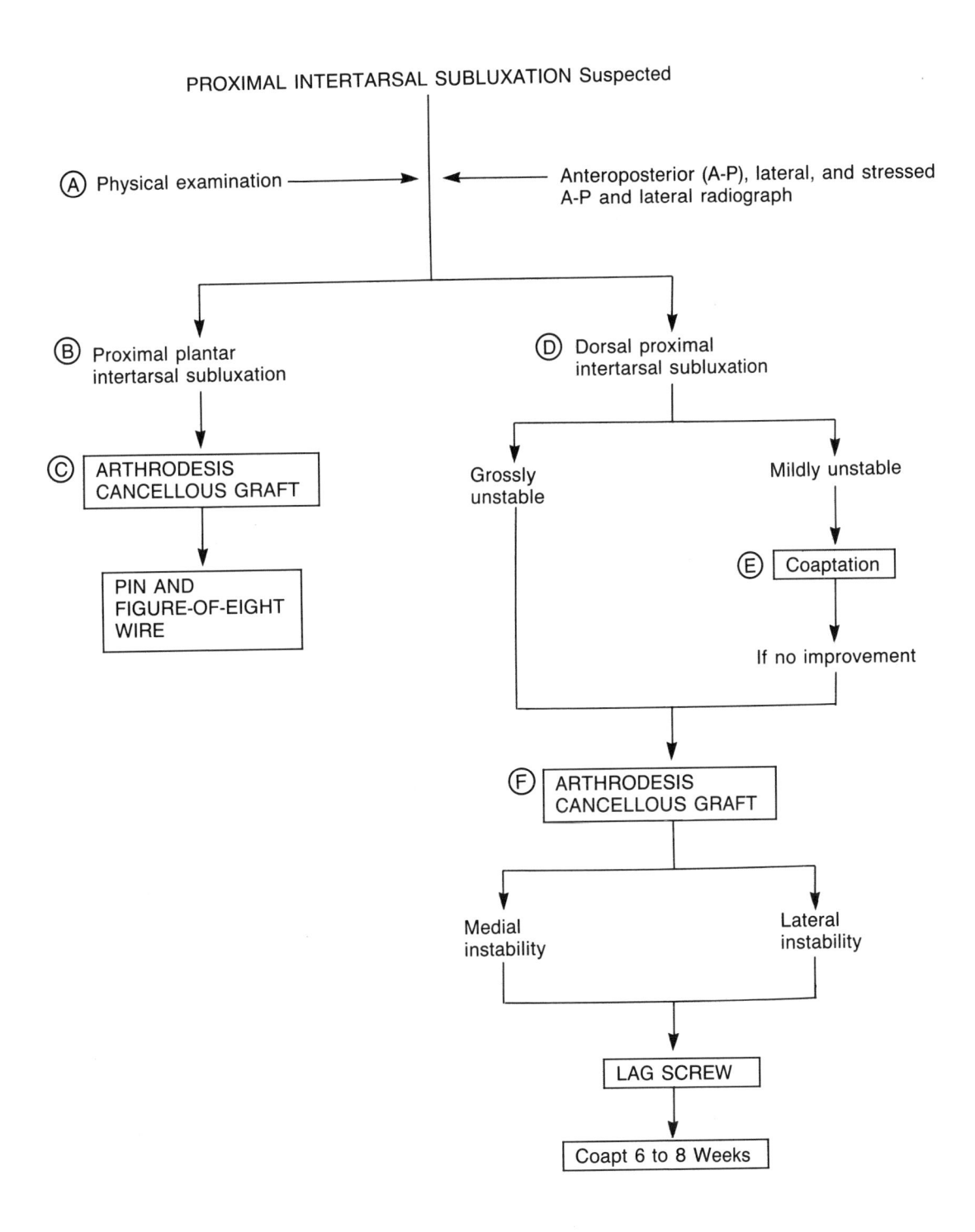

```
PROXIMAL INTERTARSAL SUBLUXATION Suspected
                    │
    ┌───────────────┴───────────────┐
Ⓐ Physical examination ──→      ←── Anteroposterior (A-P), lateral, and stressed
                                    A-P and lateral radiograph
                    │
        ┌───────────┴───────────┐
        ↓                       ↓
Ⓑ Proximal plantar      Ⓓ Dorsal proximal
  intertarsal subluxation   intertarsal subluxation
        │                   ┌───────┴───────┐
        ↓                   ↓               ↓
Ⓒ ARTHRODESIS         Grossly          Mildly unstable
  CANCELLOUS GRAFT    unstable              ↓
        ↓                               Ⓔ Coaptation
   PIN AND                                  ↓
   FIGURE-OF-EIGHT                     If no improvement
   WIRE
                            ↓
                   Ⓕ ARTHRODESIS
                     CANCELLOUS GRAFT
                      ┌─────┴─────┐
                   Medial       Lateral
                   instability  instability
                      └─────┬─────┘
                         LAG SCREW
                            ↓
                     Coapt 6 to 8 Weeks
```

References

Dee JF. Fractures in the racing greyhound. In: Bojrab MJ, ed. Patho-physiology in small animal surgery. Philadelphia: Lea & Febiger, 1981:812.

Dee JF. Injuries to the distal tibia and tarsus. Proc AAHA 1984:359.

Dee JF, Dee LG, Earley TD. Fractures of carpus, tarsus, metacarpus and phalanges. In: Brinker WO, Hohn RB, Prieur WD, eds. Manual of internal fixation in small animals. Heidelberg: Springer-Verlag, 1983:190.

Dee JF, Dee LG, Eaton-Wells RW. Injuries of high performance dogs. In: Whittick WG, ed. Canine orthopedics II. Philadelphia: Lea & Febiger, in press.

Earley TD, Dee JF. Trauma to the carpus, tarsus and phalanges of dogs and cats. Vet Clin North Am 1980; 10:717.

Earley TD, Piermattei DL, Dee JF, Weigel JP. Canine carpus and tarsus short course. Proceedings. Knoxville, Tennessee: University of Tennessee, 1981:1.

TALUS FRACTURE

Jon F. Dee

A. Even if one includes osteochondritis dissecans and dislocations of the talus, the incidence of injuries to the talus is at best uncommon. Physical signs may vary considerably from limping with localized swelling to extensive soft tissue swelling of the tarsus, accompanied by crepitation and deformity.

B. Subtle nondisplaced talar neck fractures may be successfully coapted with the tarsus in a neutral position.

C. More commonly, talar neck fractures cannot be maintained in a stable position, and they may be significantly displaced. Open reduction and rigid internal fixation offer the best opportunity for retaining function of the limb. Lag screw fixation or Kirschner wires placed across the fracture line are the most stable forms of maintaining reduction. The lag screw has the advantage of compression at the fracture site (Fig. 1).

D. Fractures of the head of the talus are predominantly dorsal slab fractures, which are associated with central tarsal bone fractures. Repair is by lag screw fixation through a dorsomedial approach.

E. Fractures of the body of the talus may involve (1) a complete separation of both condyles from the neck with no involvement of the articular surface, (2) a complete fracture of one condyle through the trochlea, or (3) an isolated fracture of a portion of one condyle. In some cases, depending on the extent and location of the fracture, an osteotomy of the appropriate malleolus may be necessary in order to gain adequate exposure. Currently the repair method of choice is countersunk Kirschner wires (Fig. 1).

F. Some subtalar dislocations may be treated by closed reduction and maintained by casting in a neutral position or in a slight varus. Those that cannot be maintained in a stable position require a positional screw into the body of the calcaneus.

G. Even when closed reduction is possible, complete peritalar dislocations are rarely stable. They may be managed by performing a talocentral arthrodesis that is stabilized by lagging a screw from the medial aspect of the neck of the talus to seat into the central and third tarsal bones. In those cases with an isolated luxation of the calcaneus, perform a similar arthrodesis at the level of the calcaneoquartal joint by lagging a screw from the lateral aspect of the calcaneus to seat in the fourth tarsal bone.

H. Osteochondritis dissecans or transchondral dome fractures most frequently involve the medial condyle of the talus and are readily apparent on anteroposterior radiographs. Lateral dome lesions are appreciated on oblique or mediolateral views. Currently most osteochondral or cartilaginous lesions are removed through medial plantar or lateral plantar approaches to the tarsus. Debride and gently curette the lesions. Although its efficacy has not yet been documented in canine lesions, drilling of all exposed subchondral bone has been reported as offering the best long-term results in human orthopaedics. A transmalleolar exposure is rarely required in the dog.

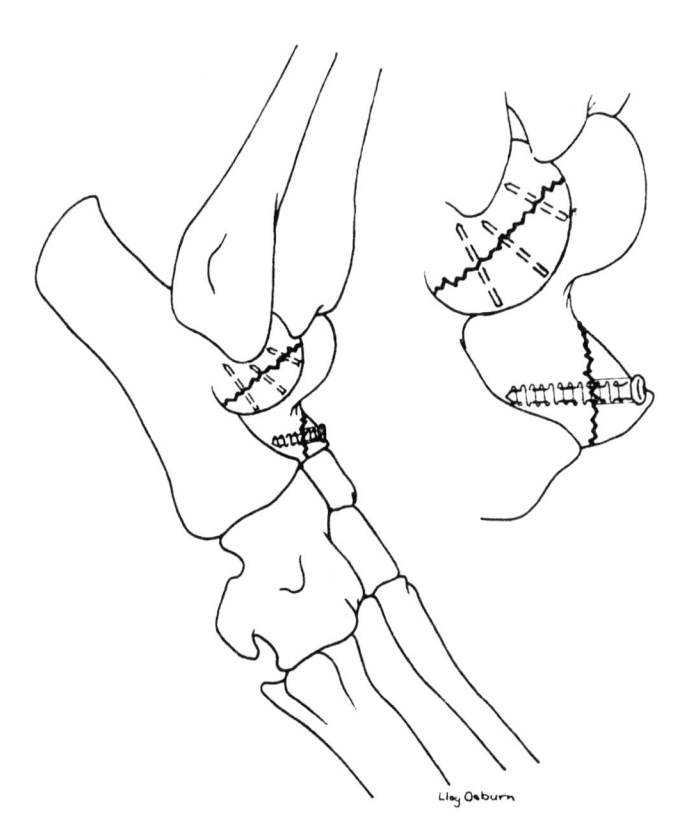

Figure 1 Fractures of the talus stabilized by means of Kirschner wires and a lag screw.

References

Alexander H, Lichtman D. Surgical treatment of transchondral talar dome fractures (osteochondritis dissecans). J Bone Joint Surg 1980; 62A:646.

Berndt A, Harty M. Transchondral fractures of the talus. J Bone Joint Surg 1959; 41A:988.

Dee JF. Injuries to the distal tibia and tarsus. Proceedings AAHA 1984; 359.

Dee JF, Dee LG, Earley TD. Fractures of carpus, tarsus, metacarpus and phalanges. In: Brinker WO, Hohn RB, Prieur WD, eds. Manual of internal fixation in small animals. Heidelberg: Springer-Verlag, 1983:192.

Earley TD, Piermattei DL, Dee JF, Weigel JP. Canine carpus and tarsus short course. Proceedings. Knoxville, Tennessee: University of Tennessee, 1981:1.

TALUS FRACTURE Suspected

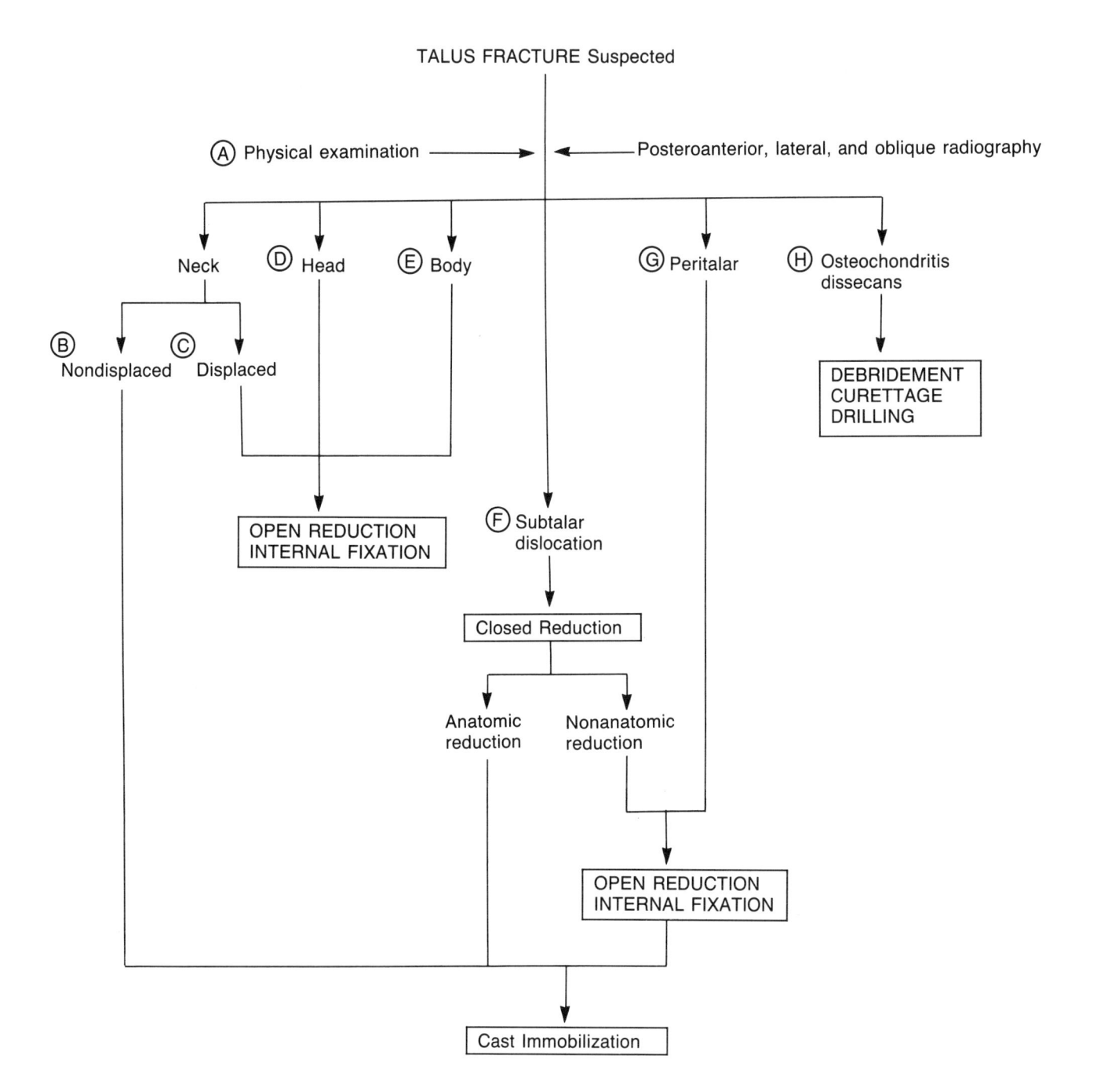

- (A) Physical examination
- Posteroanterior, lateral, and oblique radiography

Branches:
- Neck
  - (B) Nondisplaced → Cast Immobilization
  - (C) Displaced → OPEN REDUCTION INTERNAL FIXATION
- (D) Head → OPEN REDUCTION INTERNAL FIXATION
- (E) Body → OPEN REDUCTION INTERNAL FIXATION
- (F) Subtalar dislocation → Closed Reduction
  - Anatomic reduction → Cast Immobilization
  - Nonanatomic reduction → OPEN REDUCTION INTERNAL FIXATION → Cast Immobilization
- (G) Peritalar → Closed Reduction
- (H) Osteochondritis dissecans → DEBRIDEMENT CURETTAGE DRILLING

143

CALCANEUS FRACTURE

Jon F. Dee

A. The following figures show variations of calcaneal fractures that have been seen and repaired by the author either as solitary fractures or in combination with other fractures. The less severe may be characterized by local soft tissue swelling and crepitation. The more severe shaft fractures have obvious angular deformities when dorsiflexed, as well as significant soft tissue swelling.

B. These fractures are readily apparent on standard posteroanterior and mediolateral radiographs. However, the dorsal medial slab fracture of the base of the calcaneus is best localized on oblique views.

C. Avulsions of a medial or a lateral attachment of the superficial digital flexor (SDF) tendon to the tuber clacis are managed by removal of small fragments, followed by soft tissue reconstruction. Manage larger strain avulsions with internal fixation (Fig. 1).

D. Avulsions of the tuber calcis are primarily a problem of the skeletally immature. Repair is by pin and figure-of-eight tension band wire fixation (Fig. 2).

E. Manage fractures of the shaft of the calcaneus by means of pin and figure-of-eight tension band wire fixation. Comminuted shaft fractures require additional fixation in the form of lag screw and hemicerclage or cerclage wire (Fig. 3).

F. Manage lateral sagittal slab fractures of the base and shaft of the calcaneus by use of multiple lateral to medial lag screws (Figs. 4 and 5).

G. Large oblique dorsoplanter fractures of the base of the calcaneus are managed by a pin and figure-of-eight wire into the body of the fourth tarsal (T4) bone (Fig. 6).

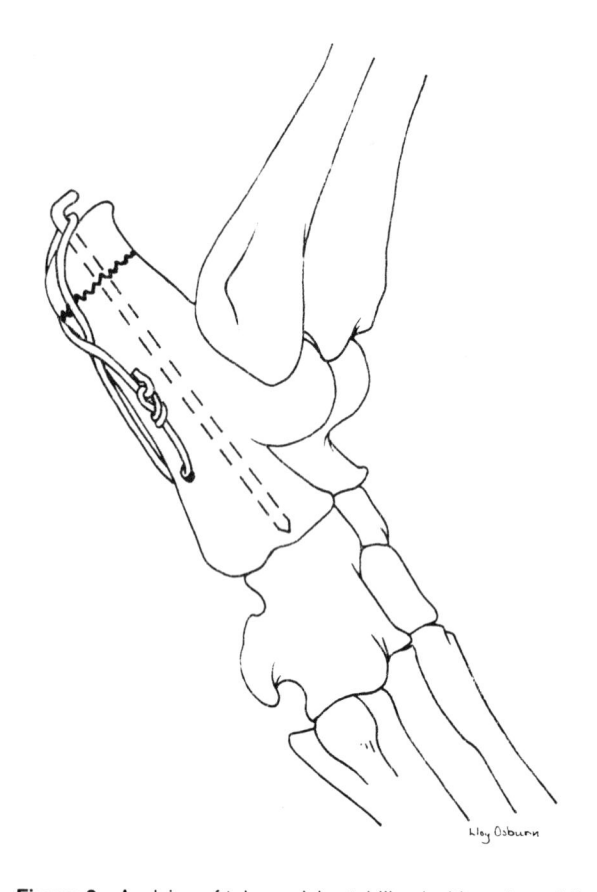

Figure 2 Avulsion of tuber calcis stabilized with a pin and figure-of-eight tension band wire.

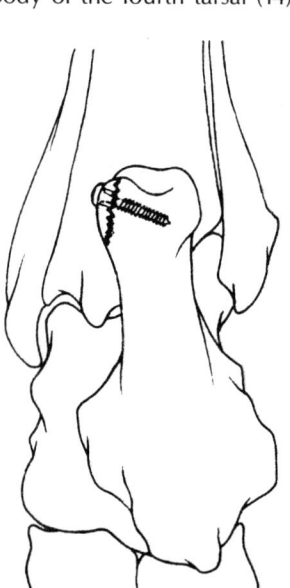

Figure 1 Fixation of a fragment of the proximal portion of the calcaneus with a screw, lagged if possible.

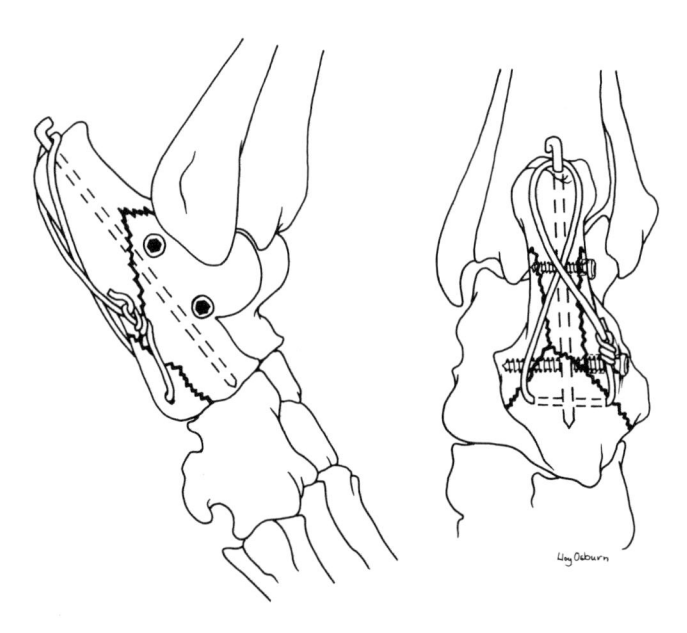

Figure 3 Comminuted (multiple) fractures of the calcaneus stabilized by means of lag screws, pin, and tension band wires.

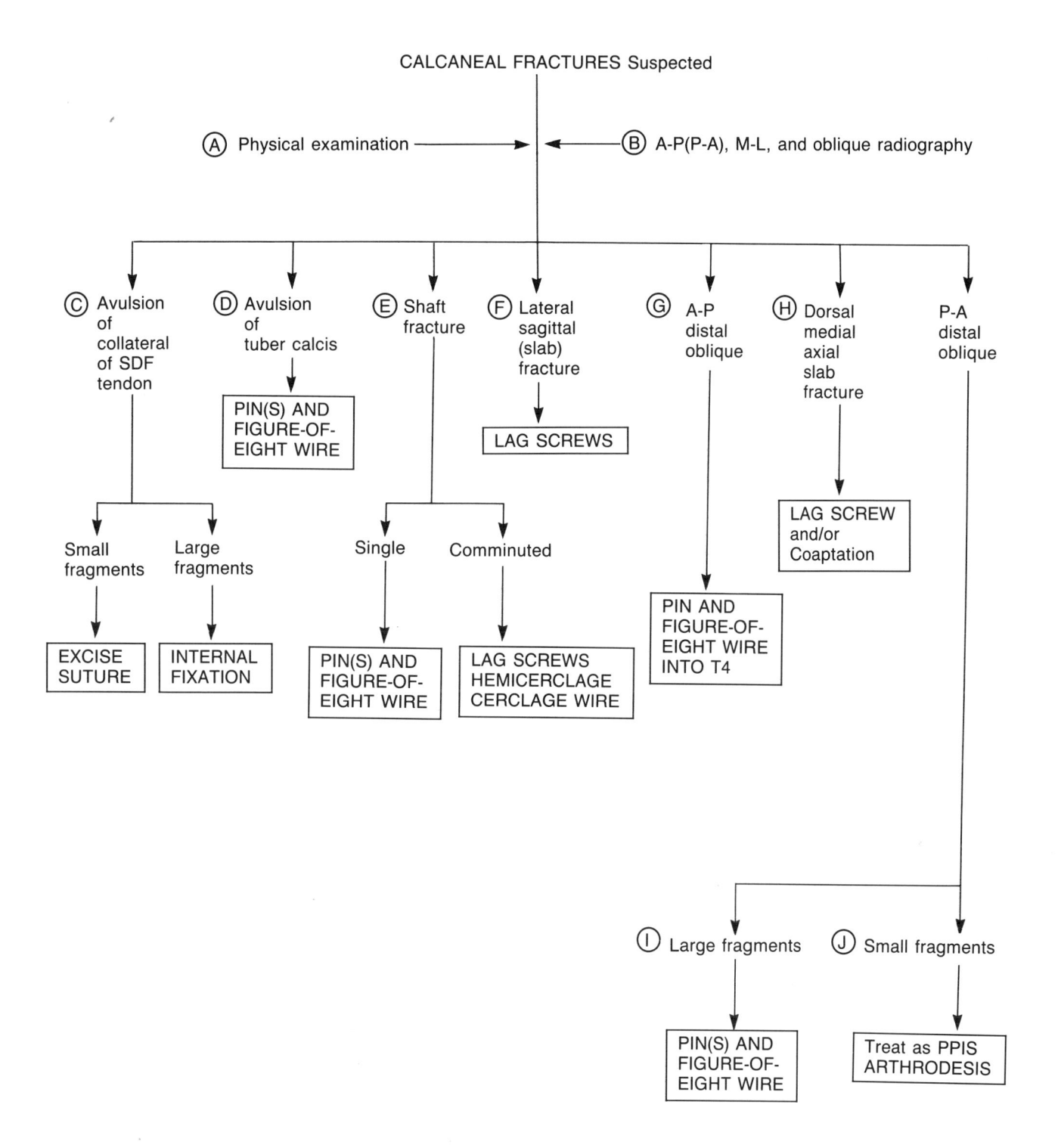

CALCANEAL FRACTURES Suspected

- **(A)** Physical examination
- **(B)** A-P(P-A), M-L, and oblique radiography

- **(C)** Avulsion of collateral of SDF tendon
  - Small fragments → **EXCISE SUTURE**
  - Large fragments → **INTERNAL FIXATION**
- **(D)** Avulsion of tuber calcis → **PIN(S) AND FIGURE-OF-EIGHT WIRE**
- **(E)** Shaft fracture
  - Single → **PIN(S) AND FIGURE-OF-EIGHT WIRE**
  - Comminuted → **LAG SCREWS HEMICERCLAGE CERCLAGE WIRE**
- **(F)** Lateral sagittal (slab) fracture → **LAG SCREWS**
- **(G)** A-P distal oblique → **PIN AND FIGURE-OF-EIGHT WIRE INTO T4**
- **(H)** Dorsal medial axial slab fracture → **LAG SCREW and/or Coaptation**
- P-A distal oblique
  - **(I)** Large fragments → **PIN(S) AND FIGURE-OF-EIGHT WIRE**
  - **(J)** Small fragments → **Treat as PPIS ARTHRODESIS**

145

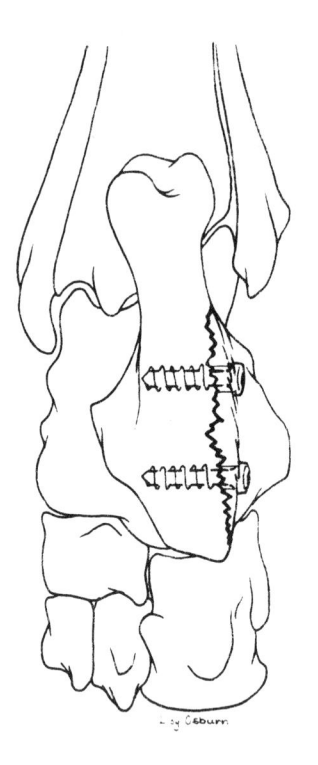

Figure 4 Lateral slab fracture of the calcaneus stabilized by means of two screws, lagged if possible.

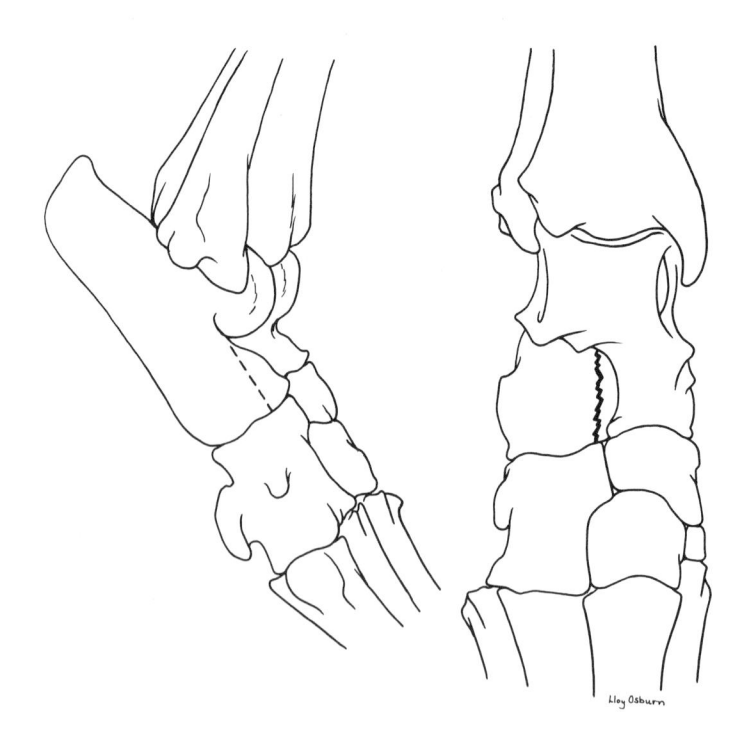

Figure 5 Dorsal medial slab fracture.

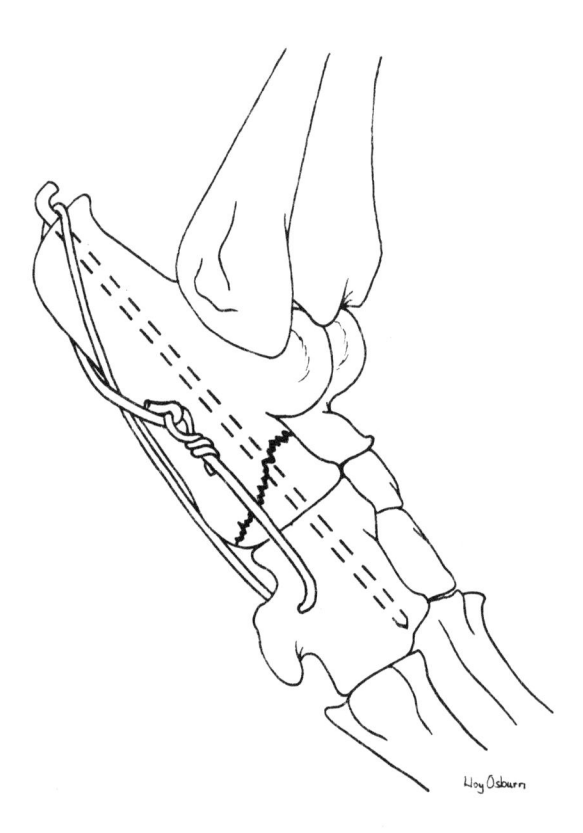

Figure 6 Distal anteroposterior fracture of the calcaneus stabilized by a pin through the site and on into fourth tarsal bone, plus a tension band wire.

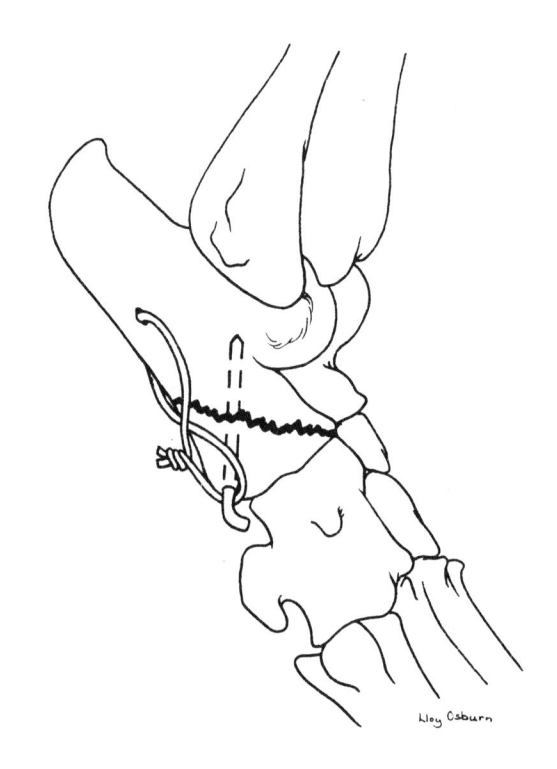

Figure 7 Posteroanterior fracture of distal calcaneus with "large" fragment stabilized by a single pin and a figure-of-eight tension band wire.

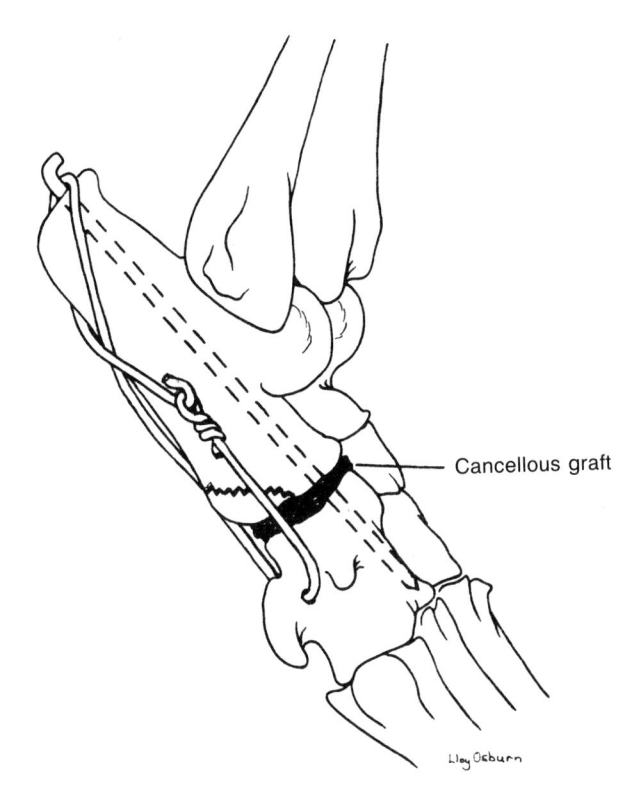

Figure 8 Posteroanterior fracture of the distal calcaneus with a "small" fragment. Arthrodesis by means of a figure-of-eight tension band wire and incorporated graft.

H. Dorsomedial slab fractures of the base of the calcaneus rarely, if ever, go to nonunion and, therefore, can be managed by lag screw fixation or coaptation.

I. Large oblique plantodistal chip fractures of the base of the calcaneus are repaired by a pin and figure-of-eight tension band wires (Fig. 7).

J. Manage small oblique plantodistal chip fractures of the base of the calcaneus as a plantar proximal intertarsal subluxation (PPIS). Support the arthrodesis of the calcaneoquartal joint by a pin and figure-of-eight wire into the fourth tarsal bone (Fig. 8).

References

Dee JF. Injuries to the distal tibia and tarsus. Proceedings AAHA 1984:359.

Dee JF, Dee LG. Fractures and dislocations associated with the racing greyhound. In: Newton CW, Nunamaker DW, eds. Textbook of small animal orthopaedics. Philadelphia: JB Lippincott, 1985:467.

Dee JF, Dee LG, Earley TD. Fractures of carpus, tarsus, metacarpus and phalanges. In: Brinker WO, Hohn RB, Prieur WD, eds. Manual of internal fixation in small animals. Heidelberg: Springer-Verlag, 1983:190.

Dee JF, Dee LG, Eaton-Wells RW. Injuries of high performance dogs. In: Whittick WG, ed. Canine orthopedics II. Philadelphia: Lea & Febiger, in press.

Ost PC, Dee JF, Dee LG, Hohn RB. Fractures of the calcaneus in racing greyhounds. Vet Surg 1987; 16:53.

INTERTARSAL SUBLUXATION

Jon F. Dee

A. The next intertarsal subluxations to be discussed involve the centrodistal joint and either the calcaneoquartal joint or the tarsometatarsal joint. Physical examination reveals instability at one or more of these joint levels. In the reduced position, the plantar support mechanism is found to be intact (Fig. 1).

B. Medially and laterally stressed radiographs in the anteroposterior projection will demonstrate the extent of the medial and/or lateral instability.

C. The most common instability involves both the centrodistal joint and the calcaneoquartal joint, with an intact plantar apparatus. Repair is by arthrodesis of the involved joints, which includes the vertical intertarsal joint between the central and fourth tarsal bone. Stabilization is maintained laterally with a seven-hole dynamic compression (DC) plate and medially with either a two-hole dynamic compression plate or a small two-hole reconstruction plate. Both medial and lateral plates are loaded in order to achieve compression (Fig. 2).

D. Occasionally a milder form of the centrodistal and calcaneoquartal instability is seen in which the lateral aspect of the tarsus is essentially stable on physical examination. In those cases in which the primary instability is at the level of the centrodistal joint, we may perform a partial arthrodesis and maintain reduction by way of a lag screw from the medial aspect of the central tarsal bone to seat in the body of the fourth tarsal bone (Figs. 3 and 4).

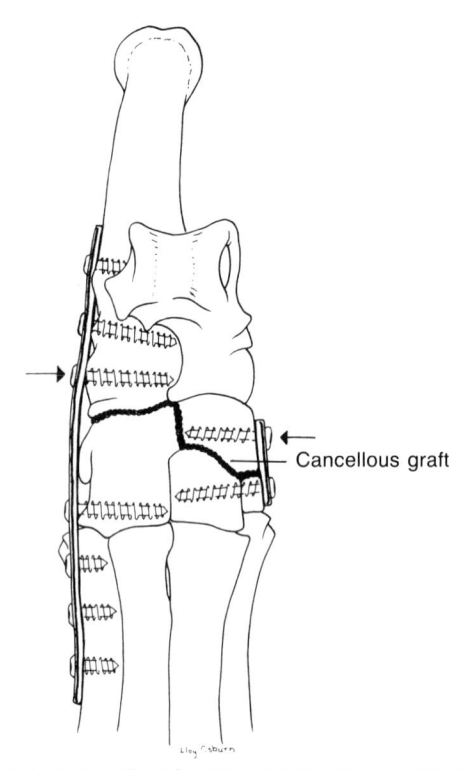

Figure 2 Total intertarsal subluxation stabilized by two DC plates and an associated graft.

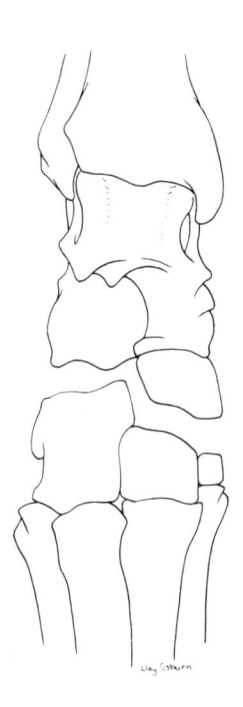

Figure 1 Intertarsal subluxation—total.

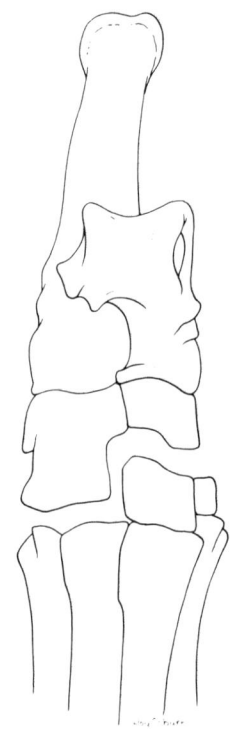

Figure 3 Intertarsal subluxation—centrodistal joint induced.

INTERTARSAL SUBLUXATION Suspected

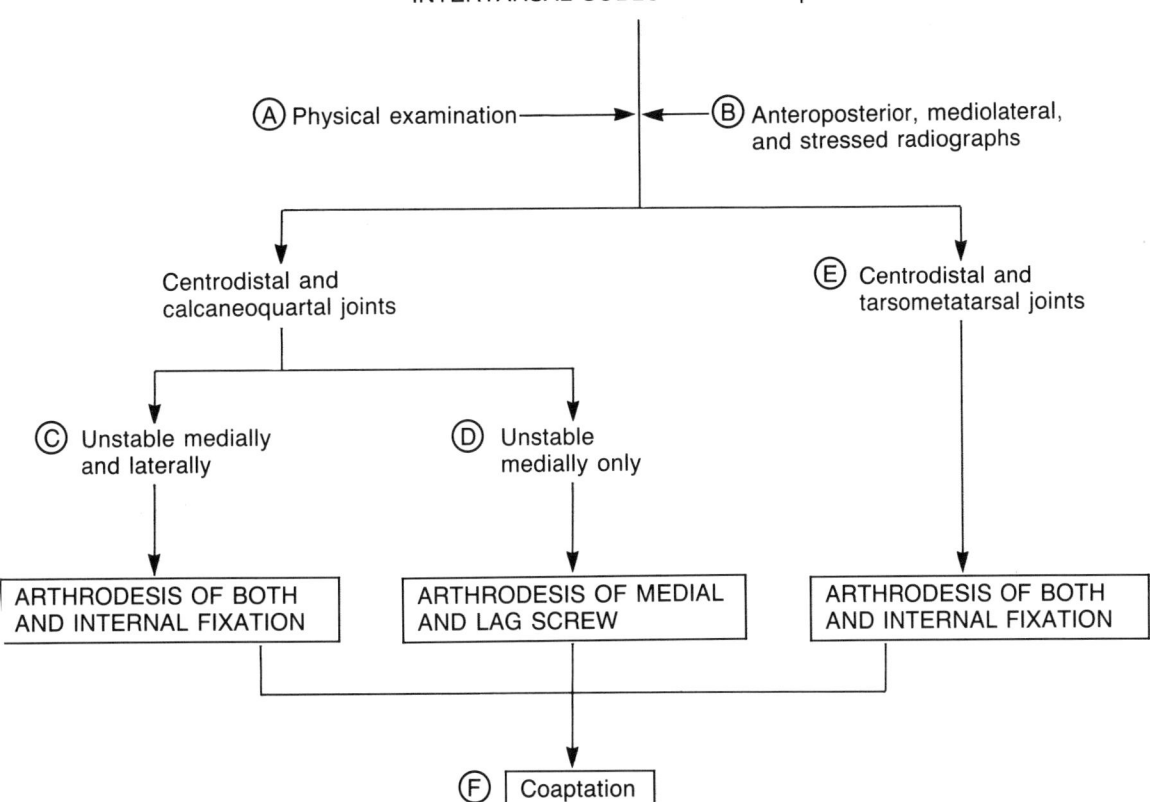

- (A) Physical examination
- (B) Anteroposterior, mediolateral, and stressed radiographs

Centrodistal and calcaneoquartal joints

(E) Centrodistal and tarsometatarsal joints

(C) Unstable medially and laterally

(D) Unstable medially only

ARTHRODESIS OF BOTH AND INTERNAL FIXATION

ARTHRODESIS OF MEDIAL AND LAG SCREW

ARTHRODESIS OF BOTH AND INTERNAL FIXATION

(F) Coaptation

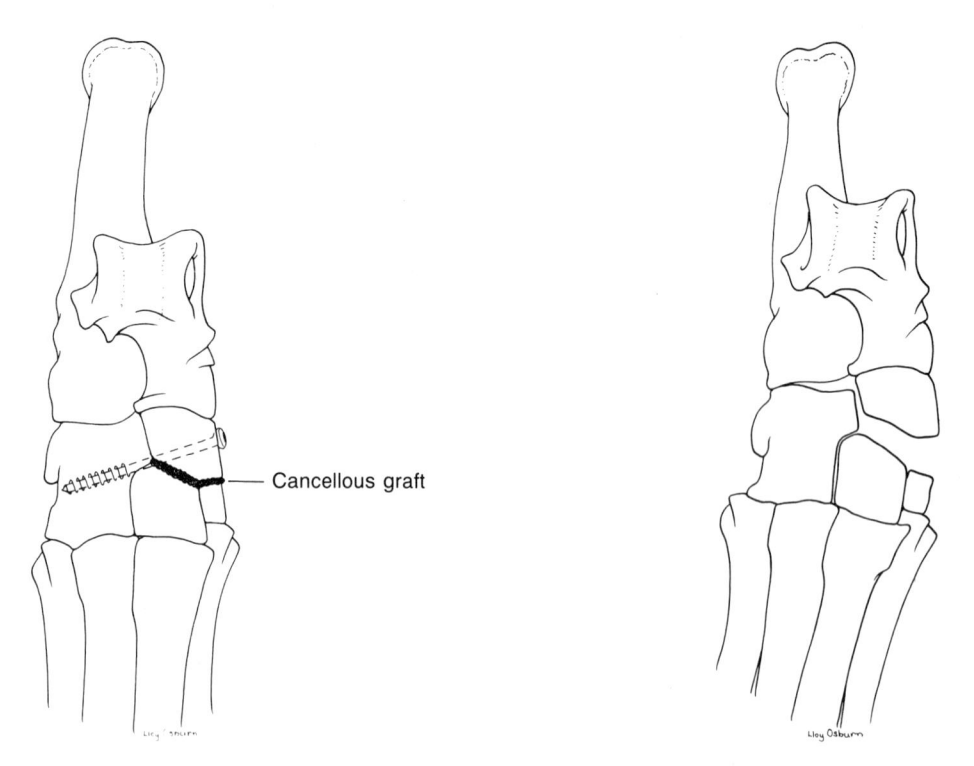

Figure 4 Centrodistal luxation stabilized by a screw and associated graft.

Figure 5 Metatarsal subluxation centrodistal (third to fourth) joint induced.

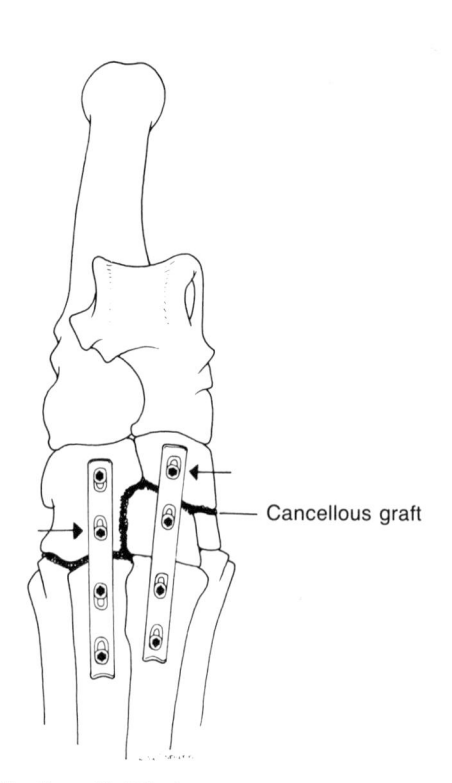

Figure 6 Stabilization with DC plates and associated graft.

E. Centrodistal tarsometatarsal subluxations involve the joint between the central tarsal bone and the distal tarsal bones and the joint between the fourth tarsal bone and the metatarsal bones (Fig. 5). These joint levels and the vertical intertarsal joint between the third and fourth tarsal bones are arthrodesed and maintained in reduction by dorsally placed bone plates (Fig. 6).

F. All of these repairs are coapted.

References

Dee JF. Injuries to the distal tibia and tarsus. Proceedings AAHA 1984; 359.

Dee JF, Dee LG, Earley TD. Fractures of carpus, tarsus, metacarpus and phalanges. In: Brinker WO, Hohn RB, Prieur WD, eds. Manual of internal fixation in small animals. Heidelberg: Springer-Verlag, 1983:190.

TARSOCRURAL ARTHRODESIS

Jon F. Dee

A. Any unstable condition of the tarsocrural joint that cannot be reconstructed successfully is an indication for tarsocrural arthrodesis. Additional indications are degenerative joint disease that is not responsive to medical therapy and unrepairable calcaneal tendon injuries.

B. Lag screw fixation of the tarsocrural joint is the least traumatic and the most commonly utilized method of arthrodesis. Approach the joint by incising the origins of the medial collateral ligaments or by performing an osteotomy of the medial malleolus. Prior to insertion of an autogenous cancellous bone graft, all articular cartilage of the distal tibia and fibula is removed, as is the articular cartilage of the condyles of the talus. With the tarsus held in the functional position for the individual patient, a screw is lagged from the dorsal medial aspect of the distal tibia through the body of the talus to seat in the lateral plantar portion of the base of the calcaneus. An additional screw may be lagged from the dorsal lateral aspect of the distal tibia through the body of the talus to seat in the head of the talus. These screws may be protected from bending by placing a positional screw from the plantar side of the tuber calcanei to engage both cortices of the distal tibia. This screw is removed when a radiograph confirms fusion (Fig. 1).

C. Plate and screw fixation of the tarsocrural joint may be accomplished on the dorsal or the plantar aspect of the dorsal tibia, tarsus, and metatarsal III. Both methods require extensive surgical exposure and, therefore, have limited application. Though more difficult to place, plantar plates have the advantage of being on the tension side of the tarsus.

D. Some form of coaptation is required until radiographic evidence of fusion is apparent.

E. Transarticular application of an external fixator is particularly useful in the management of open injuries of the tarsocrural joint that require arthrodesis. This method allows for treatment of the soft tissues while the joint is being immobilized.

References

Brinker WO, Piermattei DL, Flo GL. Handbook of small animal orthopedics and fracture treatment. Philadelphia: WB Saunders, 1983.

Dee JF, Dee LG. Fractures and dislocations associated with the racing greyhound. In: Newton CW, Nunamaker DW, eds. Textbook of small animal orthopaedics. Philadelphia: JB Lippincott, 1985:467.

Dee JF, Dee LG, Earley TD. Fractures of carpus, tarsus, metacarpus and phalanges. In: Brinker WO, Hohn RB, Prieur WD, eds. Manual of internal fixation in small animals. Heidelberg: Springer-Verlag, 1983:190.

Earley TD, Piermattei DL, Dee JF, Weigel JP. Canine carpus and tarsus short course. Proceedings. Knoxville, Tennessee: University of Tennessee, 1981:1.

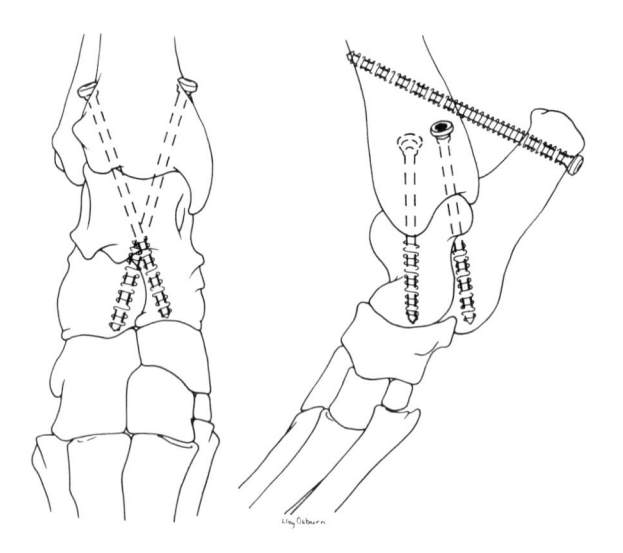

Figure 1 Arthrodesis by means of crossed lag screws and a temporary stabilizing positional screw.

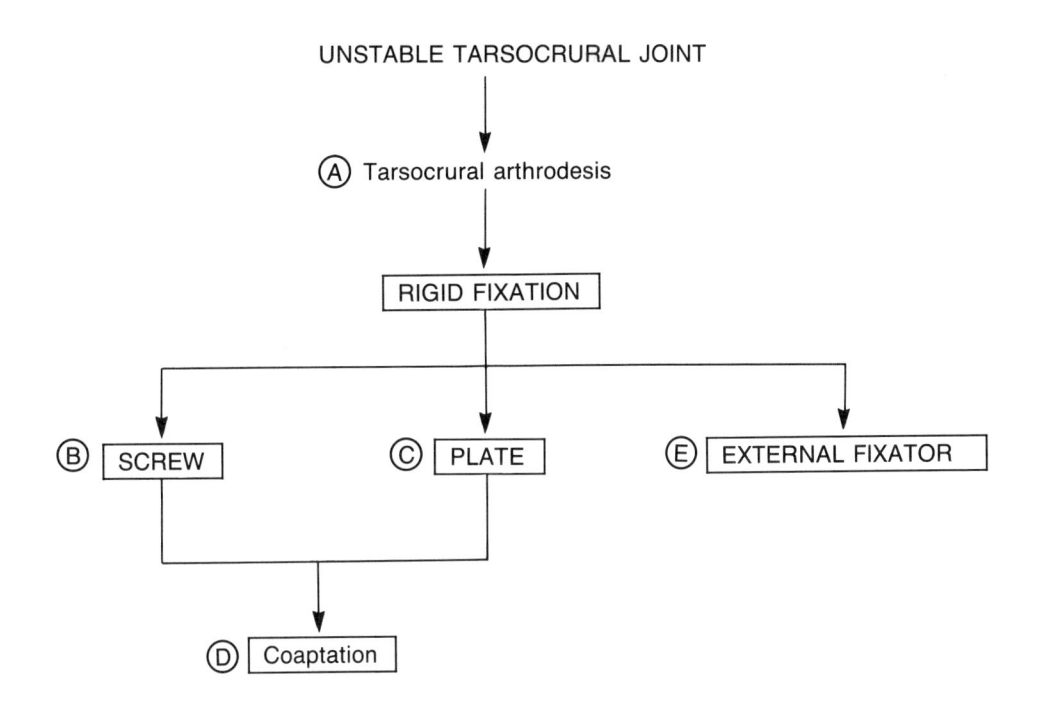

UNSTABLE TARSOCRURAL JOINT
↓
(A) Tarsocrural arthrodesis
↓
RIGID FIXATION
↓
- (B) SCREW
- (C) PLATE
- (E) EXTERNAL FIXATOR

(D) Coaptation

CENTRAL TARSAL BONE FRACTURE

Jon F. Dee

A. Fractures of the central tarsal bone are most commonly seen in the large, active, sporting or working breeds of dogs. The highest incidence occurs in the right leg of the racing Greyhound.

B. Central tarsal bone fractures are graded based upon the type of fracture and the amount of displacement present. Type I: dorsal slab fracture with no displacement; Type II: dorsal slab fracture with displacement (Fig. 1A); Type III: fracture of the sagittal plane with medial and/or dorsal displacement of the medial portion of the central tarsal bone; Type IV: dorsal displaced slab in conjunction with a larger medially displaced fragment (Fig. 1B); and Type V: severely comminuted and displaced fractures. This is a radiographic and surgical classification based upon the number and type of *displaced* fragments rather than the number of actual fragments present.

C. Type I and II fractures are associated with minimal soft tissue swelling, no crepitation, no angular deformity, a reluctance to bear weight, and point pain over the dorsal medial aspect of the central tarsal bone.

D. Occasionally a tentative diagnosis is made on physical examination and is not substantiated with radiographs. These individuals are reassessed after several days in a padded splint and treated accordingly.

E. Although Type I fractures have been coapted, optimum results are obtained in all dorsal slab fractures via cortical lag screw fixation. Type II fractures are repaired with a cortical lag screw.

F. Type III (rare), Type IV (most common of all), and Type V (uncommon) fractures have significant soft tissue swelling with obvious crepitation upon movement of the fracture site. The patient is nonweight-bearing with the tarsus in a varus and plantigrade position.

G. A true Type III fracture is reparable with a single mediolateral (M-L) screw. Although not apparent radiographically, a nondisplaced dorsal slab fracture is often present at the time of surgery and should be appropriately managed with a cortical dorsoplantar lag screw, in addition to the previously placed mediolateral lag screws (Fig. 2A, 2B).

H. Repair Type IV central tarsal bone fractures with two screws, placed mediolaterally and dorsoplantar, by using interfragmentary compression (Fig. 2A, 2B).

I. As the surgeon's learning curve flattens and the technical expertise improves, the number of Type V (unreconstructable) central tarsal bone fractures decreases. The combination of improved equipment availability and improved surgical expertise has allowed for surgical reconstruction of some of the heretofore inoperable Type V central tarsal bone fractures (Fig. 3).

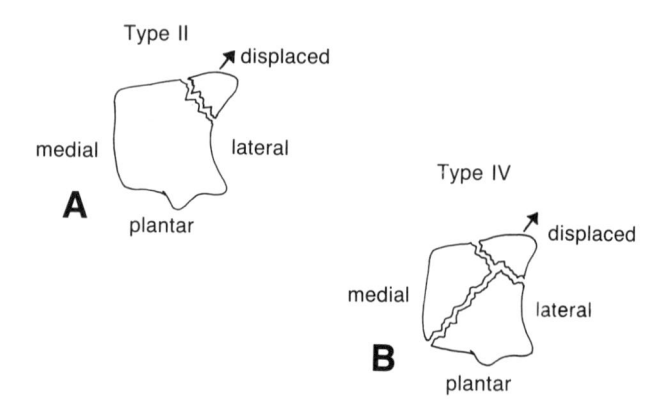

Figure 1 *A*, Type II fracture; *B*, Type IV fracture.

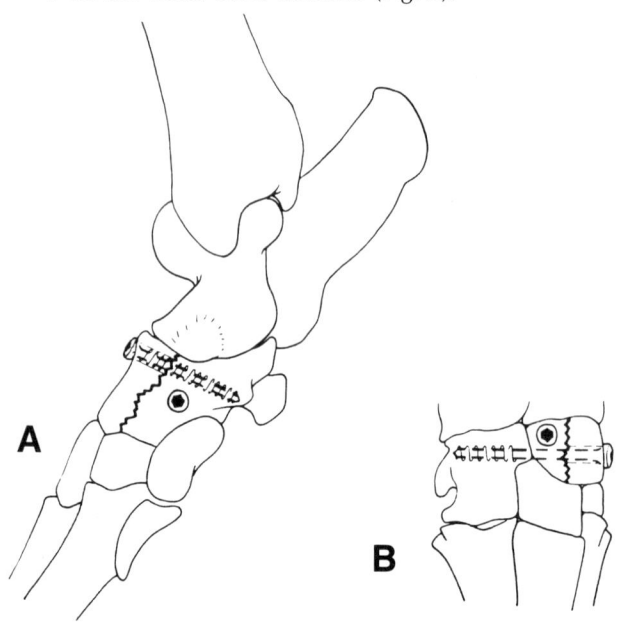

Figure 2 Fixation of central tarsal bone fracture and associated fracture of the fourth tarsal bone with screws. *A*, lateral view; *B*, anterior view.

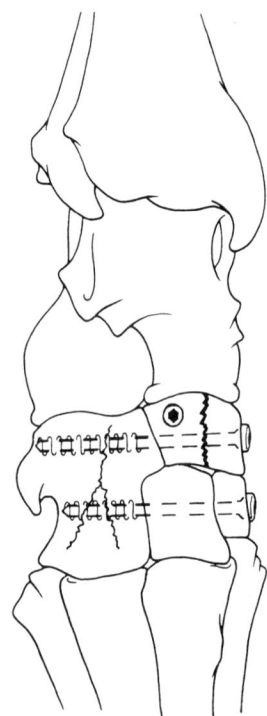

Figure 3 Fracture of the central tarsal bone stabilized by cortical lag screws.

CENTRAL TARSAL BONE FRACTURE Suspected

```
                    Ⓐ Physical examination ───→ ←─── Ⓑ Posteroanterior (P-A) and mediolateral (M-L)
                                                          radiographs
```

- Ⓒ Point pain, No crepitation
  - Ⓓ Soft tissue swelling only on radiographs → Coaptation Radiograph in 3 to 5 Days
    - No fracture → Treat as Grade I Sprain
    - Fracture → LAG SCREW A-P
  - Dorsal slab fracture → Ⓔ
    - Type I nondisplaced → Coaptation (For optimum results) → LAG SCREW A-P
    - Type II displaced → LAG SCREW A-P
- Ⓕ Crepitation with pain
  - Ⓖ Solitary medial fragment Type III (rare) → M-L LAG SCREW
  - Ⓗ Dorsal slab and a medial fragment Type IV → M-L AND A-P LAG SCREWS
  - Ⓘ Multiple displaced fragments Type V → Ⓙ
    - AUTOGENOUS GRAFT
    - SYNTHETIC REPLACEMENT
    - ALLOGRAFT

→ Postoperative Coaptation

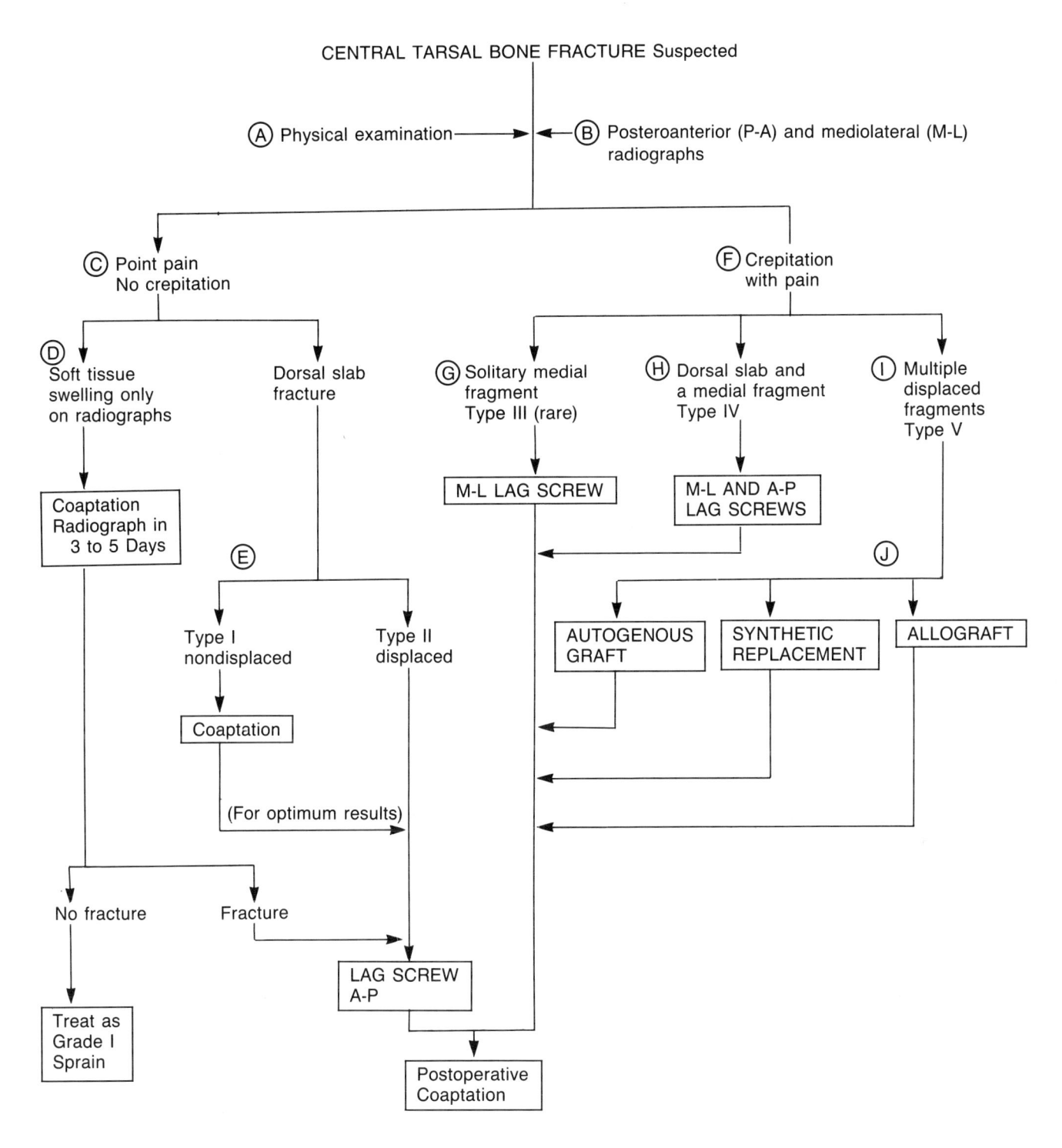

J. Those few that cannot be reconstructed by screw fixation are potential candidates for either an autogenous cortical cancellous bone graft, a synthetic replacement, or perhaps a central tarsal allograft. All of these options are in their infancy; further experience and additional numbers are needed before firm recommendations can be made. All of these require additional internal fixation for support.

References

Dee JF. Fractures in the racing greyhound. In: Bojrab MJ, ed. Patho-physiology in small animal surgery. Philadelphia: Lea & Febiger, 1981:812.

Dee JF, Dee JD, Piermattei DL. Classification, management and repair of central tarsal fractures in the racing greyhound. JAAHA 1976; 12:398.

Dee JF, Dee LG. Fractures and dislocations associated with the racing greyhound. In: Newton CW, Nunamaker DW, eds. Textbook of small animal orthopaedics. Philadelphia: JB Lippincott, 1985:467.

Dee JF, Dee LG, Earley TD. Fractures of carpus, tarsus, metacarpus and phalanges. In: Brinker WO, Hohn RB, Prieur WD, eds. Manual of internal fixation in small animals. Heidelberg: Springer-Verlag, 1983:190.

Dee JF, Dee LG, Eaton-Wells RW. Injuries of high performance dogs. In: Whittick WG, ed. Canine orthopedics II. Philadelphia: Lea & Febiger, in press.

SECOND TARSAL BONE FRACTURE

Jon F. Dee

A. Isolated injuries to the second tarsal bone are rare. Even when seen, these uncommon injuries are invariably in conjunction with a severe fracture of the central tarsal bone or a fracture of the third tarsal bone (T3). Occasionally, one may see a subluxation of the second tarsal bone (T2) in association with a centrodistal instability or with a tarsometatarsal instability.

B. Radiographic signs are subtle and generally best appreciated on the P-A (A-P) view. An increase in the intertarsal joint space between T2 and T3 is appreciated.

C. Fractures are extremely rare; subluxations are somewhat more common.

D. Screw sizes as small as 1.5 mm cortical to as large as 4.0 mm cancellous have been successfully utilized. All screws are countersunk, seated in T4 and/or T3 and left in situ. Screws in T2 fractures are lagged. Screws in T2 subluxations may be lagged or positional (Fig. 1).

E. Most repairs require some form of postoperative coaptation.

References

Dee JF. Injuries to the distal tibia and tarsus. Proceedings AAHA 1984:359.

Dee JF, Dee LG. Fractures and dislocations associated with the racing greyhound. In: Newton CW, Nunamaker DW, eds. Textbook of small animal orthopaedics. Philadelphia: JB Lippincott, 1985:467.

Dee JF, Dee LG, Eaton-Wells RW. Injuries of high performance dogs. In: Whittick WG, ed. Canine orthopedics II. Philadelphia: Lea & Febiger, in press.

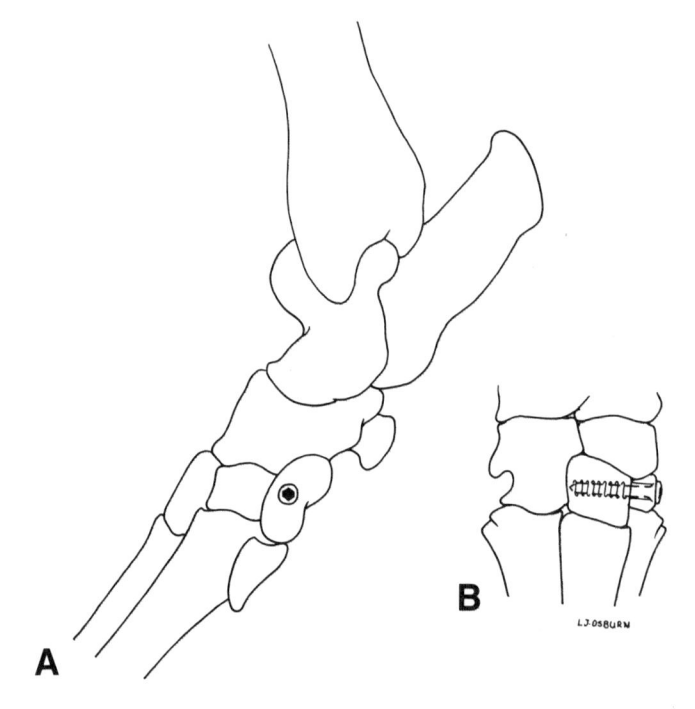

Figure 1 *A*, lateral view of lag screw fixation of a second tarsal bone fracture; *B*, cranial view of lag screw fixation of a second tarsal bone fracture.

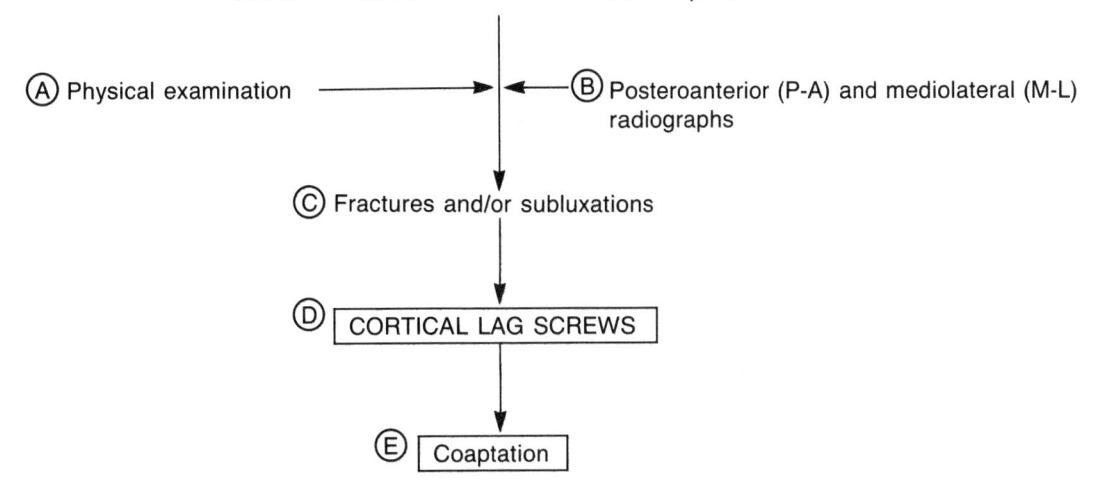

SECOND TARSAL BONE FRACTURE Suspected

Ⓐ Physical examination ⟶ ⟵ Ⓑ Posteroanterior (P-A) and mediolateral (M-L) radiographs

Ⓒ Fractures and/or subluxations

Ⓓ CORTICAL LAG SCREWS

Ⓔ Coaptation

THIRD TARSAL BONE FRACTURE

Jon F. Dee

A. Third tarsal bone fractures present as a solitary lesion, although on occasion there is an associated second tarsal bone subluxation present. If the fracture is acute, slight soft tissue swelling is present, and point pain may be elicited directly over the fracture. If it is chronic, periosteal new bone formation is palpable to the astute clinician.

B. Radiographic changes may vary from the subtle to the obvious; this is based upon the amount of displacement of the solitary dorsal slab fracture.

C. Experience has shown that whether the displacement is minimal or significant, the most predictable results with the least amount of degenerative joint disease are obtained by using countersunk cortical bone screws in a lag fashion. Screws are left in situ (Fig. 1).

D. The extremity is coapted in slight extension for approximately 6 weeks.

References

Dee JF. Fractures in the racing greyhound. In: Bojrab MJ, ed. Patho-physiology in small animal surgery. Philadelphia: Lea & Febiger, 1981.

Dee JF, Dee LG. Fractures and dislocations associated with the racing greyhound. In: Newton CW, Nunamaker DW, eds. Textbook of small animal orthopaedics. Philadelphia: JB Lippincott, 1985:467.

Dee JF, Dee LG, Earley TD. Fractures of carpus, tarsus, metacarpus and phalanges. In: Brinker WO, Hohn RB, Prieur WD, eds. Manual of internal fixation in small animals. Heidelberg:Springer-Verlag, 1983:190.

Dee JF, Dee LG, Eaton-Wells RW. Injuries of high performance dogs. In: Whittick WG, ed. Canine orthopedics II. Philadelphia: Lea & Febiger, in press.

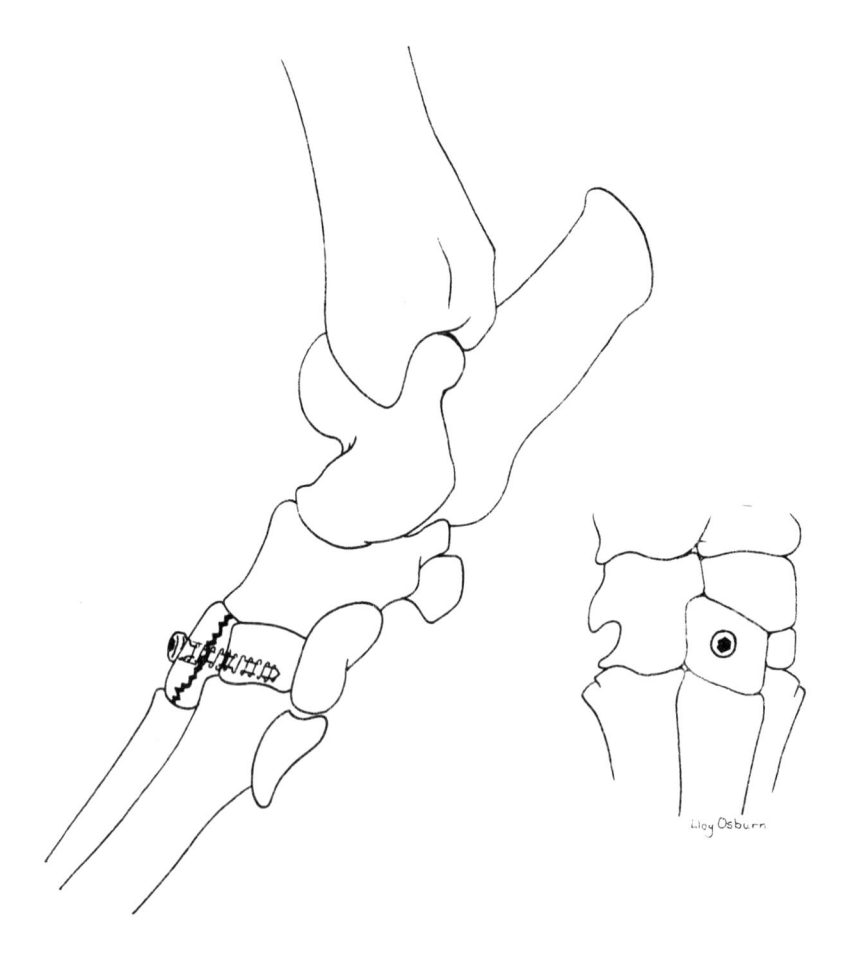

Figure 1 Slab fracture of the third tarsal bone stabilized with a lag screw.

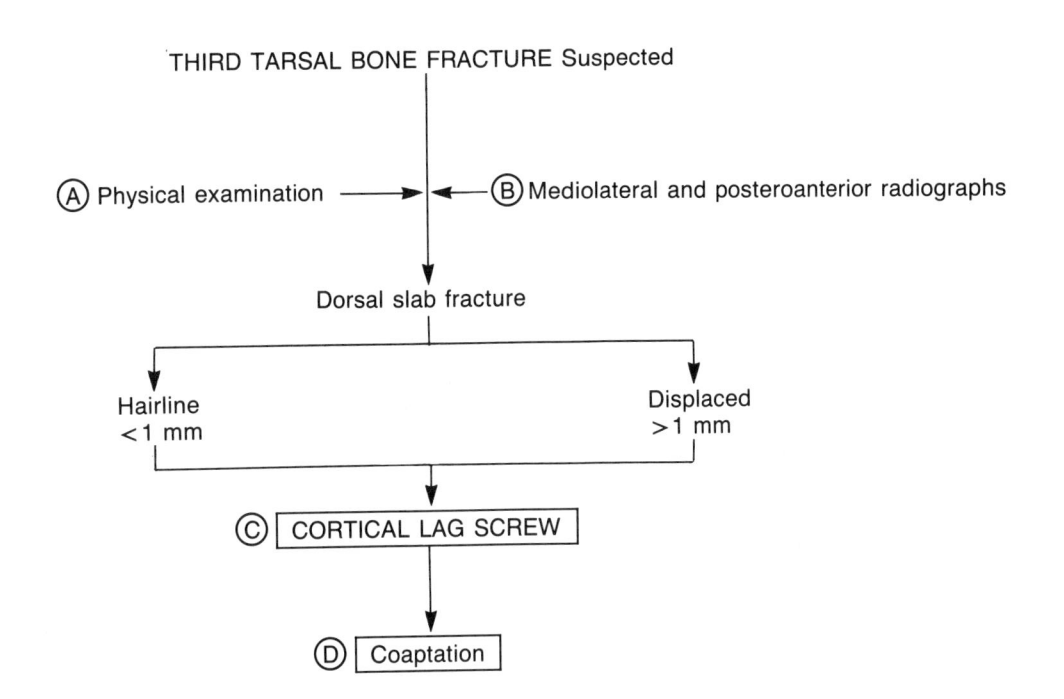

THIRD TARSAL BONE FRACTURE Suspected

Ⓐ Physical examination → ← Ⓑ Mediolateral and posteroanterior radiographs

Dorsal slab fracture

- Hairline <1 mm
- Displaced >1 mm

Ⓒ CORTICAL LAG SCREW

Ⓓ Coaptation

FOURTH TARSAL FRACTURE

Jon F. Dee

A. The physical examination reveals the presence of other fractures. Soft tissue swelling, pain, crepitation, varus deformity, and a plantigrade nonweight-bearing posture are hallmark secondary characteristics.

B. Diagnosis is made and confirmed by detail radiographs; the anteroposterior (A-P) view has the highest yield.

C. An isolated fracture of the fourth tarsal bone (T4), whether it be a compression fracture or an avulsion of the plantar process, is a rare occurrence in the canine pet or performace population.

D. These isolated fractures may be successfully coapted.

E. The vast majority of fourth tarsal bone fractures are seen in conjunction with fractures of the central tarsal bone. Approximately 40 percent of racing Greyhounds that sustain a fracture of the central tarsal bone have an associated compression fracture of the fourth tarsal bone. In the more severe (type IV) central tarsal bone fractures, the head of the talus displaces distally and medially. In its displaced position, the talus acts as a fulcrum for the calcaneus, which may either fracture or displace distally; this causes a compression fracture of the fourth bone.

F. Repair of fourth tarsal bone fractures is indirectly achieved by repairing the central tarsal bone by means of interfragmentary compression (Fig. 1). Additional support may be obtained by a second screw, which is lagged from T2 through T3 to seat in T4.

References

Boudrieau RJ, Dee JF, Dee LG. A survey of central tarsal bone fractures in the racing greyhound. A review of 114 cases. JAVMA 1984; 184:1486.

Boudrieau RJ, Dee JF, Dee LG. Treatment of central tarsal bone fractures in the racing greyhound. JAVMA 1984; 184:1492.

Dee JF, Dee LG, Earley TD. Fractures of carpus, tarsus, metacarpus and phalanges. In: Brinker WO, Hohn RB, Prieur WD, eds. Manual of internal fixation in small animals. Heidelberg: Springer-Verlag, 1983:190.

Dee JF, Dee LG, Eaton-Wells RW. Injuries of high performance dogs. In: Whittick WG, ed. Canine orthopedics II. Philadelphia: Lea & Febiger, in press.

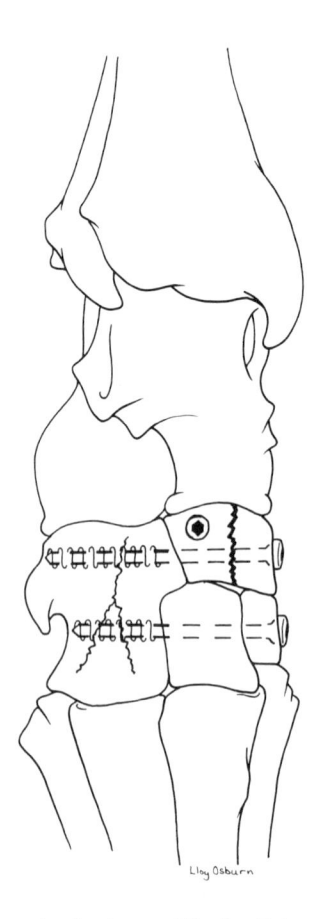

Figure 1 Compression fractures of the fourth tarsal bone. Repair is indirectly achieved by repairing the associated fractures of the central tarsal bone.

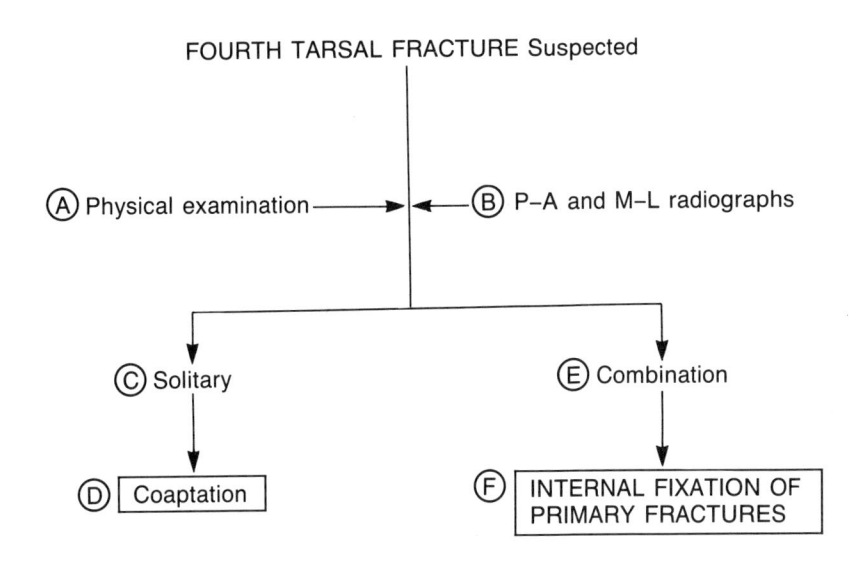

FOURTH TARSAL FRACTURE Suspected

- (A) Physical examination → ← (B) P-A and M-L radiographs
- (C) Solitary
  - (D) Coaptation
- (E) Combination
  - (F) INTERNAL FIXATION OF PRIMARY FRACTURES

TARSOMETATARSAL JOINT SUBLUXATION

Jon F. Dee

A. Tarsometatarsal joint subluxations may involve either the plantar or the dorsal surfaces (Fig. 1). The diagnosis of both is made by physical examination and verified or documented by appropriate radiographs.

B. The plantar ligaments are much thicker and stronger than those on the dorsal side of the hock. Plantar subluxations occur when the dense tarsal fibrocartilage tears from the bases of the metatarsals during severe dorsiflexion.

C. In most cases, repair consists of primary arthrodesis of the tarsometatarsal joint by pin and figure-of-eight tension band wire (Fig. 2). The wire is passed through a mediolateral hole drilled through the bases of metatarsal (MT) II through V. After the articular cartilage of the tarsometatarsal joint is removed, a cancellous graft is obtained from the ipsilateral proximal humerus. After reduction and graft placement, the appropriate pin is placed proximally from the tuber calcanei to seat in the base of MT IV. An alternate, less commonly used repair consists of a bone plate on the lateral aspect of the calcaneus that extends down the lateral aspect of MT V.

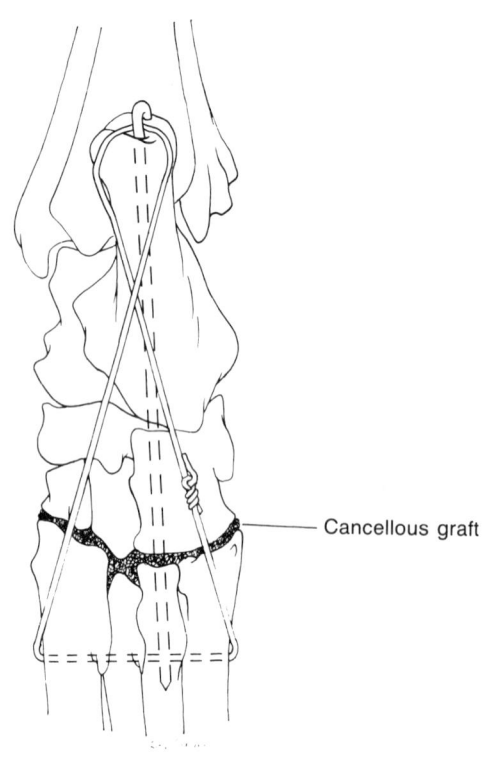

Figure 2 Arthrodesis of tarsometatarsal joint with graft, pin, and figure-of-eight tension band.

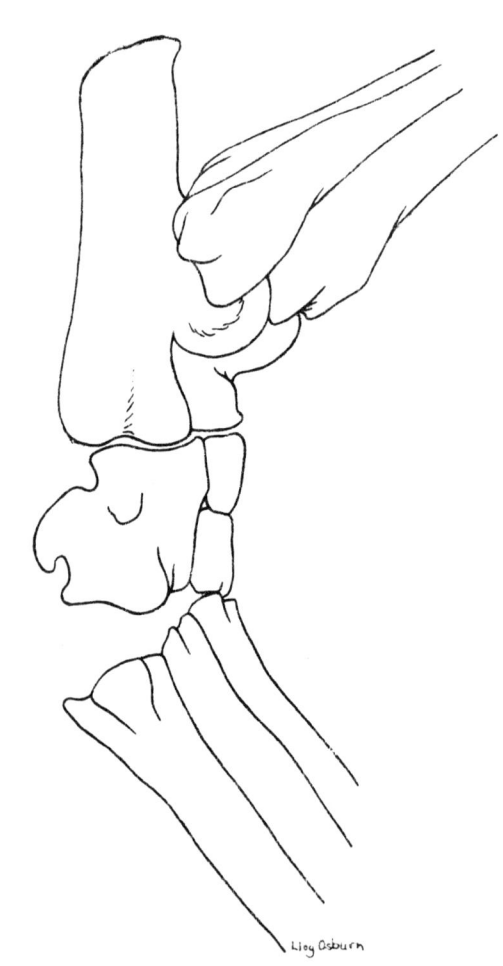

Figure 1 Plantar tarsometatarsal luxation.

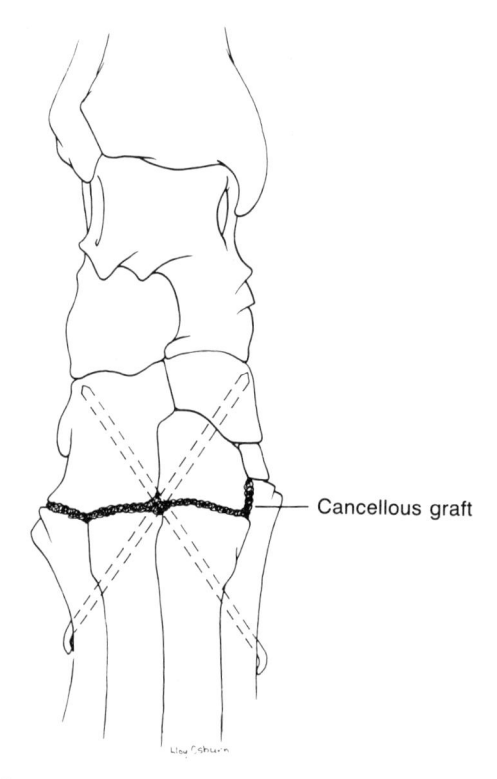

Figure 3 Arthrodesis of tarsometatarsal luxation with graft and crossed pins.

TARSOMETATARSAL JOINT SUBLUXATION Suspected

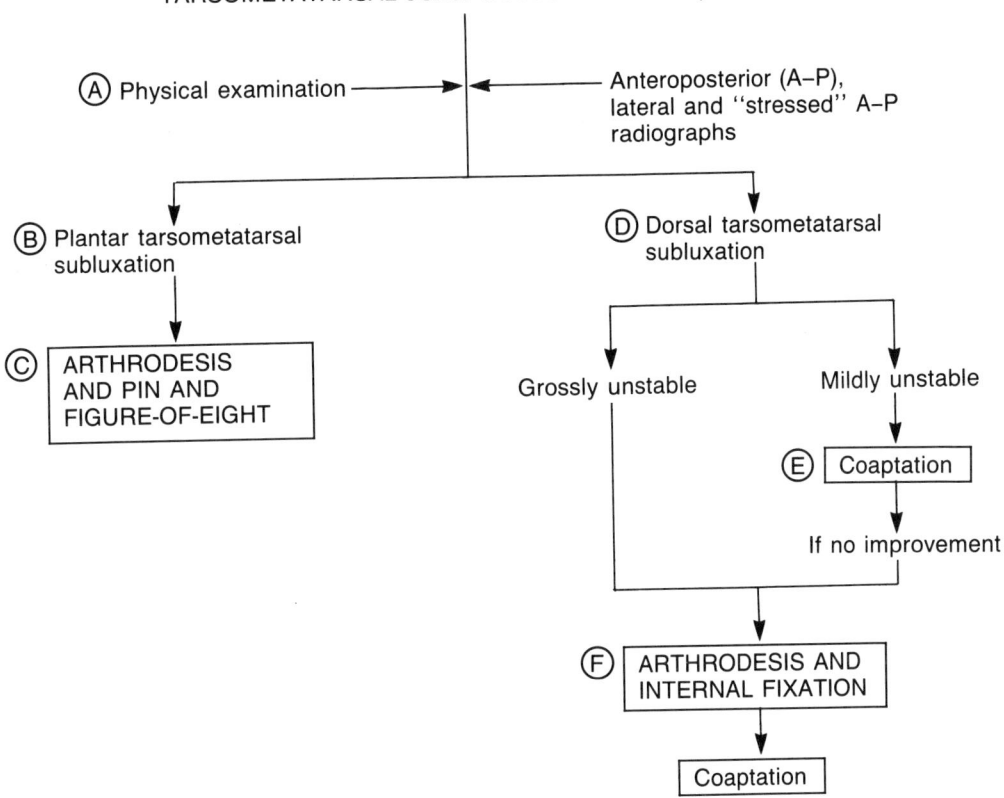

```
                    |
    (A) Physical examination ──→ ←── Anteroposterior (A-P),
                    |                  lateral and "stressed" A-P
                    |                  radiographs
        ┌───────────┴───────────┐
        ↓                       ↓
(B) Plantar tarsometatarsal   (D) Dorsal tarsometatarsal
    subluxation                   subluxation
        ↓                   ┌───────┴────────┐
(C) ┌─────────────┐    Grossly unstable   Mildly unstable
    │ ARTHRODESIS │         │                ↓
    │ AND PIN AND │         │          (E) ┌───────────┐
    │ FIGURE-OF-  │         │              │ Coaptation│
    │ EIGHT       │         │              └───────────┘
    └─────────────┘         │                ↓
                            │          If no improvement
                            ↓                ↓
                      (F) ┌─────────────────────┐
                          │ ARTHRODESIS AND     │
                          │ INTERNAL FIXATION   │
                          └─────────────────────┘
                                   ↓
                             ┌───────────┐
                             │ Coaptation│
                             └───────────┘
```

D. A dorsal tarsometatarsal subluxation is an uncommon hyperextension injury that is characterized by a self-compressing instability, which becomes more stable with weight-bearing.

E. Because of this tendency to stabilize with weight-bearing, coaption may be attempted in the milder cases.

F. In those cases in which time and coaptation have failed, and in the more severe cases, arthrodesis is performed via a dorsal arthrotomy. Because the plantar support is intact, internal fixation need consist only of a Steinmann pin down the shaft of the calcaneus to seat in the base of MT IV. Additional stabilization may be obtained in selected cases by utilizing crossed pins that are driven from the bases of metatarsals II and V and seated in the fourth and central tarsal bones respectively (Fig. 3).

References

Brinker WO, Piermattei DL, Flo GL. Handbook of small animal orthopedics and fracture treatment. Philadelphia: WB Saunders, 1983.

Dee JF, Dee LG, Earley TD. Fractures of carpus, tarsus, metacarpus and phalanges. In: Brinker WO, Hohn RB, Prieur WD, eds. Manual of internal fixation in small animals. Heidelberg: Springer-Verlag, 1983:190.

Olds RB. Arthrodesis. In: Bojrab MJ, ed. Current techniques in small animal surgery. Philadelphia: Lea & Febiger, 1975.

ATLANTOAXIAL-COMPLEX CONGENITAL LESIONS

Geoff Sumner-Smith

A. The technique of radiographic examination of these lesions is identical to that for acquired lesions (p 166).

B. The treatment depends upon the specific lesions as does the severity of symptoms. Each must be treated according to the deficiency. In all cases decompression is necessary plus stabilization of mobile segments.

C. Prophylactic fusion may be attempted in animals that have an unfused odontoid process. Lack of fusion results when the odontoid process develops from a separate center of ossification than the body of C2. Malformation of the odontoid process may require transplantation of a substantial corticocancellous bone graft.

D. Neurologic signs may develop as an animal matures. The primary condition may not have been previously diagnosed. The advent of signs requires decompression and stabilization which may be achieved by a unilateral approach in the form of a hemilaminectomy. Use of a Hall's drill and bur is an ideal method of achieving the decompression. The veterinary surgeon should consider the ethical dilemma of these cases and advise whether a particular patient should be treated or euthanized.

E. Treatment of the conditions of congenital lesion may follow those for acquired lesions described in the following chapter (p 166).

References

Chamber JN, Betts CW, Oliver JE. The use of nonmetallic suture material for stabilization of atlantoaxial subluxations. J Am Anim Hosp Assoc 1977; 13:602.

Gage ED, Smallwood JE. Surgical repair of atlantoaxial subluxation in a dog. Sm Anim Clin 1970; 65:583.

Parker AJ, Par RD. Atlantoaxial subluxation in small breeds of dogs: diagnosis and pathogenesis. Sm Anim Clin 1973; 68:1133.

Sorjonen DC, Shires PK. Atlantoaxial instability: a ventral surgical technique for decompression, fixation and fusion. Vet Surg 1981; 10:22.

```
                    CONGENITAL LESIONS OF
                    ATLANTOAXIAL-COMPLEX
                              │
                              │
                              ▼
                         Ⓐ ── Radiography series
                              │
                              ▼
                      Specific pathology
                         identified
                              │
                              ▼
                    Ⓑ  Absence of odontoid process
                                  or
                       Lack of fusion of odontoid process
                                  or
                       Malformation of odontoid process
                                  or
                          Lack of ligament support
                    ┌─────────────┴─────────────┐
                    ▼                           ▼
            No neurologic signs         Patient shows
                    │                   signs of
                    │                   acquired lesions
         ┌──────────┴──────┐           ┌─────────┴────────┐
         ▼           Ⓒ     ▼           ▼ Ⓓ                ▼
    ┌──────────┐  ┌──────────────┐  Severe paralysis    Paresis
    │Conservative│ │ PROPHYLACTIC │  Quadriplegia          │
    │ Treatment │  │   FUSION     │      │              Ⓔ   ▼
    └──────────┘  └──────────────┘  ┌───┴────┐      ┌──────────┐
         │                           ▼        ▼      │Conservative│
         ▼                        Advise  ┌────────┐ │    and    │
     No treatment               euthanasia│DECOMPRESS│ │Symptomatic│
                                          │   AND   │ │ Treatment │
                                          │STABILIZE│ └──────────┘
                                          └────────┘
```

ATLANTOAXIAL FRACTURE

Geoff Sumner-Smith

A. It is essential to ensure that the animal is able to breathe and that no further movement occurs at the fracture site as movement can readily lead to further spinal cord trauma.

B. Proper positioning of the head for radiography is vitally important. The head should rest in a normal position, neither flexed nor extended. The neck should be supported so that true lateral views are obtained. Interpretation can be difficult. If both routine views are equivocal, oblique views should be taken. Do not remove the supporting collar until major trauma has been ruled out. Because of the anatomy of the area, myelography is not likely to be helpful and is not advisable. Dorsal displacement of the axis with compression of the cord results in paresis or paralysis.

C. If the radiographs do not reveal osseous damage, unnatural movement with a history of quadrilateral gait deficit and, in the acquired case, history of trauma with local swelling and pain indicate ligament rupture.

D. Even if there is no luxation or fracture, local tissue edema may produce signs of neurologic deficit. Strain on the supporting tissue is painful and requires the support of a cervical collar to assist healing and provide comfort. The reduction of pressure on the spinal cord is of paramount importance in all but the mildest nonprogressive cases. In severe cases, surgical decompression is necessary; in mild cases, mechanical stabilization results in a diminution of local swelling.

E. If a fracture is suspected but the radiographs are equivocal, flexion and extension views may be taken, but absolute prerequisites are a conscious animal and an absence of all but the mildest neurologic signs. Mild sedation is permissible provided that muscle relaxation does not result. Palpation should be carried out with extreme care to ensure that fragments are not displaced to further traumatize the cord.

F. Arthrodesis can be extremely difficult to achieve and may require the wearing of a cervical support collar for the rest of the animal's life as the fusion is likely to be quite tenuous.

References

Gage ED. Atlantoaxial subluxation. In: Bojrab MJ, ed. Current techniques in small animal surgery. Philadelphia: Lea & Febiger, 1983.

Sorjonen D, Shires PM. Atlantoaxial instability: a ventral surgical technique for decompression, fixation and fusion. Vet Surg 1981; 10:22.

Swaim SF. Surgical approaches to spinal cord diseases of small animals. Proc Am Anim Hosp Assoc 1975; 1:317.

FRACTURE OR DISLOCATION OF THE ATLANTOAXIAL COMPLEX Suspected

- **(A)** Secure airway; Immobilize neck
- Total skeletal and neurologic examination
  - Injury to calvarum
  - No injury to calvarum
    - Anesthetize or sedate patient
    - **(B)** Radiography series: Rostro-posterior, open mouth, and lateral views; Tomography, if available
      - Specific luxation or fracture identified
      - Identification not positive
        - Flexion and extension radiography; Animal conscious; Minimal neurologic signs
          - No dislocation
            - No neurologic signs
              - **(D)** Cervical collar
            - Neurologic signs present → Reduction
          - Dislocation
            - **(E)** Rupture of ligament support; Fracture of odontoid process; Fracture of atlas or axis
              - Neurologic signs present → Reduction → **DECOMPRESS; STABILIZE**
                - Stabilization satisfactory → Cervical collar
                - Stabilization unsatisfactory → **(F) DORSAL ARTHRODESIS** → Cervical collar
              - No neurologic signs → Reduction → Repeat neurologic examination

CERVICAL SPINE FRACTURE

Geoff Sumner-Smith

A. Radiography of suspected cervical spine conditions is essential in order to differentiate the specific conditions. Traumatic situations must be differentiated from congenital lesions. An owner may report an accident and assume that the signs relate to a recent accident when in fact they relate to cervical stenosis or spondylolithesis. If an obvious fracture is not displayed, a subsequent myelography is mandatory in both flexed and hyperextended positions.

B. Restriction in a cervical collar often helps to support the area and to disperse a transient neurologic deficit.

C. Open reduction, ventral fusion, and ventral slotting are the treatment for animals with compression fractures of the cervical vertebrae impinging on the cord as well as those with cervical stenosis and lythesis. The prognosis for cases of stenosis is very poor, whereas lythesis without stenosis often responds to ventral decompression and fusion. Ventral fusion may be accomplished by inserting a corticocancellous bone graft into a slot previously undercut by means of a bur (Fig. 1A); results are equivocal. A more satisfactory stabilization may be achieved by inserting a portion of a Steinmann pin across the adjacent vertebrae (Fig. 1B) and then moulding methyl-methacrylate bone cement into the pre-prepared slot (Fig. 1C). Alternatively, following fenestration the intervertebral space may be compressed by means of a lag screw, and fusion accelerated by means of a cancellous bone graft.

D. Dorsal decompression and dorsal fusion is a difficult procedure that should be attempted only by experienced orthopaedic surgeons. Even then the prognosis is poor. The technique requires dorsosagittal dissection on each side of the ligamentum nuchae. The approach is deep, and visualization is poor. Stabilization and fusion may be attempted by bone grafting across the dorsal facets and including the remaining dorsal spines in a moulding of bone cement reinforced by Kirschner wire. Great care should be exercised to ensure that the spinal cord is protected from the exothermic heat generated as the cement polymerizes.

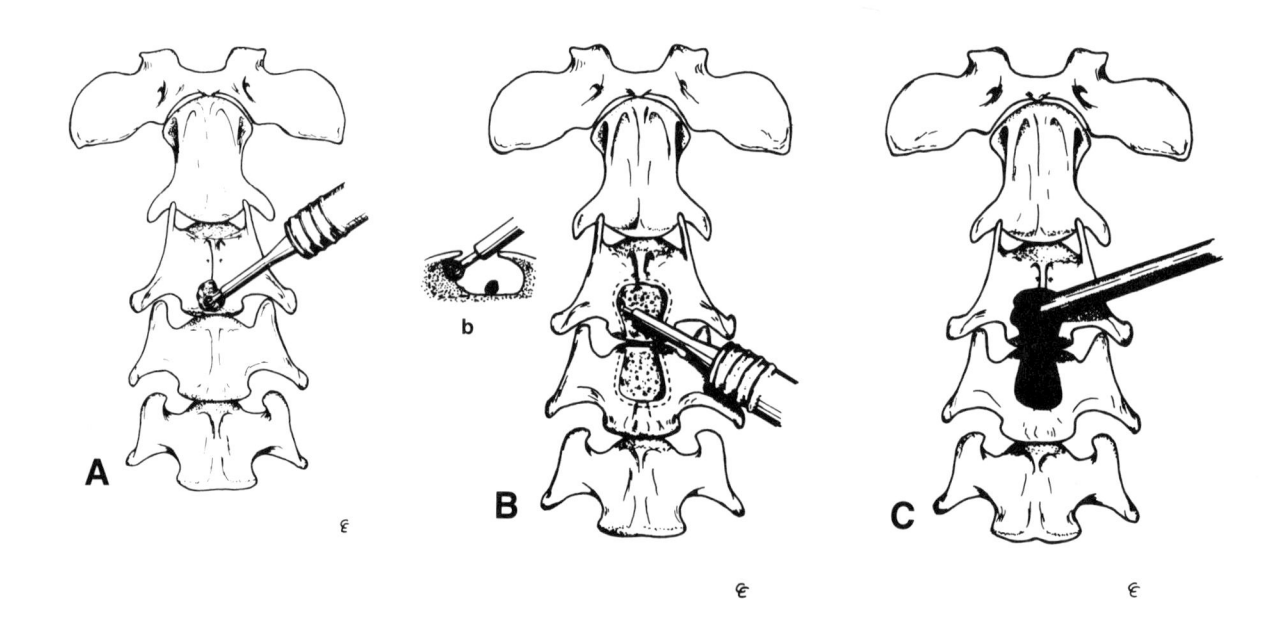

Figure 1 Ventral slotting and cement stabilization of cervical instability. *A*, initial site for burring: ventral aspect of cervical spine; *B*, burring and undercutting; *b*, insertion of Steinmann pin; *C*, insertion and tamping of bone cement.

CERVICAL SPINE FRACTURE
DISLOCATION
STENOSIS

Ⓐ Immobilize neck
- Lateral and dorsoventral radiography series
- CT scan
- Flexion/extension
- Lateral radiography (care)
- Myelography

Stable pattern (normal or minimal neurologic signs)

Unstable pattern (with or without neurologic deficit)

Ⓑ Restrict in cervical collar → Recheck radiographs

Closed reduction → Unsuccessful / Successful

Severe neurologic deficit

Ⓒ OPEN REDUCTION / VENTRAL FUSION / VENTRAL SLOTTING

Ⓓ DORSAL DECOMPRESSION / DORSAL FUSION

THORACOLUMBAR SPINE FRACTURE

Geoff Sumner-Smith

A. Suitable radiographs of the thoracolumbar area are not difficult to obtain even in large dogs. Trauma to this area is usually the result of compression forces from the rear on a rotated, flexed, or straight spine; the first results in vertebral luxation and the latter two in bursting compression fractures of the vertebral body. If the spine is flexed but not rotated, a wedge compression fracture may result. A combination of these effects may also occur producing both luxation and fracture. Radiographs of the thoracic cavity are mandatory in all cases. Those taken to evalutate the spine may be unsuitable, different radiographic factors being desirable for evaluation of the contents of the thorax.

B. Stable injuries may be treated conservatively provided that there is no deficit of spinal cord function. Instability is difficult to verify since muscle splinting may be guarding the area; hence, deep sedation or heavy analgesia is contraindicated. The presenting signs of the whole animal should govern the treatment regime. Body splinting not only aids in stabilization but eases discomfort and should be supplemented by cage rest.

C. The unstable fracture needs to be treated surgically only if marked neurologic signs are evident and/or progressive. Assessment should take into account the duration of the injury.

D. If hemorrhage around the cord appears to have ceased and signs are abating, a watching brief is desirable along with cage rest.

E. Marked neurologic signs are not always present when there is trauma to the thoracolumbar area. If present, the condition is serious, and immediate decompression is essential. It should be appreciated that minor subluxations at the time of injury may have initially suffered a greater degree of separation. Care in evaluating the neurologic signs is therefore essential. Reduction during surgery may usually be attained by grasping the superior spines and gently manipulating the vertebrae. In these cases stabilization with cross pins may be sufficient (Fig. 1A) or may require the application of double sandwich plates of steel or plastic (Lubra), (Figs. 1B and 2). The addition of methacrylate bone cement around the superior spines and implant greatly aids in stabilization (Fig. 3).

F. Open reduction, except in very mild cases, should invariably be accompanied by decompression which permits evaluation of the spinal cord. Total laminectomy is preferred in the more severe cases, but hemilaminecto-

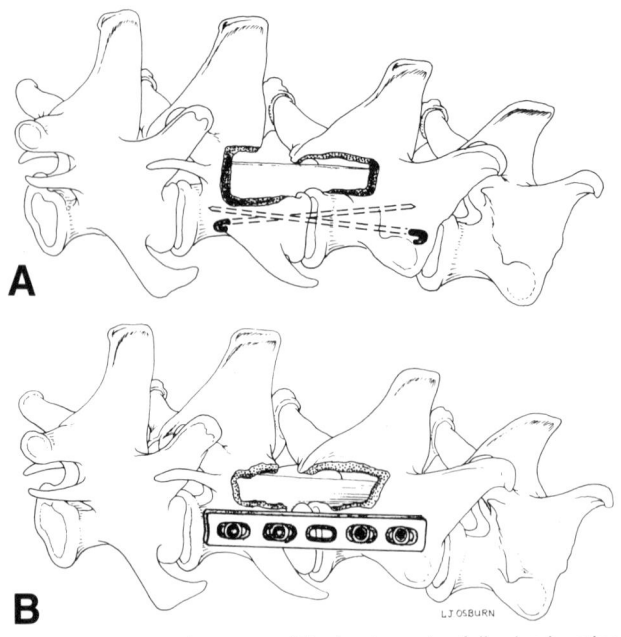

Figure 1 Hemilaminectomy of the lumbar spine following luxation. *A*, stabilization with cross pins. *B*, stabilization with a plate.

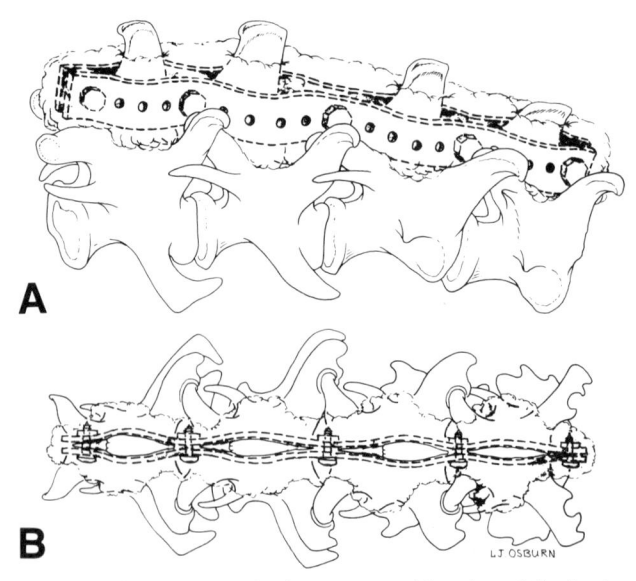

Figure 2 Stabilization of a fracture or subluxation of the lumbar spine with a Lubra sandwiching plate and superimposed bone cement. The technique may be combined with a laminectomy if, as is often the case, the latter is warranted. *A*, sideview. *B*, ventral view.

```
                    THORACOLUMBAR
                    FRACTURE AND
                     DISLOCATION
                          │
                          │ ◄── (A) A-P and lateral radiography
                          │         Body splinting
                          │         Neurologic evaluation
             ┌────────────┴────────────┐
             ▼                         ▼
       (B) Stable injuries      (C) Unstable injuries
                                      │
                          ┌───────────┼───────────────┐
                          ▼           ▼               ▼
                     Ligament    Compression    (E) Fracture of the
                     rupture     fracture           vertebral arch
                          │           │               │
                     ┌────┴────┐      │               │
                     ▼         ▼      │               │
             Undisplaced   Displaced  │               │
                     │         │      │               │
       ┌─────────────┘    ┌────┴────┐ │               │
       ▼                  ▼         ▼ │               │
  Compression       Asymptomatic  Symptomatic         │
  fracture                │         │                 │
  Process fracture        ▼         │                 │
  Ligament rupture   Body bandage   │                 │
       │              or            │                 │
       ▼              walking cast  │                 │
  (D) Conservative                  └─────┬───────────┘
      treatment                           ▼
       │                         (F) ┌─────────────────┐
       ▼                             │ OPEN REDUCTION  │
  Body splinting                     │ DECOMPRESSION   │
  Cage rest                          │ INTERNAL FIXATION│
                                     └─────────────────┘
```

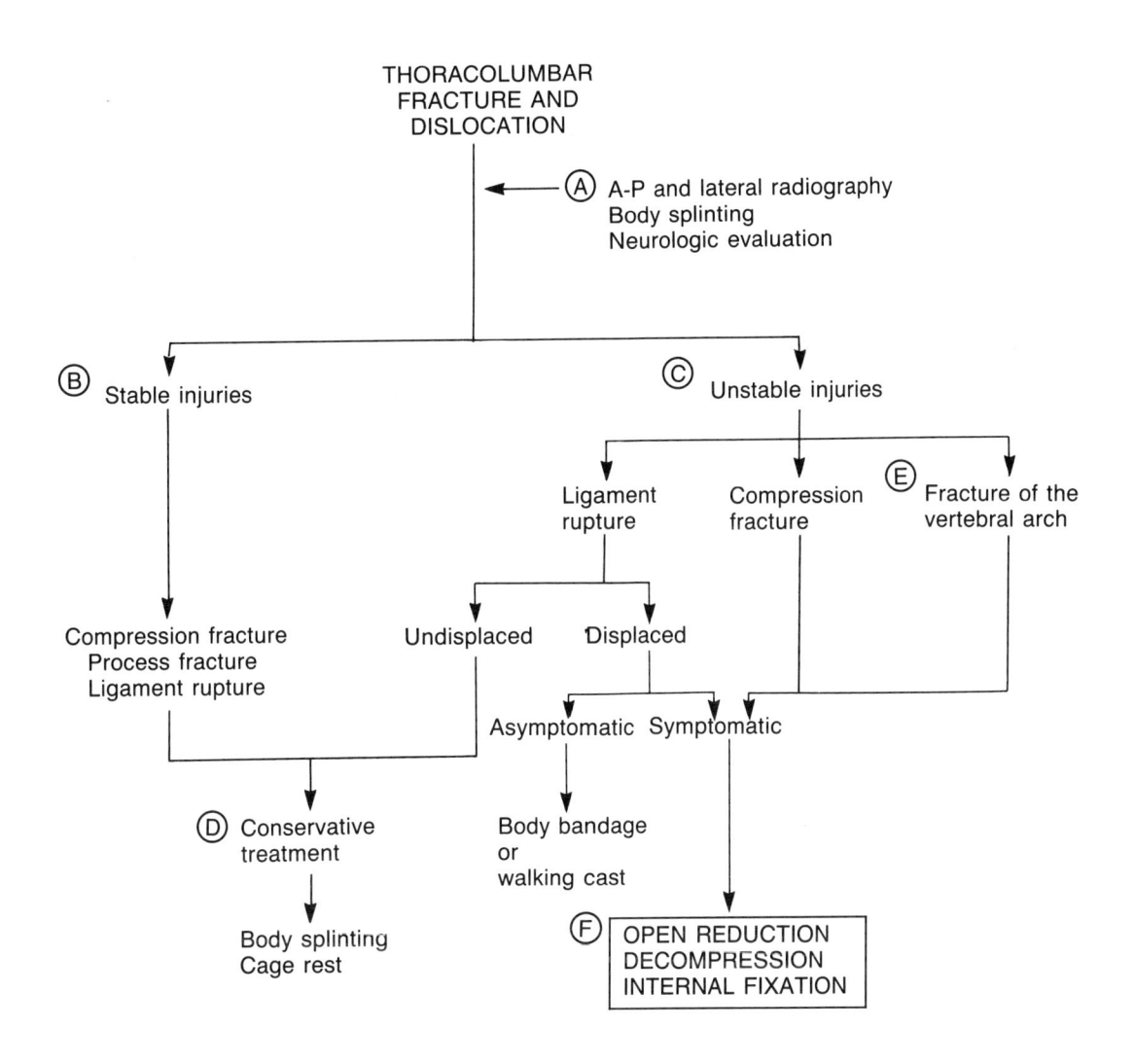

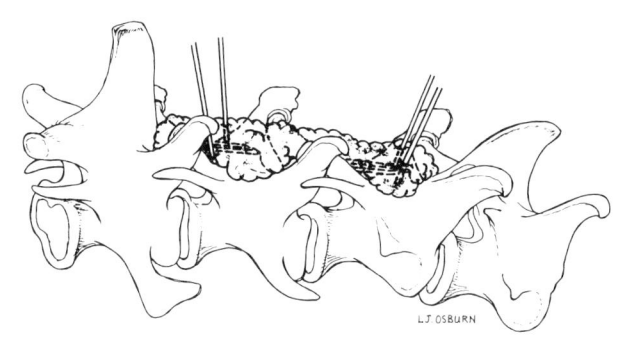

Figure 3 Stabilization of a subluxation or fracture of the lumbar spine. Following a dorsal laminectomy bone cement is modelled around preplaced pins. The spinal cord must be protected from the heat of polymerization. A fat graft will assist this.

my may be sufficient if the signs are mild and unilateral. Stabilization of severely luxated or fractured vertebrae may be achieved with dorsal spinal plates that span the gap produced by the decompression surgery. Unfortunately these plates often pull loose or break the bone, particularly in young animals. More satisfactory results may be achieved by body plating or cross pinning the vertebrae.

References

Creed JE, Ytarraspe DJ. Intervertebral disk fenestration. In: Bojrab MJ, ed. Current techniques in small animal surgery. Philadelphia: Lea & Febiger, 1981:556.

Slocum B, Rudy RL. Fractures in the seventh lumbar vertabra in the dog. J Am Anim Hosp Assoc 1975; 11:167.

SACRAL INJURIES

Joanne R. Cockshutt

A. Sacral injuries are a common result of trauma in the dog and cat. Force significant to cause a vertebral fracture often causes other bony and soft tissue injury. Neurologic deficits of the hind limbs, tail, or urinary and gastrointestinal systems may result in a confusing clinical presentation, and a thorough neurologic examination is mandatory before repair is contemplated. Injury in this region may compress or sever the cauda equina, nerve roots, or peripheral nerves. Associated inflammation may affect more cranial spinal cord segments.

B. Radiographs generally reveal the presence of a lumbrosacral sacroiliac or sacrococcygeal luxation or lumbar, sacral, or coccygeal fracture. Displacement of the sacroiliac joint is most commonly unilateral, but is always accompanied by a fracture or luxation elsewhere in the pelvic ring.

C. Lumbosacral fracture or luxation should be repaired surgically in those cases in which femoral, ischiatic, and sacral nerve function is preserved. Exploratory surgery to confirm permanent nerve damage is justified if reflexes involving those nerves are absent.

D. Sacroiliac luxations occur more commonly than sacral fractures. The ilium is usually displaced cranially, and the hemipelvis is frequently very unstable, resulting in marked discomfort. Sacral and ischiatic nerve deficits are common.

E. Coccygeal fractures and luxations, like sacral fractures, are often accompanied by irreversable neurologic deficits that affect the hind limbs, tail, and pelvic viscera.

F. Euthanasia should be considered in cases of severe neurologic deficit. Even with coccygeal fractures, avulsion injury to proximal spinal cord segments may cause permanent loss of hind limb, bowel, or urinary bladder function. Paraesthesia is not an uncommon sequel to cauda equina injury and may result in severe self multilation. Lesions that involve only the coccygeal nerves may be managed by amputation of the tail.

G. A reduction of a lumbosacral luxation is best accomplished by a dorsal approach to the sacrum. A dorsal laminectomy may be performed to assess the integrity of the cauda equina and to provide decompression. The L7 vertebra may be held in reduction by means of a transilial pin passed caudal to the dorsal spinous process of L7 (Fig. 1). A pair of dorsal spinous plates may also be used for fixation.

H. Conservative treatment of sacroiliac luxation may suffice if: (1) the dog exhibits little pain and ambulates well, (2) there is minimal pelvic displacement, and (3) no neurologic deficits. Enforced rest for 3 weeks followed by gradually increased exercise is generally adequate therapy, when combined with good nursing care and physiotherapy.

I. In most cases, if indicated by marked pelvic instability or pain, surgical stabilization of sacroiliac luxation reduces pain and provides more rapid return to function.

J. Coccygeal luxation, if only slightly displaced, may be reduced and secured by wiring the articular facets or the dorsal spinous and transverse processes.

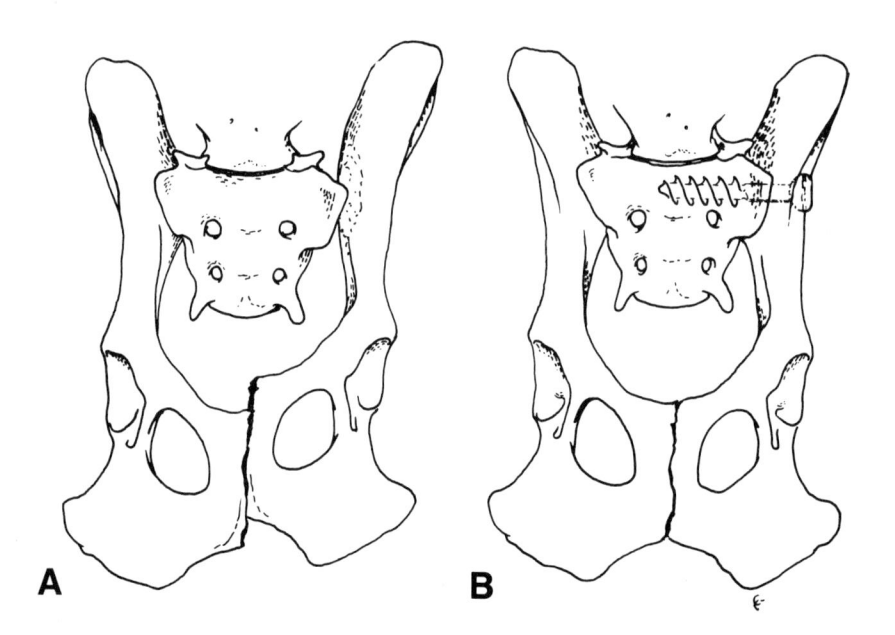

Figure 1 Sacroiliac fixation and separation of the pubic symphysis, A, stabilized, B, by lag screw fixation into the sacrum. Wherever possible a second screw should be placed into the sacrum or, alternatively, in small individuals, a Kirschner wire. For the sake of clarity these have been omitted from the diagram.

SACRAL INJURY Suspected

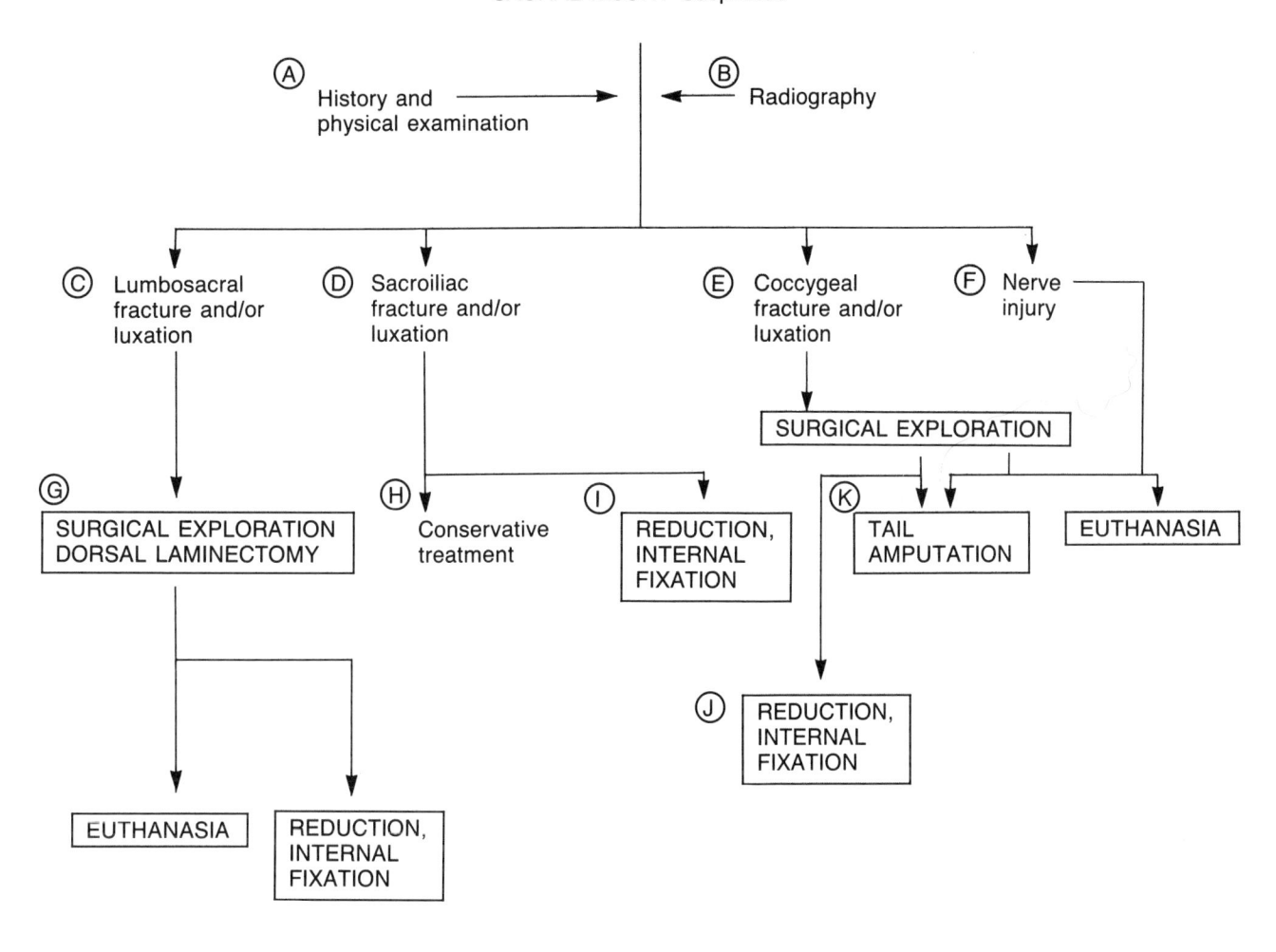

```
                    History and ──→  ←── Radiography
                    physical examination
                              │
         ┌────────────┬───────┴───────┬──────────────┐
         ▼            ▼               ▼              ▼
    Ⓒ Lumbosacral  Ⓓ Sacroiliac   Ⓔ Coccygeal    Ⓕ Nerve
      fracture       fracture        fracture        injury
      and/or         and/or          and/or
      luxation       luxation        luxation
         │                              │              │
         │                              ▼              │
         │                      SURGICAL EXPLORATION   │
         ▼              ┌──────────┐    │    │         │
    Ⓖ SURGICAL         Ⓗ         Ⓘ    Ⓚ   │         │
      EXPLORATION       Conservative REDUCTION, TAIL   EUTHANASIA
      DORSAL            treatment    INTERNAL   AMPUTATION
      LAMINECTOMY                    FIXATION
         │                                  │
    ┌────┴────┐                             ▼
    ▼         ▼                        Ⓙ REDUCTION,
  EUTHANASIA REDUCTION,                   INTERNAL
             INTERNAL                     FIXATION
             FIXATION
```

K. Tail amputation is advised if the tail is completely insensitive or if upon exploration the nerve roots are found to be severed. Amputation is also an alternative if fixation of the coccygeal fracture or luxation cannot be accomplished.

References

Bojrab MJ. Current techniques in small animal surgery. Philadelphia: Lea & Febiger, 1983.

Hulse DA et al. Sacroiliac luxations. Comp Cont Ed 1985; 7:493.

Slatter DH. Textbook of small animal surgery. Philadelphia: WB Saunders, 1985.

Taylor RA. Treatment of fractures of the sacrum and sacrococcygeal region. Vet Surg 1981; 10:119.

CRANIAL FRACTURE

Craig W. Miller

A. Physical examination of the animal with cranial fracture(s) must include a thorough neurologic examination. An exhaustive knowledge of neuroanatomy and physiology is not necessary in order to arrive at a presumptive diagnosis and a rationale for treatment. The examination should include state of consciousness, pupil size and response, posture, motor function, vision, and respiratory rate and character. The remaining cranial nerve reflexes should also be examined. Since multiple injuries often accompany severe cranial trauma, other body systems should be examined as well.

B. First aid for patients with cranial trauma consists of systemic stabilization plus the treatment of trauma that affects the central nervous system. Systemic stabilization, as in all trauma patients, should establish a patent airway, control hemorrhage, and maintain circulatory volume. The goals of medical first aid for cranial trauma patients are to minimize cerebral edema and/or hemorrhage. Dexamethasone and mannitol are the drugs most commonly used to treat cerebral edema. Corticosteroids are most effective in decreasing vasogenic edema that is caused by increased vascular permeability. Hyperosmotic solutions such as mannitol are more effective in treating cytotoxic edema that is caused by poor parenchymal perfusion. Mannitol can exacerbate intracranial hemorrhage, and it is contraindicated in cases in which hemorrhage is suspected. Occasionally, animals that are presented with cranial trauma have seizures and intravenous diazepam is indicated in order to control seizure activity.

C. Hard palate fractures often result from swan dives off apartment balconies or from road accidents. Mucosal defects of less than 2 mm heal spontaneously, but if the defect is greater than 2 mm, surgery is indicated. Wire, or pin and wire, fixation can be used to approximate the bony defect in order to allow soft tissue closure.

D. Comminuted zygomatic arch fractures may interfere with movement of the globe or temporomandibular joint function. These cases require surgical removal of interfering fragments. If comminution is minimal, internal fixation with hemicerclage wires can be accomplished. Occasionally reconstruction with small plates or a rib graft can be done for cosmetic purposes.

E. Frontal sinus fractures often present with subcutaneous emphysema caused by air leakage from the nasal passages. Resolution is often spontaneous if the fragments are small and the defect is minor. Large depressed fractures can be reduced and fixed with orthopaedic wires.

F. Conservative treatment of cranial fractures is aimed at reducing or preventing cerebral edema. As discussed under first aid, careful and continuous monitoring of these patients is essential since any deterioration may require surgical intervention. Large displaced intracranial fragments or worsening of the patient's neurologic status in the face of medical therapy are indications for surgical intervention. Depressed bony fragments should be carefully elevated. Large fragments can be fixed with orthopaedic wire, but covering the defect with the temporalis muscle is adequate. A gradually worsening neurologic status indicates extradural or subdural hemorrhage or uncontrolled brain edema. These conditions require surgical decompression. Ideally, computerized tomography could be used to locate a hematoma, but in veterinary medicine, such surgery must often be exploratory in nature.

References

de Lahunta A. Veterinary neuroanatomy and clinical neurology. Philadelphia: WB Saunders, 1983:365.

Fishman RA. Brain edema. N Engl J Med 1975; 293:706.

Newton CD, Nunamaker DM. Textbook of small animal orthopaedics. Philadelphia: JB Lippincott, 1985:287.

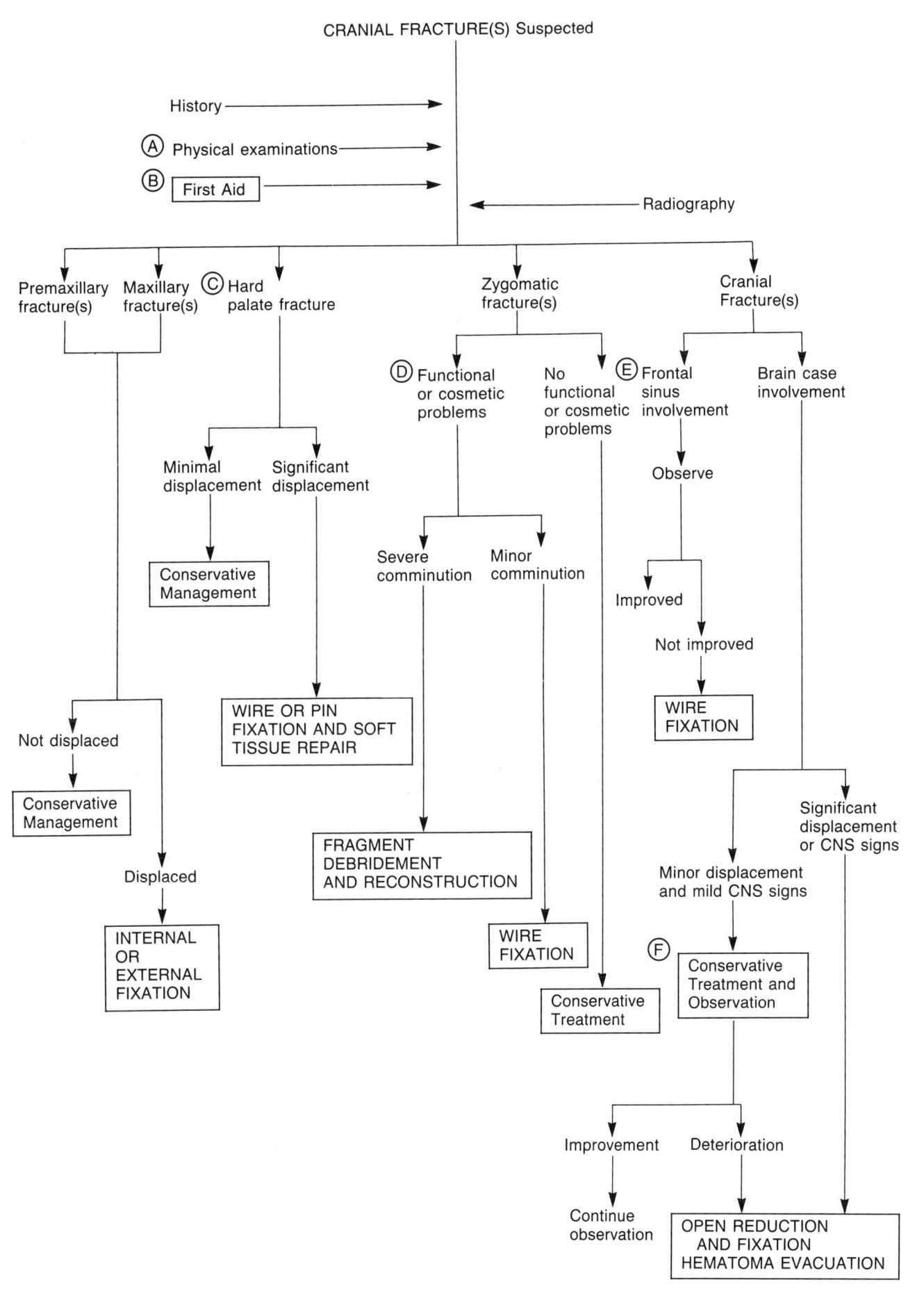

CRANIAL FRACTURE(S) Suspected

- History →
- (A) Physical examinations →
- (B) First Aid →
- Radiography ←

Branches:

Premaxillary fracture(s)
- Not displaced → Conservative Management
- Displaced → INTERNAL OR EXTERNAL FIXATION

Maxillary fracture(s)

(C) Hard palate fracture
- Minimal displacement → Conservative Management
- Significant displacement → WIRE OR PIN FIXATION AND SOFT TISSUE REPAIR

Zygomatic fracture(s)
- (D) Functional or cosmetic problems
  - Severe comminution → FRAGMENT DEBRIDEMENT AND RECONSTRUCTION
  - Minor comminution → WIRE FIXATION
- No functional or cosmetic problems → Conservative Treatment

Cranial Fracture(s)
- (E) Frontal sinus involvement → Observe
  - Improved
  - Not improved → WIRE FIXATION
- Brain case involvement
  - Minor displacement and mild CNS signs → (F) Conservative Treatment and Observation
    - Improvement → Continue observation
    - Deterioration → OPEN REDUCTION AND FIXATION HEMATOMA EVACUATION
  - Significant displacement or CNS signs → OPEN REDUCTION AND FIXATION HEMATOMA EVACUATION

MANDIBULAR FRACTURE

Geoff Sumner-Smith

Fractures of the mandible vary considerably from simple separations, commonly seen in cats, to multiple fragmented bilateral fractures seen in giant dogs.

A. Digital and visual examination often reveals as much as or more than radiographs and can resolve those difficulties of radiographic interpretation caused by superimposition.

B. If the animal appears to be able to cope with the fracture without distress, conservative treatment is preferred. Initially the mandible may be supported by a soft tape muzzle, which should be loosened for the animal to feed. As strength returns to the jaw, the muzzle is removed, but the patient should only receive soft food until it is judged, either clinically or radiographically, that the fracture or fractures have healed. Hard food should be witheld for at least 12 weeks.

C. Dental occlusion takes preference over fracture reduction. Elaborate techniques are not desirable, provided occlusion and fair stability can be obtained.

D. Elaborate attention to detail, removal of small avascular fragments, and debridement are necessary. Larger bone fragments should be retained if they will accept a wire or screw since they act as an autograft. Alternatively an external fixator may be applied, although these devices tend to catch on surrounding objects. Repair must be carried out with the mouth taped closed and the anesthetic administered via a tracheal tube inserted through a pharyngostomy incision. Postoperative feeding via pharyngostomy tube is usually not necessary if good stability has been obtained.

E. Temporomandibular joint luxation may occur in association with fractures or on its own. It may be either unilateral or bilateral. Reduction is undertaken with the animal anesthetized; a fulcrum is inserted across the teeth, level with the last molar teeth. Closure of the mouth then usually permits forceful reduction of the joint.

References

Renegar WR, Olds RB. The use of the Kirschner-Ehmer splint in clinical orthopaedics. Comp Cont Ed 1982; 4:381.

Sumner-Smith G, Dingwall JS. The plating of mandibular fractures in the dog. Vet Rec 1971; 88:595.

Withrow SJ. Taping of the mandible in treatment of mandibular fractures. J Am Anim Hosp Assoc 1981; 17:27.

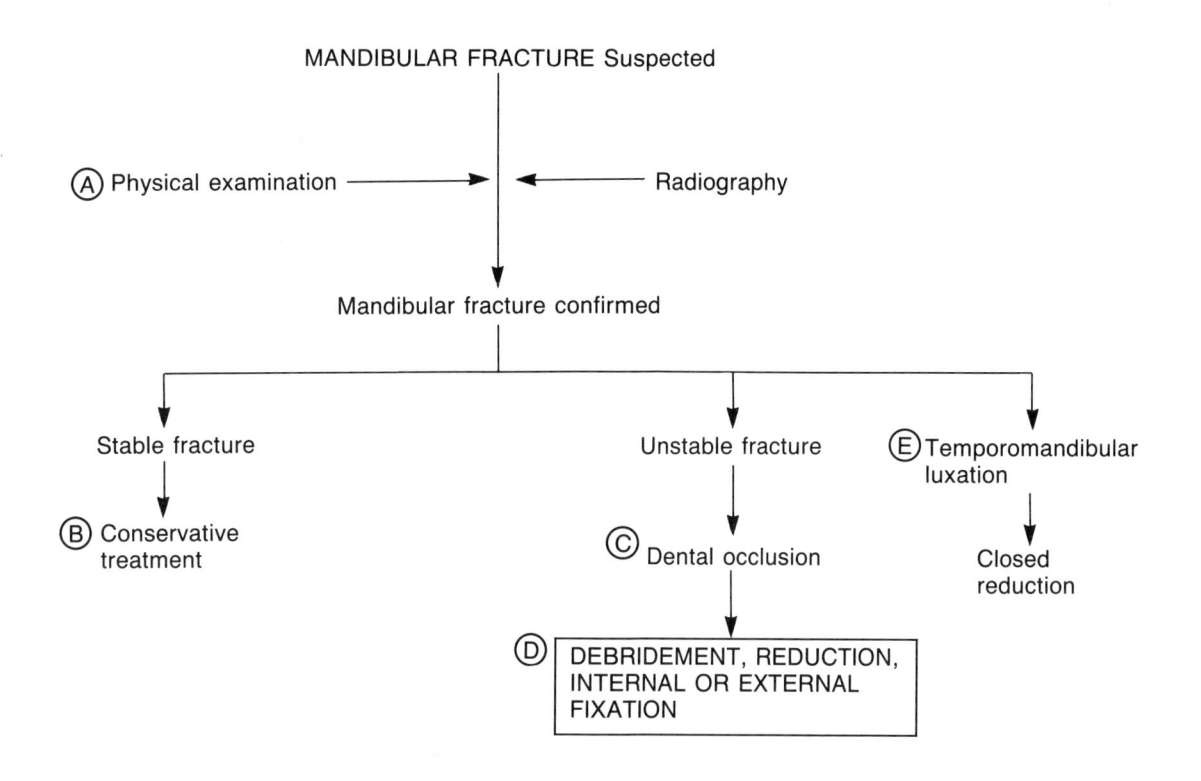

MANDIBULAR FRACTURE Suspected

(A) Physical examination → ← Radiography

↓

Mandibular fracture confirmed

- Stable fracture
  - (B) Conservative treatment
- Unstable fracture
  - (C) Dental occlusion
  - (D) **DEBRIDEMENT, REDUCTION, INTERNAL OR EXTERNAL FIXATION**
- (E) Temporomandibular luxation
  - Closed reduction

CONDITIONS OF THE MANDIBLE

Geoff Sumner-Smith

A. Initially, pain in the mandible is difficult to differentiate from pain within the mouth or from associated conditions of the temporomandibular joint (TMJ), but careful examination indicates the route to be taken. If the pain appears to originate from the bone and the oral cavity itself is normal, radiographs should be ordered. While the animal is sedated or anesthetized, a more detailed examination is undertaken.

B. Most dogs suffering from craniomandibular osteopathy (CMO) are presented with fever, depression, and pain associated with opening the mouth; differentiation of the condition from problems within the temporomandibular joint is necessary. Radiographs of the area typically display dense lesions within the bone. The condition can extend to the TMJ, causing bony fusion of that joint. Euthanasia is often elected, but if the animal retains some mobility of its joint, resolution usually occurs at the time of skeletal maturity.

C. Fistulas draining from the mandible may be the result of a sequestrum from a previous fracture or from an apical abscess of an adjacent tooth.

D. Changes in the consistency of the mandible bone may require a full biochemical profile as well as radiographs. The changes may be reversible with proper medication and dietary control or irreversible in cases of renal failure.

References

Alexander JW. Orthopaedic diseases. In: Slatter DH, ed. Textbook of small animal surgery. Philadelphia: WB Saunders, 1985:2312.

Cavanagh PG. Secondary renal hyperparathyroidism. In: Bojrab MJ, ed. Pathophysiology in small animal surgery. Philadelphia: Lea & Febiger, 1981:681.

Krock L. Nutritional secondary hyperparathyroidism in the dog. 18th Gaines Symposium, 1968:27.

CONDITIONS OF THE MANDIBLE

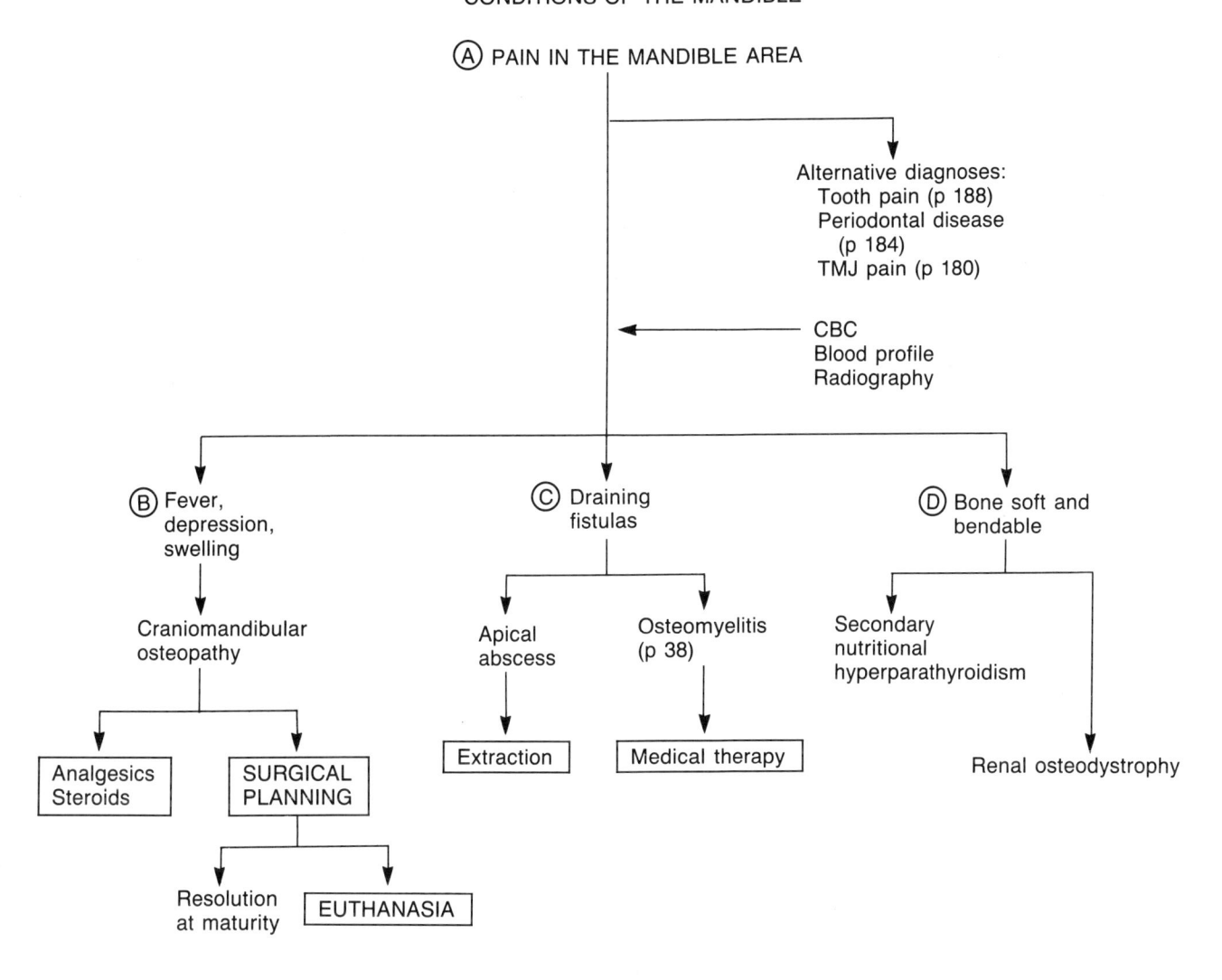

Ⓐ PAIN IN THE MANDIBLE AREA

→ Alternative diagnoses:
 Tooth pain (p 188)
 Periodontal disease (p 184)
 TMJ pain (p 180)

CBC
Blood profile
Radiography

Ⓑ Fever, depression, swelling
→ Craniomandibular osteopathy
 → Analgesics / Steroids
 → SURGICAL PLANNING
  → Resolution at maturity
  → EUTHANASIA

Ⓒ Draining fistulas
 → Apical abscess → Extraction
 → Osteomyelitis (p 38) → Medical therapy

Ⓓ Bone soft and bendable
 → Secondary nutritional hyperparathyroidism
 → Renal osteodystrophy

TEMPOROMANDIBULAR JOINT PAIN

Geoff Sumner-Smith

A. Spasm of the masseter muscles caused by various forms of myositis may well give the impression of a problem with the temporomandibular joint (TMJ). Muscle biopsy aids in differential diagnosis. The myositis may be degenerative, for which a poor prognosis must be given, or eosinophilic, which may respond to anti-inflammatory treatment.

B. Fracture of the joint is not common and, when it does occur, is usually subcondyloid. In the larger animal, internal fixation is possible, but exposure may require osteotomy of the zygomatic arch. Luxations may have a congenital component, i.e., shallowness of the temporomandibular joint predisposes to the condition.

C. If the animal opens its mouth to its full extent, displacement of the mandible laterally may cause the coracoid process to lock under the zygomatic arch. This may be the result of temporary neuropraxia of the mandibular branch of the trigeminal nerve. Most cases respond to loose muzzling for up to 3 weeks. Resection of the zygomatic arch is required if the condition persists (Fig.1).

D. The TMJ may cease to function and appear to be "locked" because of the intense pain that accompanies a retrobulbar abscess. Although protrusion of the eye is not always present, an apparent increase in intra-ocular pressure occurs caused by the retrobulbar swelling. Under anesthesia intrabulbar swelling is usually palpable via the mouth, and the abscess may be drained from that approach.

E. The early signs of tetanus in the dog may include pain on attempting to open the mouth; the condition progresses to an inability to open the mouth, and the rigidity extends to other muscle groups.

References

Robins GM. Dropped jaw - mandibular neuropraxia in the dog. J small Anim Pract 1976; 17:753.

Stewart WC et al. Temporomandibular subluxation in the dog. J small Anim Pract 1975; 16:345.

Thomas RE. Temporomandibular joint dysplasia and open mouth locking in a basset hound. J small Anim Pract 1979; 20:697.

Tomlinson J, Presnell KR. Mandibular condylectomy. Effect in normal dogs. Vet Surg 1983; 12:148.

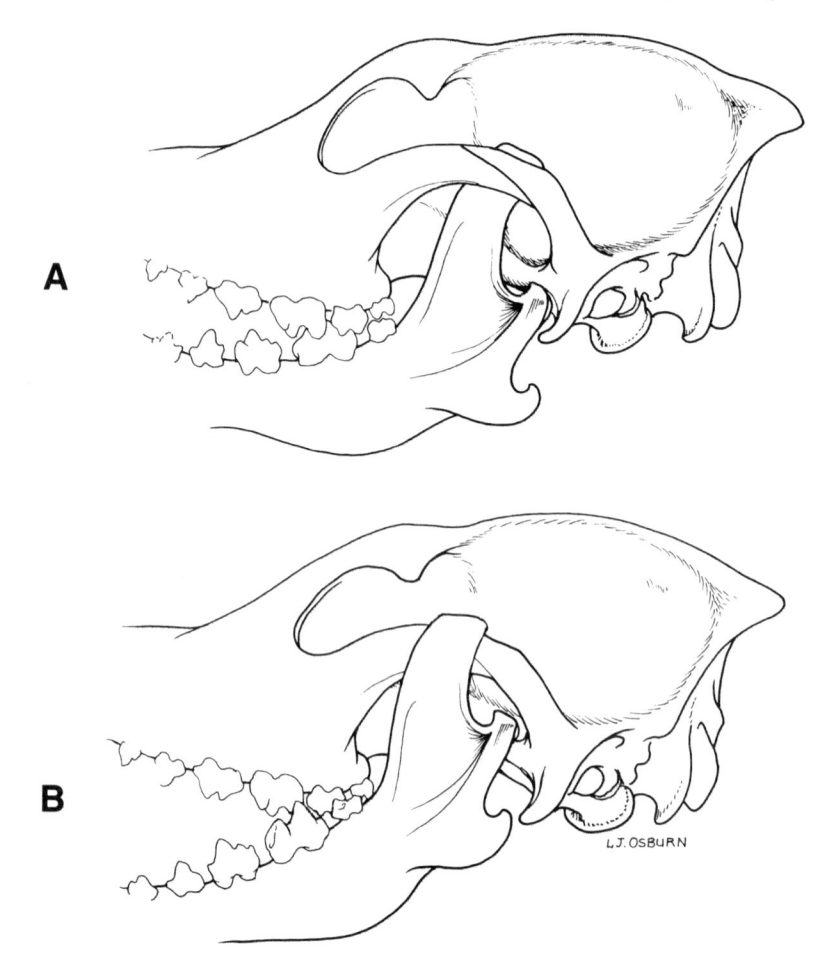

Figure 1 Diagrams displaying *A*, Normal position and *B*, positions of the mandible and the process following a major displacement laterally.

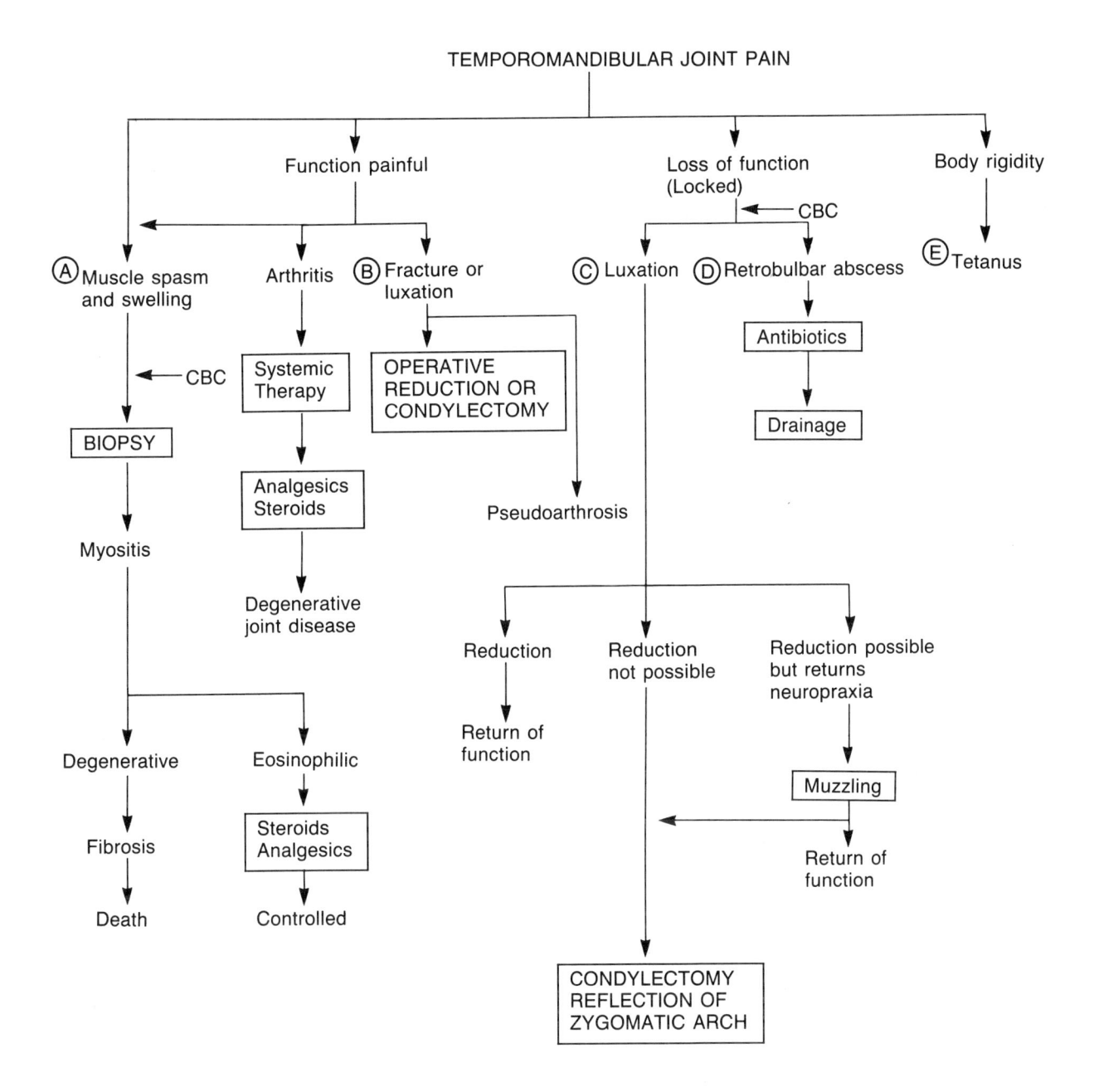

TEMPOROMANDIBULAR JOINT PAIN

- Function painful
  - Ⓐ Muscle spasm and swelling ← CBC
    - BIOPSY
    - Myositis
      - Degenerative
        - Fibrosis
        - Death
      - Eosinophilic
        - Steroids Analgesics
        - Controlled
  - Arthritis
    - Systemic Therapy
    - Analgesics Steroids
    - Degenerative joint disease
  - Ⓑ Fracture or luxation
    - OPERATIVE REDUCTION OR CONDYLECTOMY
- Loss of function (Locked) ← CBC
  - Ⓒ Luxation
    - Pseudoarthrosis
      - Reduction → Return of function
      - Reduction not possible
      - Reduction possible but returns neuropraxia
        - Muzzling → Return of function
    - CONDYLECTOMY REFLECTION OF ZYGOMATIC ARCH
  - Ⓓ Retrobulbar abscess
    - Antibiotics
    - Drainage
- Body rigidity
  - Ⓔ Tetanus

CONDITIONS OF GROWING TEETH

Geoff Sumner-Smith

Growing teeth may suffer from abnormal conditions that may result from abnormal eruption or are a sequel to normal eruption of either the deciduous or permanent dentition.

A. Abnormal eruption of the teeth may result in malocclusion (p 180) and is considered to be "normal" in some breeds, e.g., Bulldog, Pekinese, etc. Various abnormal forms of eruption may require treatment to ensure that the animal does not develop a painful oral condition or to improve the function of the teeth. Treatment should not be employed to correct abnormal occlusion that has no effect on the animal's health.

B. Loose deciduous teeth may adhere to the gingiva and turn to the transverse position. Deciduous teeth are commonly retained, particularly in the toy breeds; the canine teeth are most often involved in this situation. The retention of teeth may or may not have an effect on the eruption of subsequent local permanent teeth. Extraction of the retained teeth is recommended, particularly if the puppy has attained the age of 6 months and the teeth are still present. Impacted teeth are seen only rarely in dogs and require surgical exposure and realignment, provided that the retained teeth are radiographically normal. Otherwise, they should be extracted. Such impacted teeth may give the impression of oligodontia and may not cause the animal any distress. Diagnosis may only occur if the area is radiographed for some other reason.

C. According to the particular condition involved, surgical intervention may take various forms that range from extraction to resection of the surrounding gingiva and bone with associated orthodontic correction of the malalignment as the impacted tooth erupts.

D. The presence of supernumerary permanent teeth may vary from the presence of a single "extra" tooth to that of a total second set of teeth. Careful examination should confirm that the extra teeth are not retained deciduous elements. Surgical extraction should be carried out if the extra teeth cause problems, such as impaction of food and malalignment with kissing trauma to the tongue and buccal mucosa.

E. Hypoplasia of the enamel may be the result of embryonic edema of the pulp or hypoplasia of the enamel organ. Additionally, if the dog suffers a severe febrile illness during eruption of the teeth, particularly at 4 and 5 months of age when mineralization of the crowns is occurring, multiple enamel hypoplasia may occur with associated discoloration of the enamel and dentine. Treatment of enamel hypoplasia prevents further deterioration. Following proper grinding and preparation of the area, minor defects are treated with a filling using an amalgam or composite material (Fig. 1). However, these techniques should only be used in nonaggressive dogs and animals that are not inclined to chew everything in sight. More severe defects may be treated by flat filling or, if the owners are willing to go to the expense, by crowning. Severe hypoplasia of the canine teeth should be treated by amputation, followed by a flat filling.

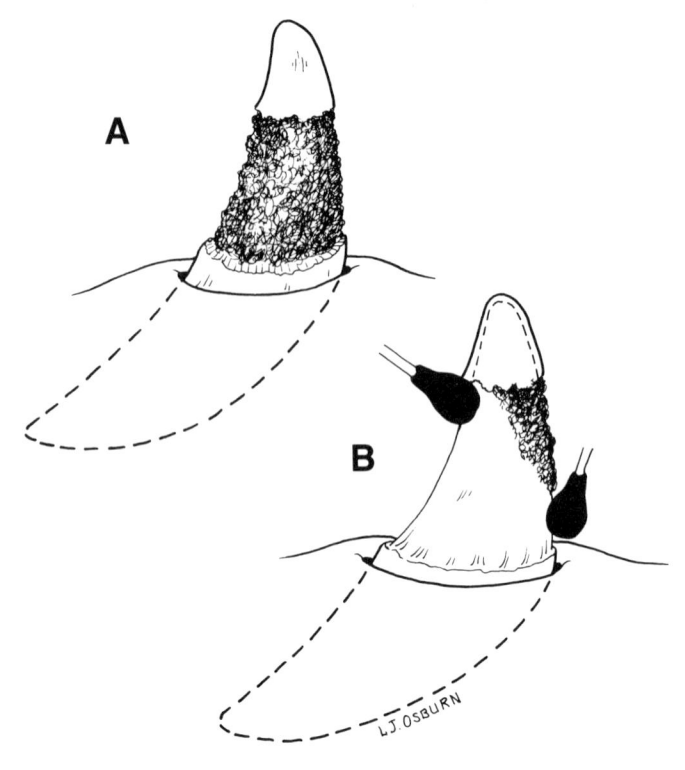

Figure 1 Enamel hypoplasia: *A*, The remaining enamel is removed. *B*, A shallow, circular, rounded groove is cut in the dental neck with a pear-shaped bur. (Redrawn after Eisenmengar E, Zetner K. Veterinary dentistry. Philadelphia: Lea & Febiger, 1985).

F. Normal eruption is usually followed by the formation of arcades of normal teeth. However, such normal teeth may be discolored a yellowish orange if the animal has received tetracycline medication during puppyhood. Apparently normal enamel may in fact be very thin, quickly developing a hypoplastic appearance, possibly caused by early malnutrition. Inflammation of the pulp capillary may result in a subsequent grey discoloration and later death of a tooth. Root canal therapy may be called for in such circumstances (p 188).

G. Neoplasia of teeth is not common in the canine patient; when it does occur it is usually teratoidal in origin.

H. Ameloblastoma behave as locally invasive malignant tumors by causing pressure atrophy of the surrounding soft tissue and bone with loosening and displacement of adjacent teeth. The condition may not be diagnosed until it is well advanced as proliferation is towards the oral cavity and is covered by ulcerating mucosa. Extraction of the teeth is necessary, and the operation should also include judicious resection of the surrounding bone to ensure all portions of the tumor have been removed.

I. Odontoma are tumors of the dental papilla and contain cement and enamel, whereas cementoma are tumors of the cement alone, which commence during the embryonic development of the tooth.

CONDITIONS OF GROWING TEETH

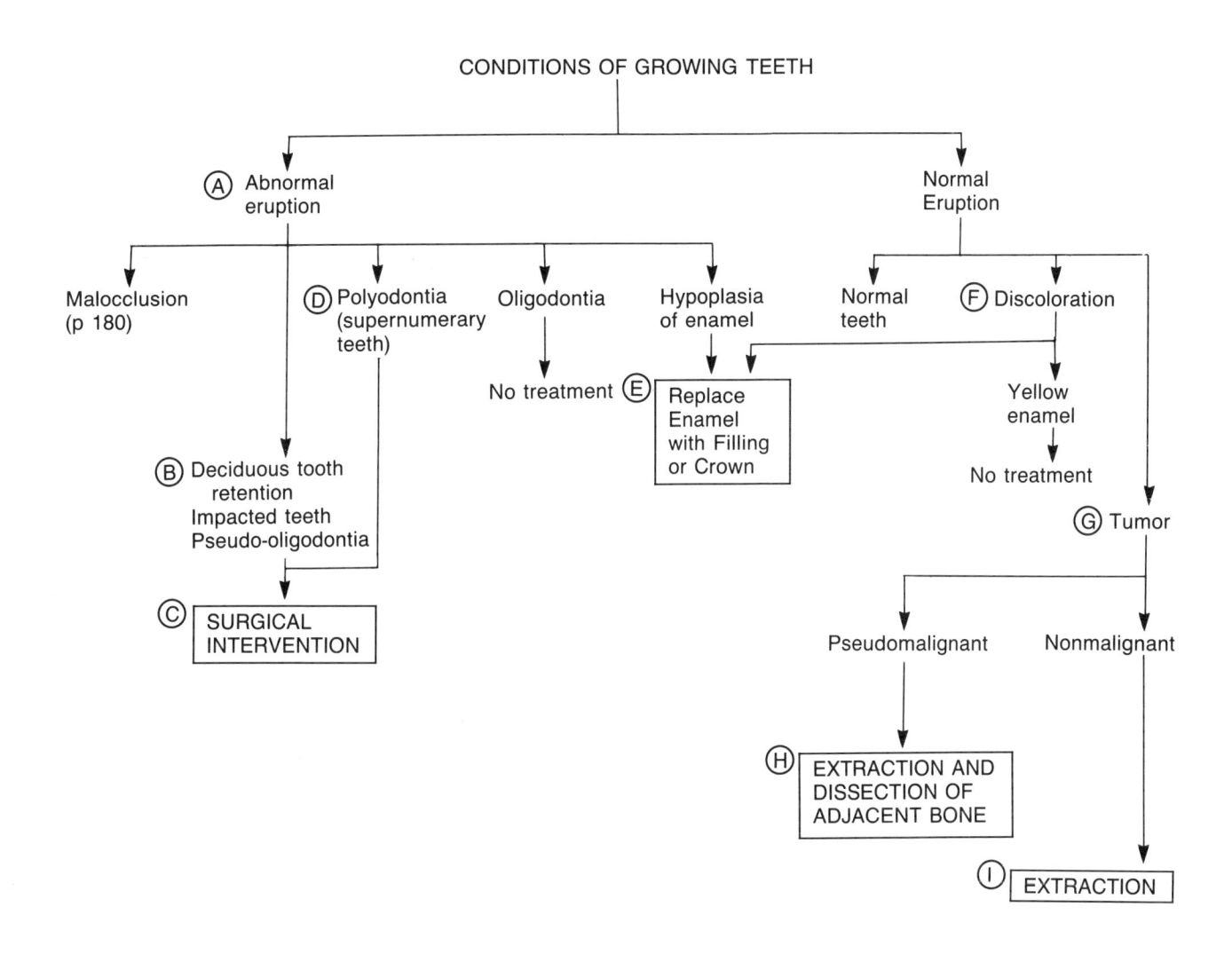

- (A) Abnormal eruption
  - Malocclusion (p 180)
  - (D) Polyodontia (supernumerary teeth)
    - (B) Deciduous tooth retention
      Impacted teeth
      Pseudo-oligodontia
      - (C) **SURGICAL INTERVENTION**
  - Oligodontia
    - No treatment
  - Hypoplasia of enamel
    - (E) **Replace Enamel with Filling or Crown**
- Normal Eruption
  - Normal teeth
  - (F) Discoloration
    - Yellow enamel
      - No treatment
    - (E) Replace Enamel with Filling or Crown
  - (G) Tumor
    - Pseudomalignant
      - (H) **EXTRACTION AND DISSECTION OF ADJACENT BONE**
    - Nonmalignant
      - (I) **EXTRACTION**

References

Eisenmenger E, Zetner K. Veterinary dentistry. Philadelphia: Lea & Febiger, 1985.

Harvey CE. Veterinary dentistry. Philadelphia: WB Saunders, 1985.

Tholen MA. Concepts in veterinary dentistry. Kansas: Veterinary Medicine Publication Co, 1983.

PERIODONTAL TISSUE DISEASE

Geoff Sumner-Smith

Although separate conditions, gingivitis and periodontitis, are described in this chapter, it should be appreciated that they often appear together in varying degrees caused by plaque build-up.

A. Inflamed gingiva are common in the dog. The condition may exist on its own or concomitantly with other conditions described in this chapter. The animal may not display any signs in the early stages, but as the condition rapidly progresses, halitosis develops. The gingiva become swollen and spongy. Usually correction of the diet, teeth cleaning, and antibiotic therapy ameliorate the condition.

B. If these measures fail to do so, this may indicate involvement of the deeper tissues, and more correctly, the condition should be termed periodontitis. Successful treatment then requires a gingivectomy and, in advanced cases, gingivoplasty. If the frenulum is hyperplastic, resection is required. Oral antiseptics are useful in reducing the bacterial flora once the tissue has been dealt with. Loose teeth may require extraction, but if they are only slightly loose, they should be left in place; following treatment they often restabilize. Primary periodontosis (degenerative periodontal disease) occurs occasionally in association with periodontitis. Apart from treating the periodontal disease, stabilization of the teeth is achieved by glass-fiber splinting.

C. Plaque is the build-up of food and debris around the teeth. *Bacteroides asaccarolyticus* and *Fusobacterium nucleatum* are especially important in the development of subsequent periodontal disease. Build-up is particularly apparent around the canine teeth. Early identification of and subsequent attention to plaque is facilitated by the use of plaque-disclosing agents, such as sodium flourescin, which adheres to the plaque and fluoresces a bright greenish yellow when illuminated by ultraviolet light.

D. If plaque is allowed to accumulate it becomes very thick and calcifies as tartar (calculus). Mechanical removal of the tartar is necessary as is attention to the adjacent gingiva, which is invariably inflamed. Chlorhexidine dental ointment is useful in reducing the bacterial flora; when applied to the gingival margins, its effect lasts up to 12 hours.

E. Overzealous use of an ultrasonic scale for mechanical removal of the tartar may cause etching of the teeth, which because of its roughened surface, predisposes to future plaque formation.

    Following removal of tartar from the exposed neck of a tooth or exposed portion of the root, the surface of the tooth should be smoothed by planing in order to delay tartar formation. Odontoplasty, removal of the enamel ridge around the margin of the neck, delays the collection of food debris within the furrow between the ridge and the gingiva, and the teeth are more readily self cleaned.

References

Barvasser P, Hill TJ. The effect of hard and soft diets on the gingival tissues of the dog. J Dent Res 1939; 18:389.

Egelberg J. Cellular elements in gingival pocket fluid. Acta Odont Scand 1963; 21:283.

Eisenmenger E, Zetner K. Veterinary dentistry. Philadelphia: Lea & Febiger, 1985.

Lindhe J et al. Influence of topical application of chlorhexidine on chronic gingivitis and gingival wound healing in the dog. Scand J Dent Res 1970; 78:471.

DISEASES OF THE PERIODONTAL TISSUE

- (A) Gingivitis
- (B) Periodontitis
- (C) Plaque
- (D) Tartar
- Swelling over tooth root → Neoplasia
- Swelling under eye → Tooth root abscess

Periodontitis → Antibiotic Pretreatment → Chemotherapy → Stabilization EXTRACTION

Plaque → Fluorescent staining

Tartar → MECHANICAL REMOVAL

Tooth root abscess → EXTRACTION Drainage

(E) MECHANICAL REMOVAL
ROOT PLANING
ODONTOPLASTY

GINGIVECTOMY
FRENECTOMY
GINGIVOPLASTY

MALOCCLUSION

Geoff Sumner-Smith

A. Congenital malocclusion is seen in specific breeds and is considered "normal" for these breeds, i.e., the prognathism of the Bulldog and Boxer. Treatment is not required unless the malocclusion causes malfunction of the mandible. Malocclusion in breeds that normally have good occlusion may be the result of an autosomal recessive gene inheritance pattern; such as prognathism in Long-haired Dachshunds. Extraction of individually displaced teeth is the usual method of treating the condition. If the malocclusion is not severe, wiring to reposition the teeth may be attempted. Alternatively, burring with associated filling of exposed dentine may make it possible to attain a satisfactory occlusion. Should the malocclusion be observed early in the development of the teeth, extraction of specific individual teeth prior to their eruption often permits the remaining teeth to grow into place without overcrowding.

B. Malocclusion following trauma results from a tooth or teeth being displaced. Extraction is a simple remedy to this form of malocclusion, but may not be acceptable to the owner, particularly if the animal is a show specimen. If the tooth itself is fractured, remaining displaced fragments should be removed. The remaining portion of the tooth is then filled or the crown may be built up, or in an extreme situation, a prosthesis manufactured and fitted in place.

C. Fracture of the supporting bone may take two forms, which are: (1) loss of support from alveolar fracture or (2) total fracture of the supporting bone (mandible, premaxilla, or maxilla). The determination of the severity of the fracture plays an important part in deciding upon the line of treatment to be followed. If the gingiva is still supporting the fragments of the alveolus and the tooth is still attached within the alveolus, replacement of the elements and wiring of the tooth to adjacent teeth often results in it reseating itself and becoming stable. It is essential to maintain the animal on a soft diet until the tooth is firm. Malocclusion caused by more extensive fractures of the supporting bone is dealt with on p 176. A careful assessment should be made before damaged teeth are extracted; too hasty a decision to extract may result in a loss of supporting elements needed to return the occlusion to normal or to support implants used to stabilize extensive fractures.

References

Grunberg H, Lea AJ. An inherited jaw anomaly in long-haired dachshunds. J Genet 1940; 39:285.

Leighton RL. Surgical correction of prognathous inferia in the dog. Vet Med Small Anim Clin 1977; 72:401.

Weigel JP, Dorn AS. Diseases of the jaw and abnormal occlusion. In: Harvey CF, ed. Veterinary dentistry. Philadelphia: Lea & Febiger, 1985:106.

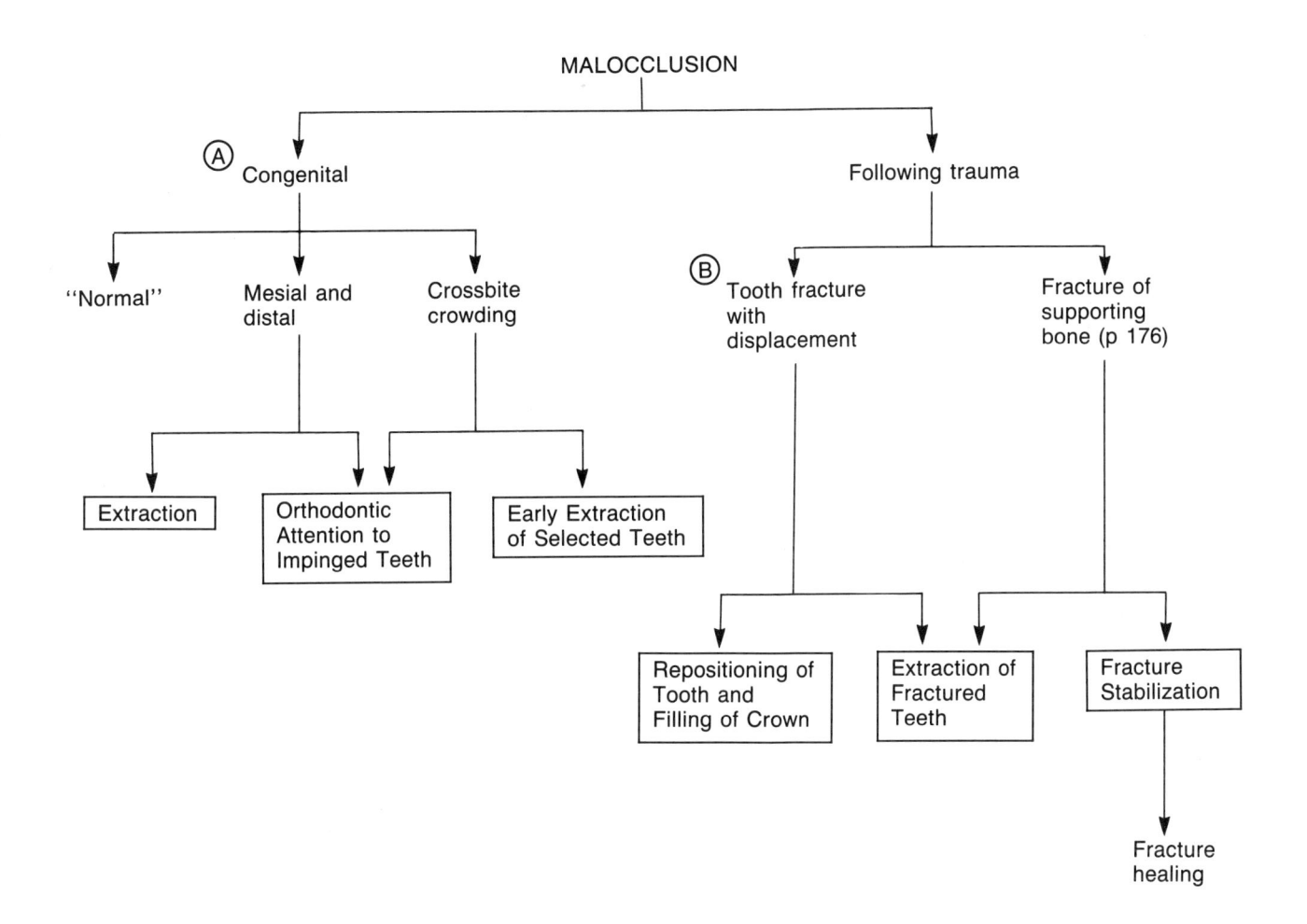

```
                          MALOCCLUSION
                               │
          ┌────────────────────┴────────────────────┐
        Ⓐ Congenital                          Following trauma
          │                                        │
    ┌─────┼─────┐                          Ⓑ ┌─────┴─────┐
"Normal"  │     │                     Tooth fracture   Fracture of
     Mesial and Crossbite             with             supporting
     distal     crowding              displacement     bone (p 176)
          │     │                          │                │
     ┌────┤     ├────┐                ┌────┴────┐      ┌────┴────┐
     ▼    ▼     ▼    ▼                ▼         ▼      ▼         ▼
┌─────────┐ ┌────────┐ ┌──────────┐ ┌──────────┐ ┌─────────┐ ┌──────────┐
│Extraction│ │Orthodontic│ │Early Extraction│ │Repositioning│ │Extraction│ │Fracture  │
└─────────┘ │Attention to│ │of Selected Teeth│ │of Tooth and │ │of Fractured│ │Stabilization│
            │Impinged Teeth│ └──────────┘    │Filling of Crown│ │Teeth    │ └──────────┘
            └────────┘                       └──────────┘   └─────────┘       │
                                                                              ▼
                                                                         Fracture
                                                                         healing
```

DISEASES OF THE TEETH

Geoff Sumner-Smith

In examining teeth a structured protocol sheet is helpful (Fig. 1).

A. Although not as commonly as in man, caries does occur in canine teeth. Approximately 4 percent of animals presented for dental work have caries in one or more teeth; the molars are most commonly involved, but caries of the neck of the canine teeth is also seen. Provided that a tooth is not loose, drilling and preparing a cavity, which is then lined and filled with amalgam, is preferable to extraction. If deemed necessary, a "visible" tooth may be filled with a composite that is the same color as the tooth.

ORAL EXAMINATION AND TREATMENT

General Medical Findings: _____
_____
_____

1. Habits: Bone chewing—Ball fetching—Rock chewing—Frisbee catching—Other

2. Nutrition: a. Staple diet (sugar content) _____
   b. Treats_____

3. Oral Cavity: a. Lips_____
   b. Cheeks: Mucosa _____
   c. Frenum: Supply _____ Information _____
   d. Palate: Shape _____ Mucosa _____
   e. Maxilla: Palpation _____
   f. Mandible: Palpation _____
   g. Tongue: Dorsum _____ Sides _____ Floor of mouth _____
   h. Lymph glands of head and neck _____

4. Occlusion: Correct _____ Discrepancies _____
   Missing teeth _____ Supernumerous teeth _____
   Retained teeth _____

5. Periodontic Findings
   a. Mucous membrane_____
   b. Gingiva: color _____ appearance _____ puffy _____
      knife-sharp edge _____ depth of pockets _____
      tooth mobility _____ bifurcation _____

Services Required

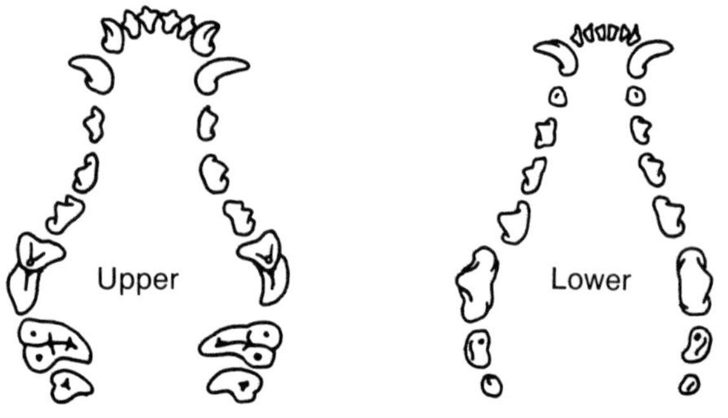

Upper   Lower

Use reverse side for continuation

Figure 1 Structural protocol sheet for examining canine teeth.

DISEASES OF THE TEETH

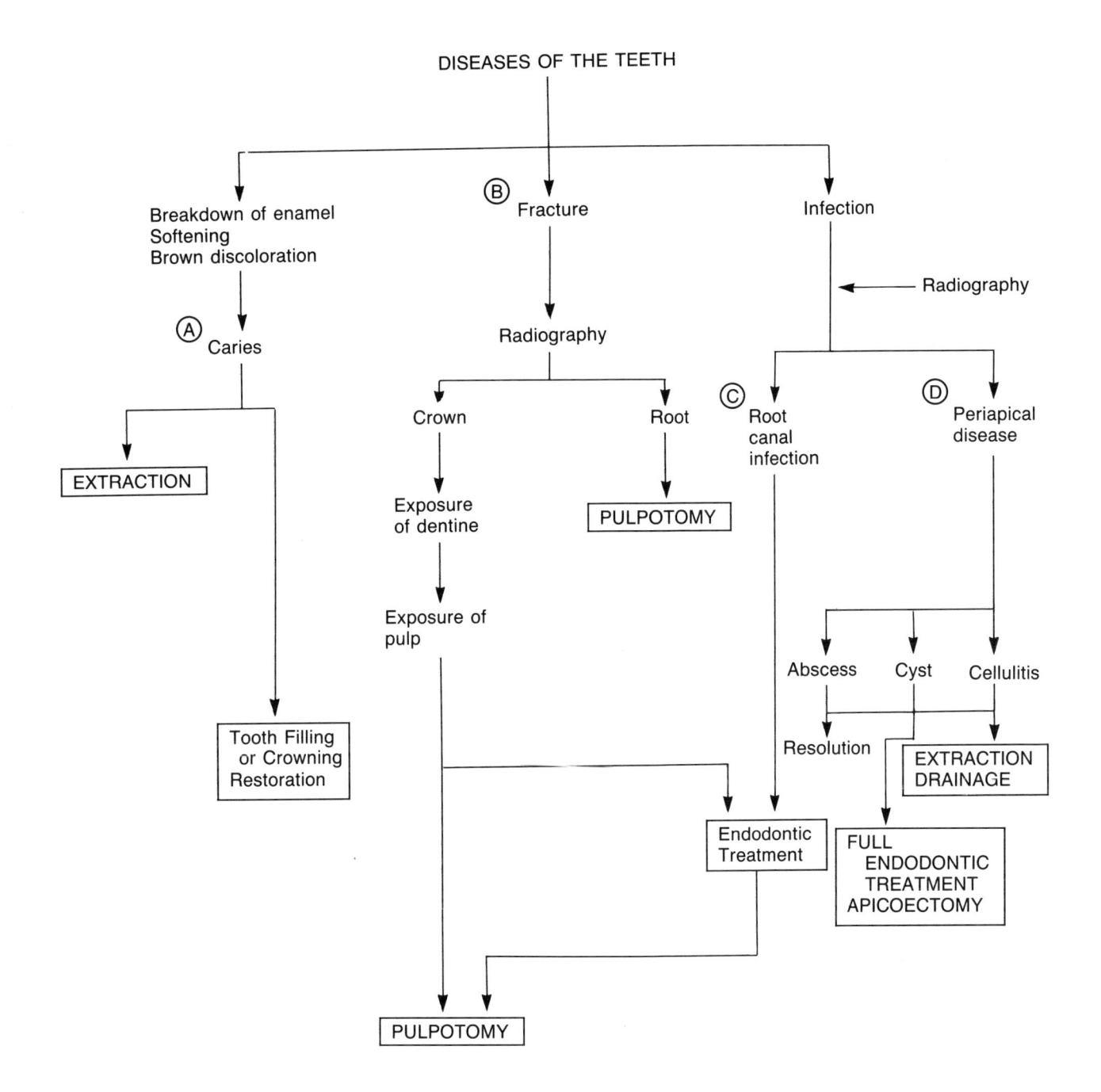

```
DISEASES OF THE TEETH
├── Breakdown of enamel / Softening / Brown discoloration
│      └── (A) Caries → EXTRACTION
│                    → Tooth Filling or Crowning Restoration
├── (B) Fracture → Radiography
│      ├── Crown → Exposure of dentine → Exposure of pulp → PULPOTOMY
│      └── Root → PULPOTOMY
└── Infection → Radiography
       ├── (C) Root canal infection → Endodontic Treatment
       └── (D) Periapical disease
              ├── Abscess → Resolution
              ├── Cyst → FULL ENDODONTIC TREATMENT / APICOECTOMY
              └── Cellulitis → EXTRACTION DRAINAGE
```

B. Fracture of the teeth is common and is either the result of a violent accident or of chewing on very hard objects. Depending on the damage that has been caused, the tooth may be extracted or repaired by orthodontic treatment. In dogs, crowns must be custom made and therefore are very expensive. Restoration is a more practical process, provided that the animal is not subsequently allowed to chew on hard materials.

C. Extensive caries, or tooth fracture with exposure of the pulp, results in infection that is beyond recovery. The exposed pulp cannot be covered by a restoration (amalgam or composite) as such material interferes with the blood supply and autolysis. If the animal is presented soon after exposure of the pulp has occurred, pulpotomy may be attempted; otherwise full endodontic therapy must be performed. Apicoectomy is recommended if it proves impossible to gain total access to the pulp cavity via the crown of the tooth.

D. Extension of infection in the periapical area of the tooth varies according to the site. It tends to limit itself to local swelling except in the case of the third upper premolar (malar) tooth, wherein infection may tract into the sinus. Extraction is usually followed by drainage and healing. Antibiotics should be used in all cases where infection is anticipated or is present.

References

Ross DL. Veterinary dentistry. In: Ettinger SJ, ed. Textbook of veterinary internal medicine. Philadelphia: WB Saunders, 1975.

Rossman LE, Garber DA, Harvey CF. Disorders of teeth. In: Harvey CF, ed. Veterinary dentistry. Philadelphia: Lea & Febiger, 1985.

BITE WOUNDS

Geoff Sumner-Smith

A. The history of the bite is not always available. Most fights occur when animals are left unattended, but if the history is known, it can have a marked bearing on the course of action that is subsequently followed. Tissue damage may be extensive, and the patient may be in critical shock. Stabilization of the animal's general condition is of first concern.

B. In acute cases thorough debridement of the wound, along with pressure lavage with either a solution of chlorhexidine or an iodine-containing solution, is strongly recommended. The regimen of treatment must then be determined by the extent of local tissue injury and the possibility of rabies infection. The latter is influenced by whether the aggressor is a wild carnivore, is unknown, or is a healthy domestic animal. If the aggressor is a domestic pet, the availability of an up-to-date vaccination history is relevant.

C. Contrary to the situation in human patients, chronic bite wounds are commonly presented for treatment; the canine patient may have suffered a bite sometime before it is either noticed or the animal returns home. An accumulation of pus must be released, and gentle irrigation of abscess is acceptable except in cases of cellulitis; wherein infection may be forced into fascial planes if the wound is irrigated. Drainage should be established and maintained.

D. Protection of the patient by a booster vaccine is advisable and, if the possibility of rabies is high, a full course is recommended. The long incubation period of rabies should be borne in mind. Positive cases have occurred more than 9 months following initial exposure.

E. Should the animal become ill, local, as well as State and Federal, health regulations should be followed. In most cases, euthanasia of a suspected rabies case is not permitted without the permission of the appropriate government officer. The responsibilities of a veterinary clinician to the general public who may have been exposed to the diseased animal must be remembered and, if deemed appropriate, the local Medical Officer of Health informed.

F. Primary closure of bite wounds is rarely desirable; in fact, penetrating wounds may even be held open for up to 12 to 24 hours. Drains should be used and closure delayed for 5 to 8 days. Ampicillin or penicillin are the drugs of choice as *Pasteuralla* is the most common organism involved. Once sensitivity test results are available a decision may be made whether to change to another drug.

References

Gross A, Cutright DE, Bhaskar SN. Effectiveness of pulsating water jet lavage in treatment of contaminated crush wounds. Am J Surg 1972; 124:373.

Howry B, Rodenheaver G, Versko J. Debridement—an essential component of traumatic wound care. Am J Vet Surg 1978; 135:278.

Neal TM, Key JC. Principles of treatment of dog bite wounds. JAAHA 1978; 12:657.

Rodenheaver GT, Bellamy W, Kody M. Bacterial activity and toxicity of iodine–containing solutions in wounds. Arch Surg 1982; 117:181.

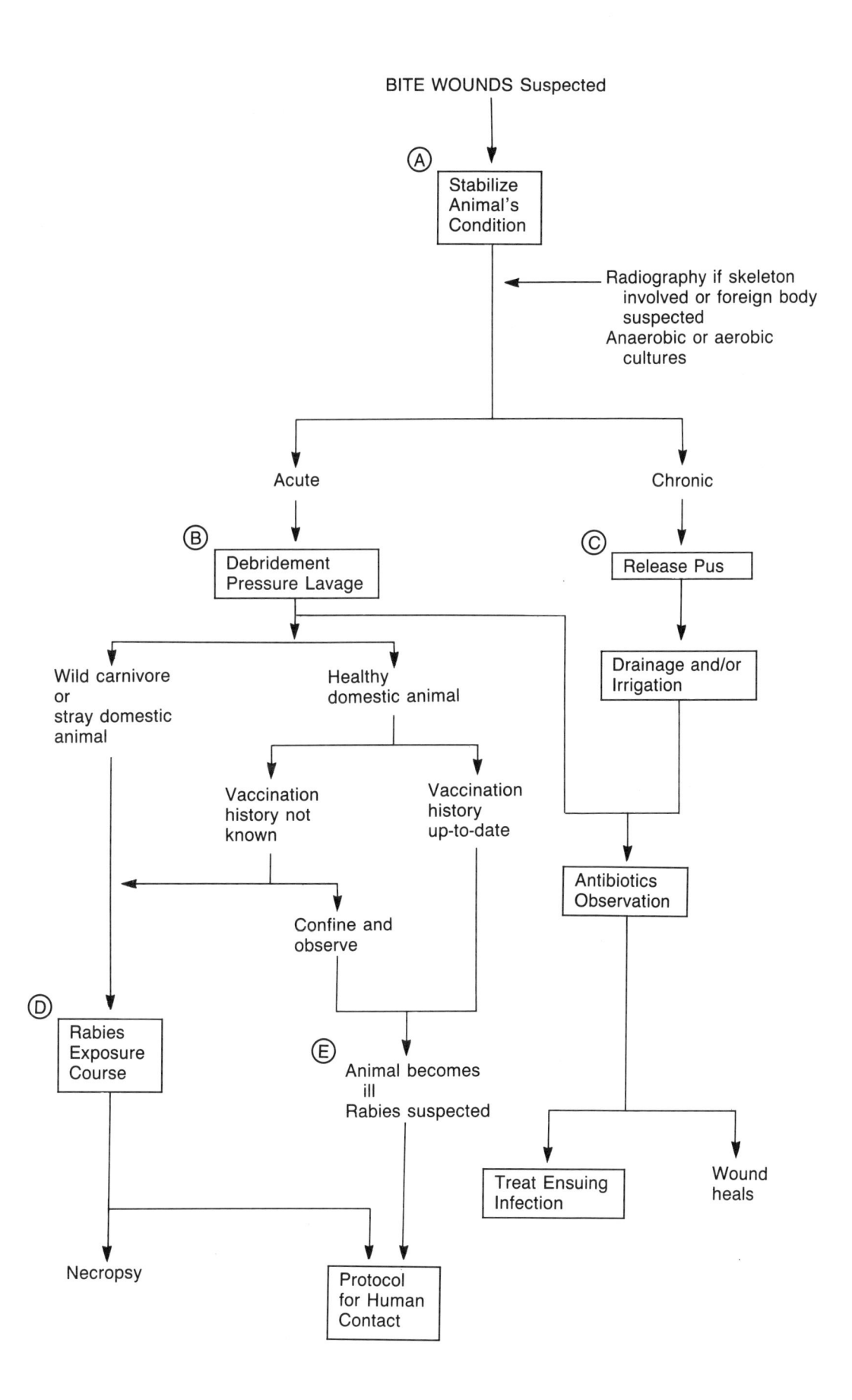

```
                    BITE WOUNDS Suspected
                              │
                              ▼
                        ┌───────────┐
                    (A) │ Stabilize │
                        │ Animal's  │
                        │ Condition │
                        └───────────┘
                              │
                              │  ← Radiography if skeleton
                              │    involved or foreign body
                              │    suspected
                              │    Anaerobic or aerobic
                              │    cultures
                      ┌───────┴───────┐
                      ▼               ▼
                    Acute          Chronic
                      │               │
                ┌─────────────┐   ┌──────────┐
            (B) │ Debridement │(C)│ Release  │
                │ Pressure    │   │ Pus      │
                │ Lavage      │   └──────────┘
                └─────────────┘         │
                      │                 ▼
         ┌────────────┴────────┐   ┌───────────────┐
         ▼                     ▼   │ Drainage and/or│
    Wild carnivore       Healthy   │ Irrigation    │
    or                   domestic  └───────────────┘
    stray domestic       animal            │
    animal                 │               │
                    ┌──────┴──────┐        │
                    ▼             ▼        │
               Vaccination    Vaccination  │
               history not    history      │
               known          up-to-date   │
                    │             │        │
                    │             ▼        │
                    │         Confine and  │
                    │         observe      │
                    │             │        ▼
         ┌──────────┐             │   ┌─────────────┐
     (D) │ Rabies   │             │   │ Antibiotics │
         │ Exposure │             │   │ Observation │
         │ Course   │         (E) │   └─────────────┘
         └──────────┘       Animal becomes   │
              │             ill              │
              │             Rabies suspected │
              ▼                   │     ┌────┴────┐
          Necropsy                │     ▼         ▼
                                  │  Treat    Wound
                              ┌───────────┐ Ensuing heals
                              │ Protocol  │ Infection
                              │ for Human │
                              │ Contact   │
                              └───────────┘
```

GUNSHOT WOUND TO THE LIMB

Geoff Sumner-Smith

In the rural setting, those breeds of dogs with the natural hunting instinct are often shot, either in error or by owners protecting their stock. In the urban setting, dogs may fall prey to people with sick minds who derive pleasure from the use of a gun on a moving target. The kinetic energy and therefore the wound potential of a missile vary with the square of its velocity. Low-velocity gun shots are defined as having a muzzle velocity of less than 600 to 700 m per second. Most civilian handguns and rifles, including 22-, 38-, 32-, 25-, and 45-caliber weapons, inflict low-velocity injuries. Only certain hunting and military rifles have muzzle velocities over 700 m per second, and they are classified as high-velocity weapons. In addition to the type of missile tract damage caused by a low-velocity bullet, a high-velocity bullet inflicts extensive wound cavitation and distant tissue necrosis. Depending on the missile involved, the fracture may, although multiple, be quite simple; alternatively the velocity may be such that the part of the bone impacted by the missile may totally explode.

A. Stabilization of the animal's general condition is of first concern. Emergency treatment includes wound attention, antibiotics, and radiography to assess bone damage.

B. The soft tissue damage from low-velocity rifles and handguns is minimal, and it is only by chance that the skeleton is injured. If the fragmentation is considerable, the bone fragments themselves further damage the tissue as they are split apart. The fracture should be stabilized as soon as the animal's general condition permits and the wound treated by local debridement and general care. The missile may or may not be still imbedded. If it is readily available it should be removed, but an extensive search should not be made. Subsequent deep wound infection may occur, but is not necessarily the rule.

C. If a joint has been traversed by the bullet, the consequences are more serious as lead intoxication may be a sequel to the bullet being bathed in synovial fluid. Additionally, if a fracture is compound to the joint, careful reconstruction of the articular surface with associated irrigation and drainage of the hemarthrosis is necessary in order to minimize the incidence of septic arthritis.

D. Occasionally animals are injured at close range by a shotgun and, in such circumstances, the result is similar to that produced by a high-velocity bullet. Debris and hair permeate the wound when the range is less than 10 m.

E. Once the patient has been stabilized, major debridement of soft tissue and devitalized bone is necessary. Repair of injured tendons and nerves should be delayed until infection is completely controlled. In order to properly debride and inspect all of the soft tissue damage, exploratory incisions may be necessary elsewhere in the limb.

F. Splinting of the limb should be undertaken as early as possible. Once the animal's condition permits, the application of an external fixator adds considerably to the stability of the bones and the ability of the clinician to treat the soft tissue wound. Early internal fixation is contraindicated as it may aid in the spread of infection. Once the latter has been controlled, internal fixation may be considered, but as primary union is not possible in such cases, continued use of a fixateur external should be considered.

G. Long-range shotgun injuries do not often result in serious damage to the skeleton, although they may be fatal to vital organs. A pellet may lodge in a joint and thereby require surgical attention. Occasionally pellets enter the spinal column via an intervertebral foramen with disastrous consequences to the spinal cord.

References

Chirife J, Scarmato G, Herszage L. Scientific basis for use of granulated sugar in treatment of infected wounds. Lancet 1982; 1:561.

Dilman R, Brook C, Lidskym M. Lead poisoning from gunshot wound. Am J Med 1979; 66:509.

Carr C, Stevenson C. The treatment of missile wounds of the extremities. Instructional Course Lectures of the American College of Orthopaedic Surgeons, 1954; 11:189.

Sumner-Smith G, Waters EH. The adjunctive use of methylmethacrylate bone cement with stabilization of multiple fracture. JAAHA 1976; 12:778.

Swaim SF. Etiology of skin trauma and defects. In: Swaim SF, ed. Surgery of traumatized skin: management and reconstruction in the dog and cat. Philadelphia: WB Saunders, 1980:55.

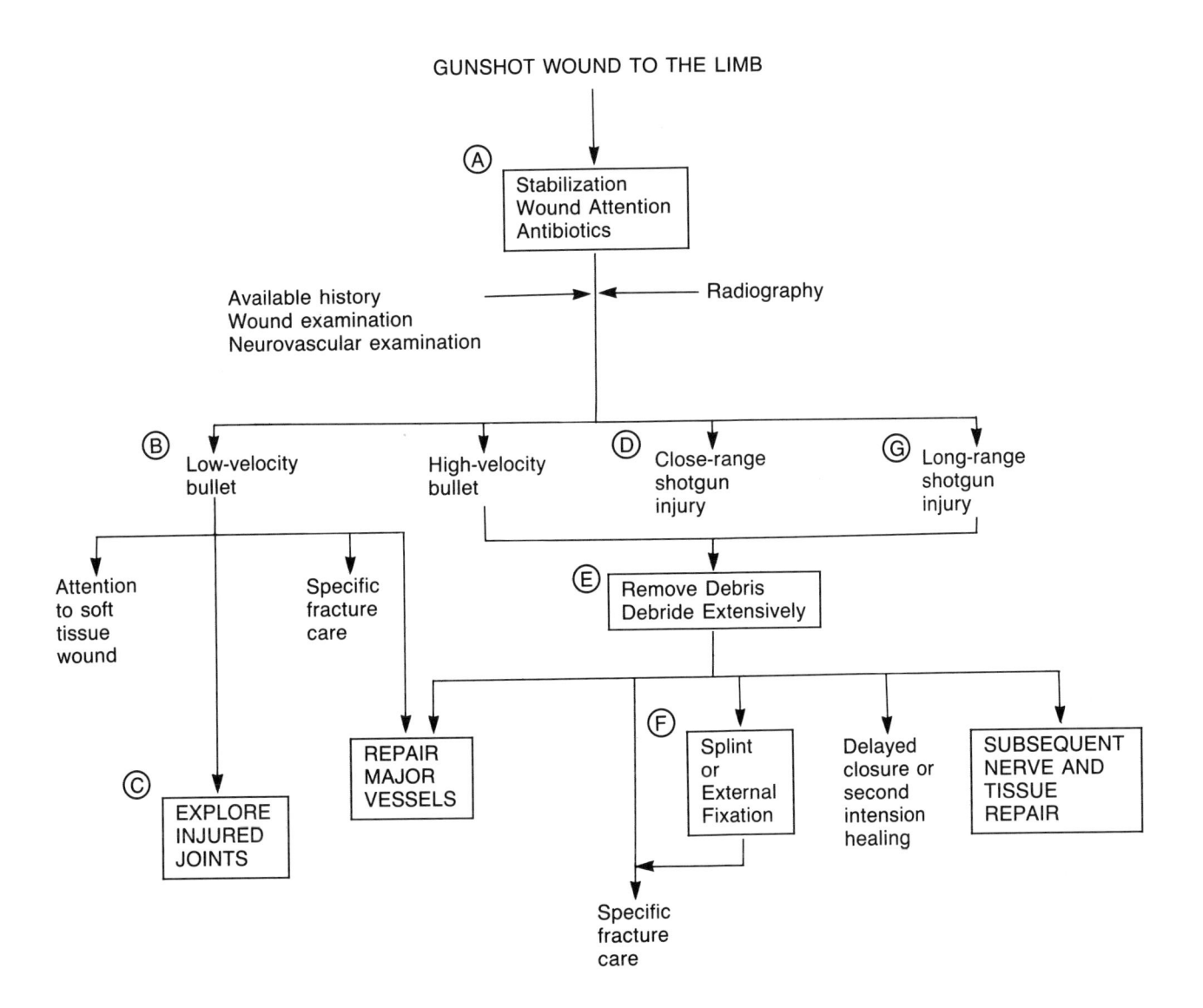

```
                    GUNSHOT WOUND TO THE LIMB
                                │
                                ▼
                      ┌──────────────────┐
                   Ⓐ  │ Stabilization    │
                      │ Wound Attention  │
                      │ Antibiotics      │
                      └──────────────────┘
                                │
     Available history  ───────►│◄─────── Radiography
     Wound examination          │
     Neurovascular examination  │
                                │
        ┌───────────────┬───────┴───────┬───────────────┐
     Ⓑ  ▼               ▼            Ⓓ ▼               ▼ Ⓖ
    Low-velocity   High-velocity   Close-range      Long-range
    bullet         bullet          shotgun          shotgun
                                   injury           injury
```

Low-velocity bullet			High/Close/Long-range

- Attention to soft tissue wound
- Ⓒ **EXPLORE INJURED JOINTS**
- Specific fracture care
- **REPAIR MAJOR VESSELS**
- Ⓔ **Remove Debris / Debride Extensively**
- Ⓕ Splint or External Fixation → Specific fracture care
- Delayed closure or second intension healing
- **SUBSEQUENT NERVE AND TISSUE REPAIR**

TENDON INJURY

Geoff Sumner-Smith

A. Injuries to flexor tendons may, on account of their close proximity, also involve injuries to neighboring vessels and nerves. An early assessment of nerve function is important in order that any injured nerves may receive attention at the same time as the tendons are treated. In examining the wounded area, careful attention to individual tendon function aids in assessing the severity of the injury. Animals require the return of tensile strength to injured tendons more than they require functional gliding; they do not perform finely controlled movements, but do exert sudden and violent loads, requiring a maximum possible strength of all tendons. The clinician involved in repair and treatment of tendon injuries should always bear these facts in mind.

B. A "clean" laceration usually results from a cut by a sharp object; the skin and tissues have not been torn, but have been cleanly incised, and there is minimal contamination. Repair by end-to-end anastomosis is possible up to 3 weeks after the injury, but the longer the delay, the greater the contraction of the attendant muscle belly and, hence, the greater the necessity for supporting stay sutures. The inclination not to treat individually severed single digital flexor tendons is inadvisable; this may well result in dorsal displacement of the toe with subsequent malwear of the toe pad and a lever effect on the elongated toenail. Repair to tendons requires meticulous patience; whenever possible, tendon sheaths should be closed separately. The pattern of sutures employed is more important than the actual material (Fig. 1).

C. An "untidy" laceration has the appearance of contusion and prevents primary closure of the wound. The wound should be considered contaminated and treated accordingly (p 196). Commonly the patient is presented many hours after the injury, and in such cases, even if the skin edges are relatively cleanly cut, the area should be considered "untidy" and treated as such prior to attempting delayed primary repair.

D. Judicious debridement and care of untidy wounds may well make it possible to repair the tendons by end-to-end anastomosis; with subsequent split support, the long-term prognosis can be quite good.

E. When there has been substantial loss of tendon, there is inadequate tissue coverage, and primary repair is not possible. Although some animals may function reasonably well following granulation tissue ingrowth, there is always a strong possibility of poor function and extension of related joints. Consequently tendon reconstruction is recommended—either by grafting, by a flap, or by implanting a prosthetic tendon.

F. Midsubstance rupture is occasionally seen in the athletic individual. More commonly the tendon is partially ruptured, and the animal is said to have "broken down". Splint support is the method of choice in treating such injuries and an exercise regimen is of paramount importance.

G. Tendons of origin or insertion are commonly involved in avulsion injuries. Such injuries may be of three types: (1) rupture of the tendon from its insertion into the bone, (2) avulsion of fractures, and (3) avulsion of small pieces of bone with the tendon. The two latter conditions are dealt with in the appropriate chapters. The normally-encountered avulsion injuries are of the tendon of origin of the long digital extensor, of the origin of the popliteus muscle, of the head of the lateral or medial gastrocnemius muscle, of the origin of the biceps tendon, or of the gastrocnemium tendon from the tuber calcanei. Repair of all of the above injuries requires the use of specific suture patterns to reattach the tendon by employing the tension band principle. Whichever method is employed to treat tendon injuries, support by splintage is important. The removal of the support should be gradual and not commenced until at least 6 weeks post repair. Careful exercise and physiotherapy should be introduced gradually.

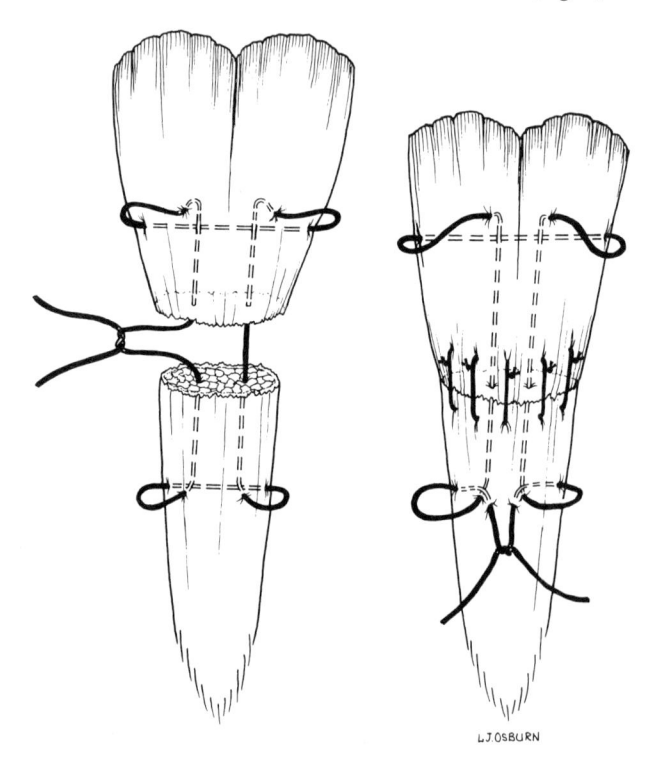

Figure 1 Suture pattern for tendon repair (modified Kessler).

References

Bernhart MA. Superficial digital flexor tendon injuries in the dog. Can Vet J 1977; 18:105.

Bloom M. Muscle and tendons. In: Slatter DH, ed. Textbook of small animal surgery. Philadelphia: WB Saunders, 1985; 2331.

Borne LC, Edward GB. The use of carbon fiber (Grafil) for tendon repair in animals. Vet Rec 1978; 102:287.

Hickman J. Greyhound injuries. J small Anim Pract 1975; 16:455.

Vaughan LC. Tendon injuries in dogs. Calif Vet 1980; 34:15.

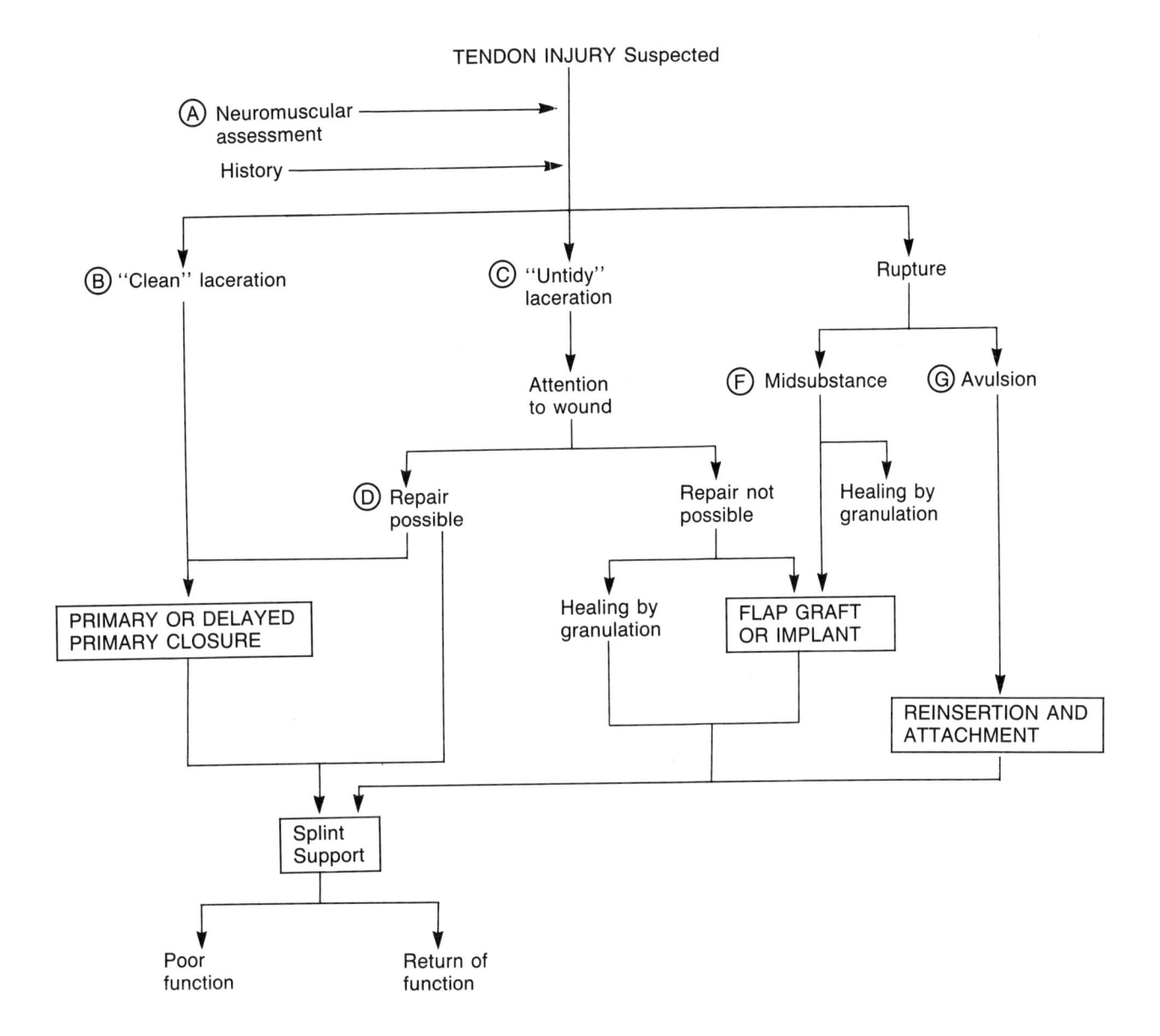

```
                    TENDON INJURY Suspected
                              │
    Ⓐ Neuromuscular ──────────→│
       assessment              │
       History ───────────────→│
                              │
        ┌─────────────────────┼─────────────────────┐
        ↓                     ↓                     ↓
   Ⓑ "Clean" laceration  Ⓒ "Untidy"            Rupture
                           laceration              │
                              │              ┌─────┴─────┐
                              ↓              ↓           ↓
                         Attention       Ⓕ Midsubstance  Ⓖ Avulsion
                         to wound            │
                              │         ┌────┴────┐
                    ┌─────────┴─────┐   │    Healing by
                    ↓               ↓   │    granulation
               Ⓓ Repair        Repair not│
                 possible      possible  │
                    │           ┌────┴───┐│
        ┌───────────┘           ↓        ↓↓
        ↓                   Healing by  FLAP GRAFT
   PRIMARY OR DELAYED      granulation  OR IMPLANT
   PRIMARY CLOSURE              │           │
        │                       │           │      REINSERTION AND
        │                       │           │      ATTACHMENT
        │                       │           │           │
        └───────┬───────────────┴───────────┘           │
                ↓                                       │
            Splint  ←──────────────────────────────────┘
            Support
              │
        ┌─────┴─────┐
        ↓           ↓
      Poor       Return of
      function   function
```

THE SEVERELY INJURED PATIENT: PART I

Geoff Sumner-Smith

A. No matter what emergency measures are instituted, the patient will die if the airway is blocked. If the obstruction is deeper in the pulmonary tree, a crisis may not emerge, as only a portion of the lung collapses. However, with obstruction of the larynx, trachea, or bronchial division, emergency surgery is required if the foreign material cannot be dislodged by upending the patient. As the spinal column may be injured, care should be exercised in this dislodging procedure.

B. In all cases of severe trauma, the thorax must be radiographed. Paradoxical breathing occurs as the result of flail-type segmental damage to the chest wall. One part of the rib cage moves in the opposite direction from the rest of the chest, being drawn in when the rest expands and expanding when the rest is drawn in. Temporary stabilization of the area may be supplied by means of a supporting bandage. Chest splinting should be followed by intermittent positive-pressure ventilation in order to avoid pneumonia.

C. Air within the pleural cavity restricts expansion of the lungs and heart. It gains entrance either via a wound in the chest wall or via a breakdown in the lung parenchyma. The soft tissue acts as a one-way valve, and relief of the situation requires the establishment of a one-way valve system in the other direction (Heimlich or underwater).

D. Immediately following the establishment of aeration, an intravenous access should be established and fluids administered at a fast rate. If there has been severe blood loss, whole blood administration via a separate venous access is necessary. If the venous pressure is low, a cutdown to the vein may be necessary to place the catheter.

E. In order to maintain vascular tone, adequate analgesia must be produced; reduce and immobilize all fractures as quickly as possible. The administration of intravenous steroids may be commenced in order to combat adrenocortical insufficiency, provided that other causes of shock have been excluded. Specific treatment is required for toxicemic and septic shock, which may not occur at the immediate time of injury. *The routine administration of corticosteroids to the severely injured patient is still equivocal.*

F. Heart failure is not a common finding in the acutely injured patient unless preexisting heart disease is present. In this case, the additional insult of a low BP may bring about inadequate myocardial oxygenation with resulting cardiac arrest.

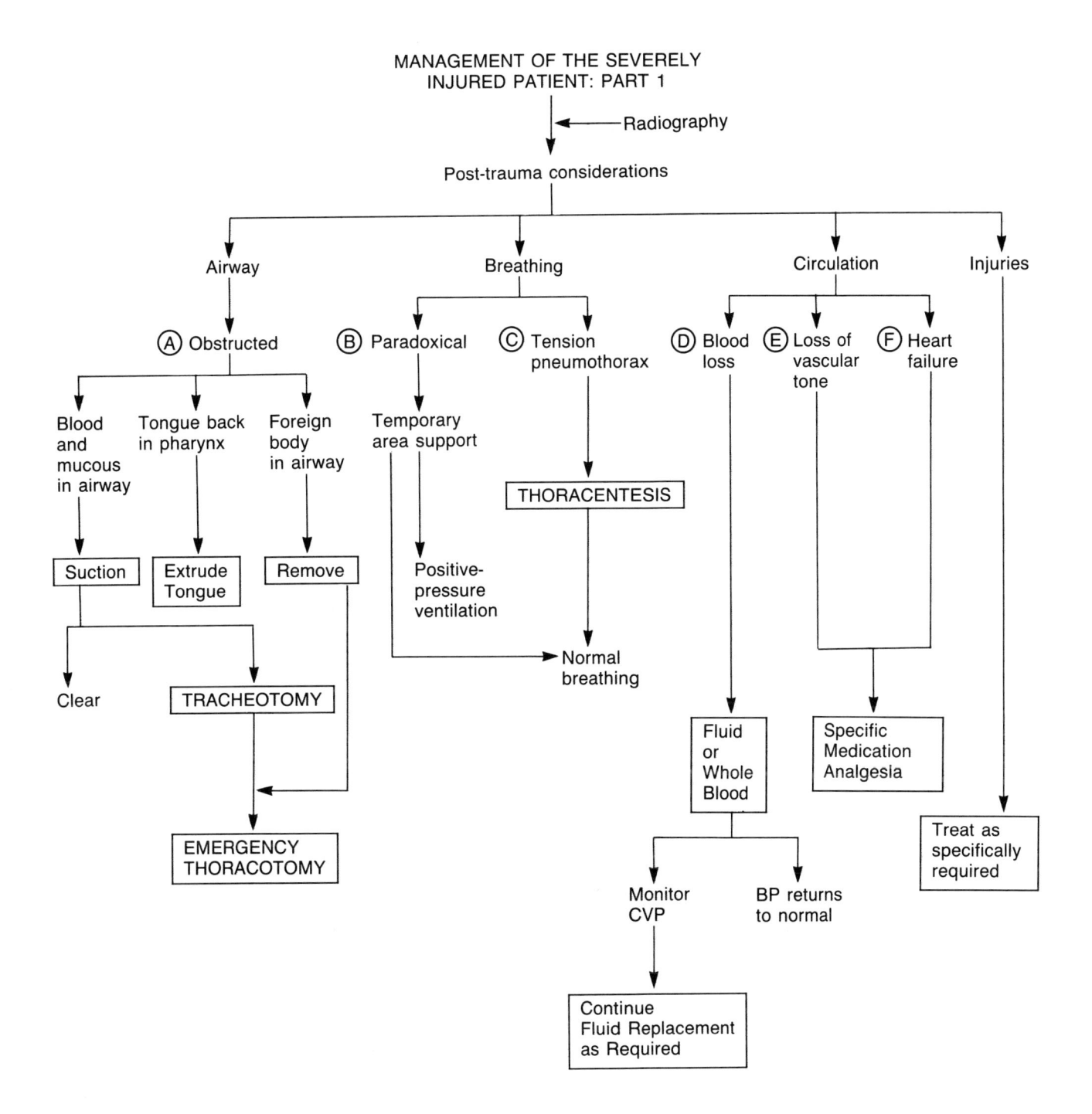

MANAGEMENT OF THE SEVERELY INJURED PATIENT: PART 1

Radiography → Post-trauma considerations

Airway

- **(A) Obstructed**
  - Blood and mucous in airway → Suction → Clear
  - Tongue back in pharynx → Extrude Tongue → TRACHEOTOMY
  - Foreign body in airway → Remove → TRACHEOTOMY
  - → EMERGENCY THORACOTOMY

Breathing

- **(B) Paradoxical** → Temporary area support → Positive-pressure ventilation → Normal breathing
- **(C) Tension pneumothorax** → THORACENTESIS → Normal breathing

Circulation

- **(D) Blood loss** → Fluid or Whole Blood
  - Monitor CVP → Continue Fluid Replacement as Required
  - BP returns to normal
- **(E) Loss of vascular tone** → Specific Medication Analgesia
- **(F) Heart failure** → Specific Medication Analgesia

Injuries

→ Treat as specifically required

197

THE SEVERELY INJURED PATIENT: PART II

Geoff Sumner-Smith

A. When there has been a history of an injury to the head, or if the animal has been unconscious, the skull should be radiographed. Intensive monitoring is required as the animal's condition can change very rapidly; carry out a physical examination and assessment at frequent intervals. Deterioration of the animal's condition may precipitate emergency decompression surgery. Supportive medical therapy is essential and may take the form of diuretics, steroids, and antibiotics. *Good nursing care is essential.*

B. The results of trauma to the spine may be apparent on presentation, but signs may worsen if there is a slow hemorrhage within the elements of the spinal cord. Deteriorating signs also necessitate surgical decompression (p 170).

C. Hemorrhage into the abdominal cavity may be slow and insidious. As such it may prove to be extremely dangerous, not being recognized until the patient is in critical collapse. Injuries to the skeleton, because they are often more obvious, may take precedence in the mind of the clinician, and important deficiencies in the circulation may be overlooked. Tapping both the thorax and the abdomen is a valuable procedure in order to determine whether or not hemorrhage is occurring.

References

Archibald J, Holt JC, Sokolovsky V, Catcot E, eds. Management of trauma in dogs and cats. Santa Barbara: American Veterinary Publishing, 1981.

Brasmer TH. Shock: basic pathophysiology and treatment. Vet Clin North Am 1972; 2:219.

Levy MN. The cardiovascular physiology of the critically ill patient. Surg Clin North Am 1975; 55:483.

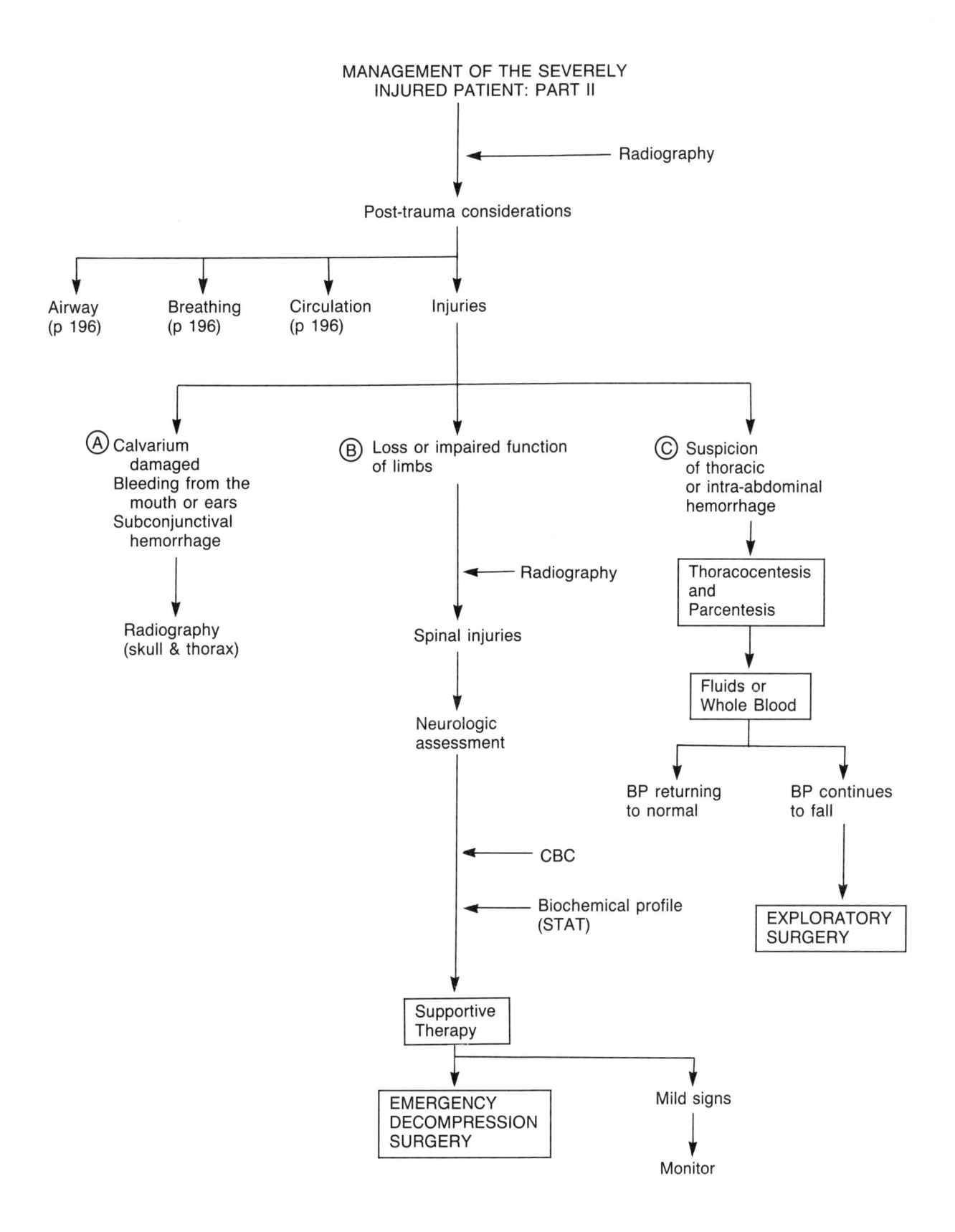

MANAGEMENT OF THE SEVERELY INJURED PATIENT: PART II

Radiography → Post-trauma considerations

Post-trauma considerations branches into:
- Airway (p 196)
- Breathing (p 196)
- Circulation (p 196)
- Injuries

Injuries branches into:

Ⓐ Calvarium damaged / Bleeding from the mouth or ears / Subconjunctival hemorrhage → Radiography (skull & thorax)

Ⓑ Loss or impaired function of limbs → (Radiography) → Spinal injuries → Neurologic assessment → (CBC) → (Biochemical profile (STAT)) → Supportive Therapy → **EMERGENCY DECOMPRESSION SURGERY** / Mild signs → Monitor

Ⓒ Suspicion of thoracic or intra-abdominal hemorrhage → Thoracocentesis and Parcentesis → Fluids or Whole Blood →
- BP returning to normal
- BP continues to fall → **EXPLORATORY SURGERY**

199

Appendix I Clinical Pathology of Synovial Fluid

TABLE 1 Synovial Fluid Changes in Various Types of Canine Arthritis

Condition	Appearance	Nucleated Cells/ml	Differential % Mononuclears	Differential % Neutrophils	Mucin Clot	Ig and C3 Inclusions	Synovial Cells
	Clear Translucent	0 to 2,900 (430)	88 to 100 (98) same proportions as peripheral blood	0 to 12 (2) same proportions as peripheral blood	normal 1	Absent	(−)
Degenerative Degenerative	Cloudy yellow to red	0 to 3,470 (990)	88 to 100 (96) lymphocytes vary in size—monocytes large and vacuolated	0 to 12 (4) nontoxic hypersegmented	Normal 1 to fair 2	Absent	(+)
Erosive Rheumatoid-like	Clear to turbid	3,000 to 38,000 (13,600)	20 to 80 (45) lymphocytes vary in size—Monocytes increase with chronicity and are vacuolated	20 to 80 (55) moderate toxic change, pyknotic	Poor 3	Present	(+++) in papillary clumps
Nonerosive Lupus erythematosus-like	Clear to turbid	4,000 to 371,000 (66,300)	5 to 58 (27) lymphocytes variable and reactive	15 to 95 (73) moderate toxic change, pyknotic	Fair 2 to poor 3	Absent to rare	(++)
Septic	Flocculent to pale yellow	110,000 to 267,000 (173,560)	1 to 10 (4) reactive chromatin rimming, toxic vacuolations	90 to 99 (96) marked cytoplasmic vacuolation and karyolysis	Very poor 4	Not tested	(+) to (++)
Traumatic	Clear to red	5,000 to 24,000 (7,200)	10 to 30 (14)	70 to 90 (86)	Normal 1 to fair 2	Not tested	(+)

The chart is derived from the work of Drs. D.C. Sawyer, E.O. Valli, N.C. Pederson, J.B. Miller, et al.

Appendix II Growth Plate Closure

TABLE 1 Variation in Ages of Growth Plate Fusion in the Dog

	Forelimb			Hind limb	
	Earliest Fused	Latest Unfused		Earliest Fused	Latest Unfused
Scapular tuberosity	12w*	5m	Great trochanter	6m	9m
Proximal humerus	10m*	10m	Proximal femur	6m	9m
Distal humerus	5m	8m	Lesser trochanter	9m	10m
Proximal ulna	5m	8m	Distal femur	6m	8m
Proximal radius	6m	9m	Proximal tibia	6m	11m
Distal radius	6m	9m	Proximal fibula	6m	10m
Distal ulna	6m	8m	Distal tibia	5m	8m
Accessory carpal	10w	5m	Distal fibula	5m	8m
Metacarpal	5m	7m	Tuber calcis	11w	7m
Proximal phalanx	16w	5m	Metatarsal	5m	7m
Middle phalanx	16w	5m	Proximal phalanx	16w	7m
			Middle phalanx	16w	5m

* w = weeks, m = months
G. Sumner-Smith. Growth plate fusion in the appendicular skeleton of the dog. Fellowship Thesis. R.C.V.S. London, 1964.

Appendix III

Radiologic observations in growth plate closure in the dog. (Redrawn with permission: Smith RN. Radiological observations on the limbs of young greyhounds. J small Anim Pract 1961; 1:84.)

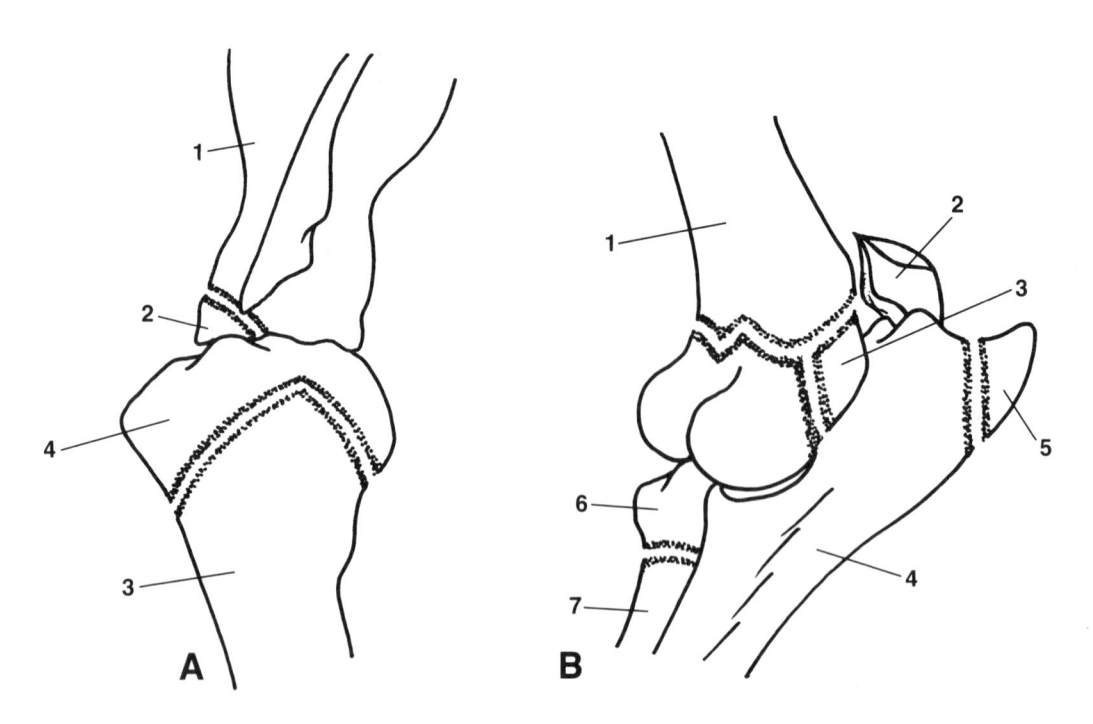

In tracings of radiographs of paws, only one digit is shown.

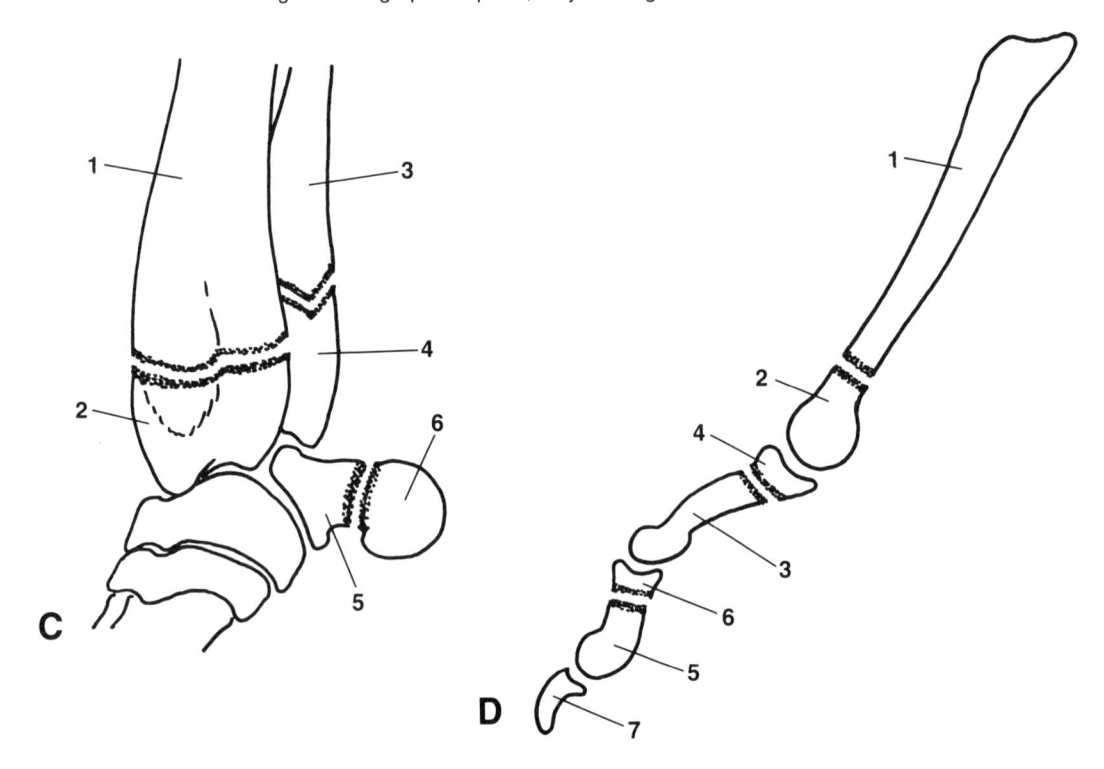

Figure 1 TRACINGS OF RADIOGRAPHS AT 3 MONTHS are as follows—*A*, Lateral view of shoulder: 1, scapula; 2, epiphysis for scapular tubercle; 3, humerus, diaphysis (shaft); and 4, humerus, proximal epiphysis; *B*, Lateral view of elbow: 1, humerus, diaphysis; 2, humerus, medial epicondyle; 3, humerus, distal epiphysis; 4, ulna, diaphysis; 5, ulna, proximal epiphysis; 6, radius, diaphysis; and 7, radius, proximal epiphysis; *C*, Lateral view of carpus: 1, radius, diaphysis; 2, radius, distal epiphysis; 3, ulna, diaphysis; 4, ulna, distal epiphysis; 5, accessory carpal bone (pisiform), body; and 6, accessory carpal bone, epiphysis; *D*, Lateral view of forepaw: 1, metacarpal, diaphysis; 2, metacarpal, epiphysis; 3, first phalanx, diaphysis; 4, first phalanx, epiphysis; 5, second phalanx, diaphysis; 6, second phalanx, epiphysis; and 7, third phalanx.

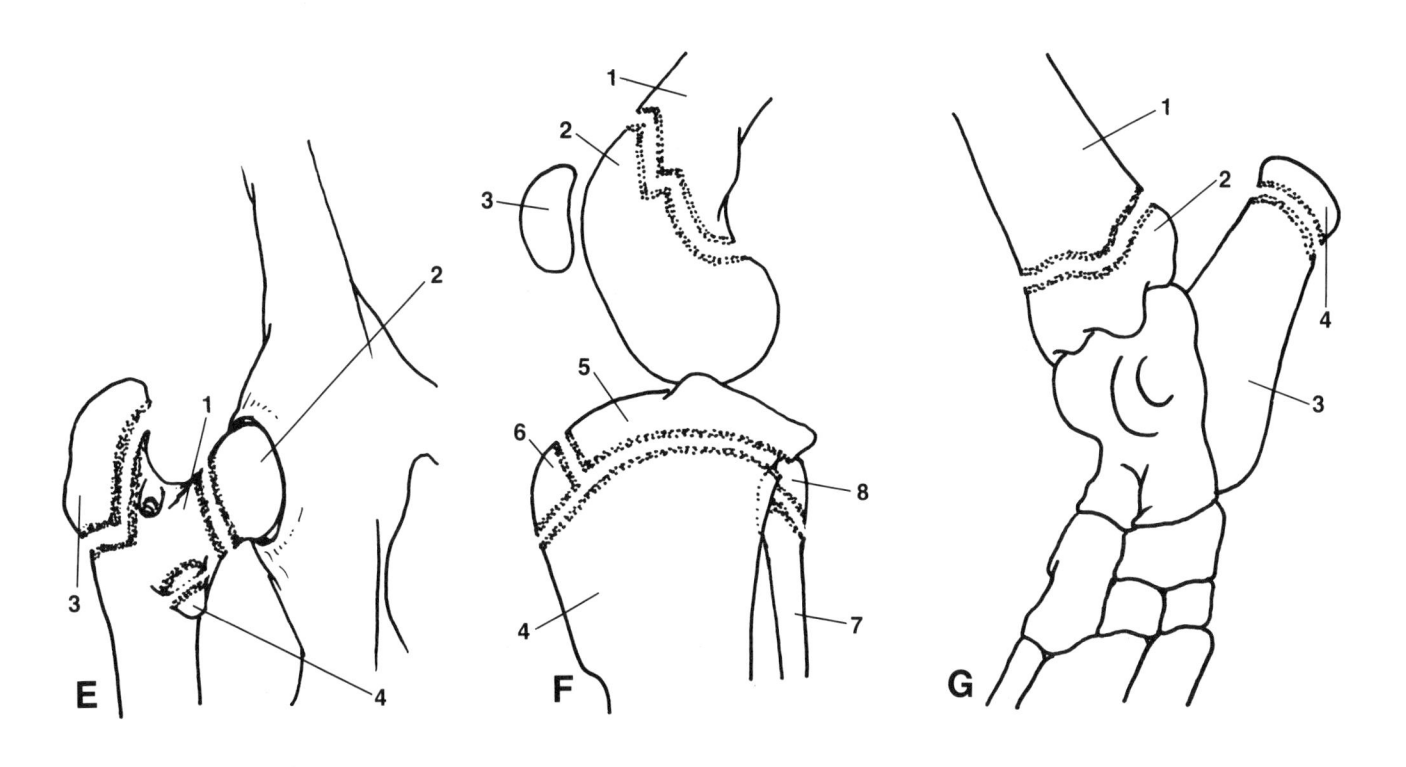

Figure 1 (Continued) *E*, Dorsal view of hip: 1, femur, diaphysis; 2, femur, proximal epiphysis; 3, femur, greater trochanter; and 4, femur, lesser trochanter; *F*, Lateral view of stifle: 1, femur, diaphysis; 2, femur, distal epiphysis; 3, patella; 4, tibia, diaphysis; 5, tibia, proximal epiphysis; 6, tibia, epiphysis for tubercle; 7, fibula, diaphysis; and 8, fibula, proximal epiphysis; *G*, Lateral view of hock: 1, tibia, diaphysis; 2, tibia, distal epiphysis; 3, fibular tarsal bone (os calcis), body; and 4, fibular tarsal bone, epiphysis; *H*, Lateral view of hind paw: 1, metatarsal, diaphysis; 2, metatarsal, epiphysis; 3, first phalanx, diaphysis; 4, first phalanx, epiphysis; 5, second phalanx, diaphysis; 6, second phalanx, epiphysis; and 7, third phalanx.

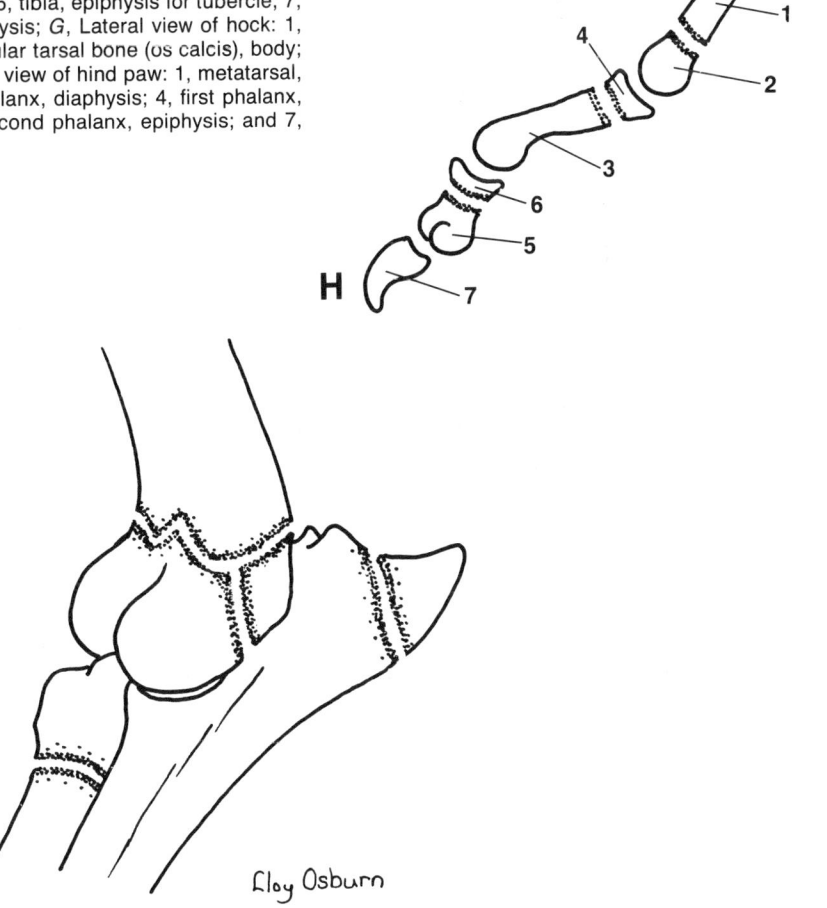

Figure 2 TRACING OF LATERAL RADIOGRAPH OF ELBOW AT 5 MONTHS.

203

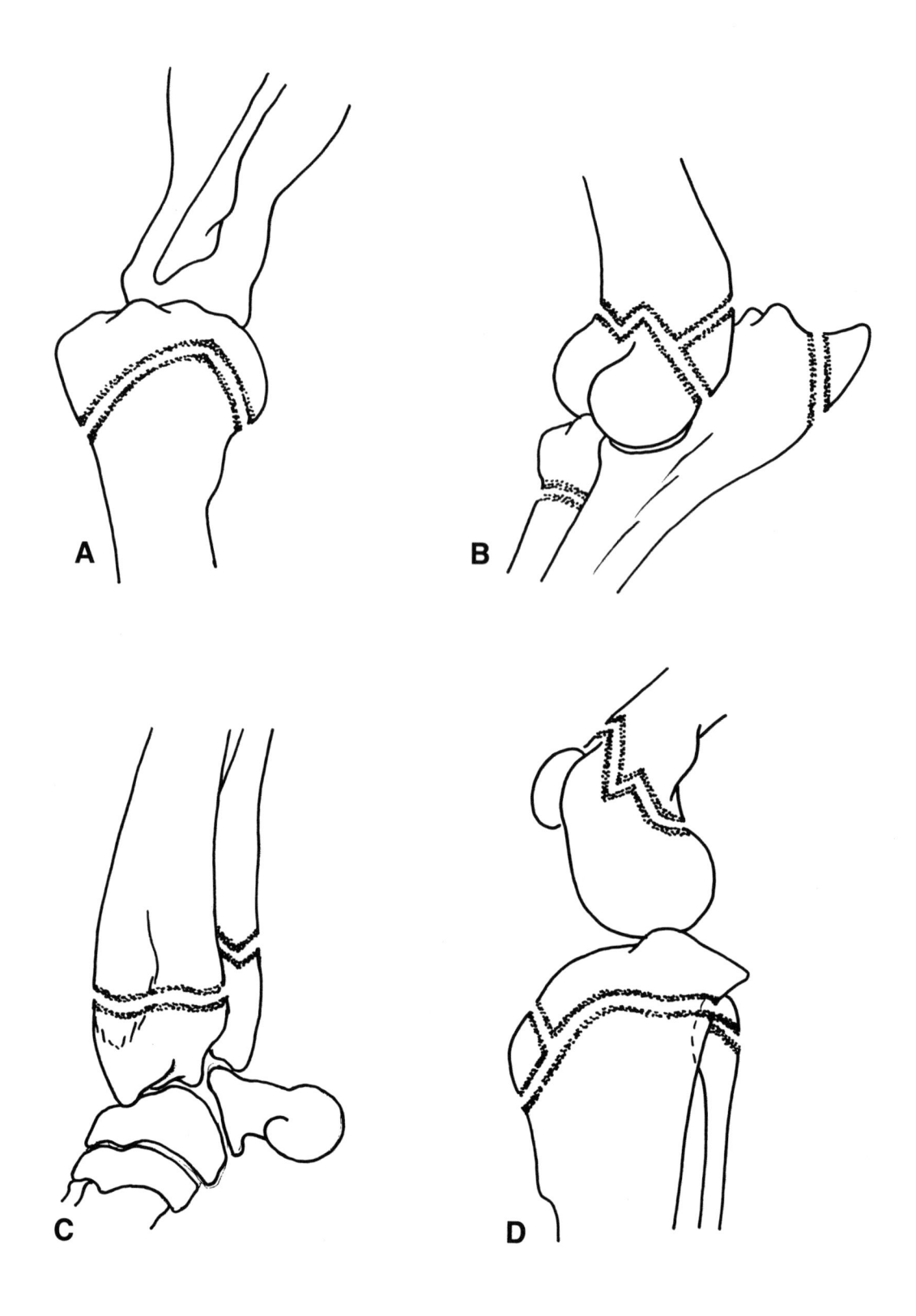

Figure 3 TRACINGS OF LATERAL RADIOGRAPHS AT 6 MONTHS: *A*, shoulder; *B*, elbow; *C*, carpus; and *D*, stifle.

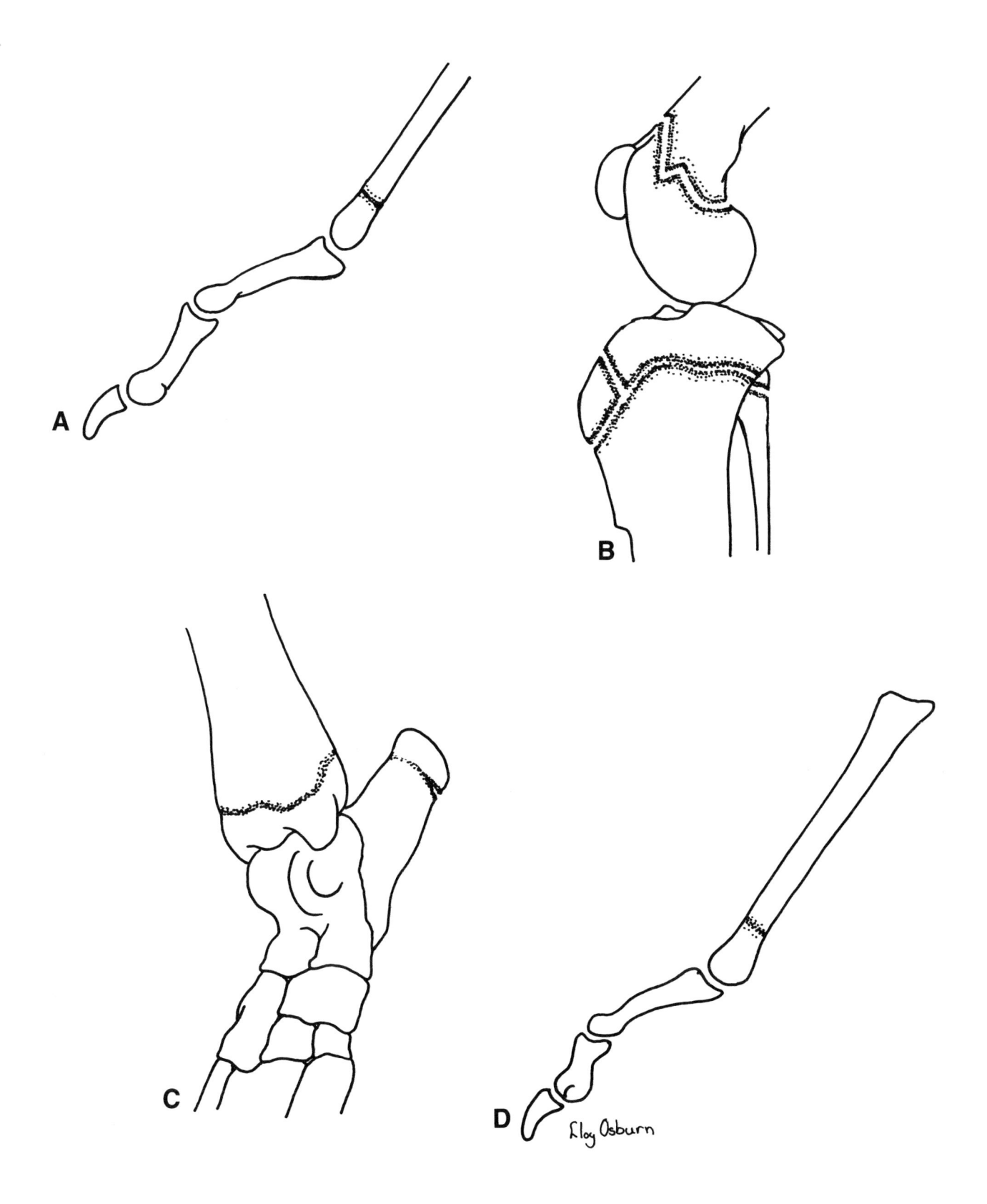

Figure 4 TRACINGS OF LATERAL RADIOGRAPHS AT 7 MONTHS: *A*, forepaw; *B*, stifle; *C*, hock; and *D*, hind paw.

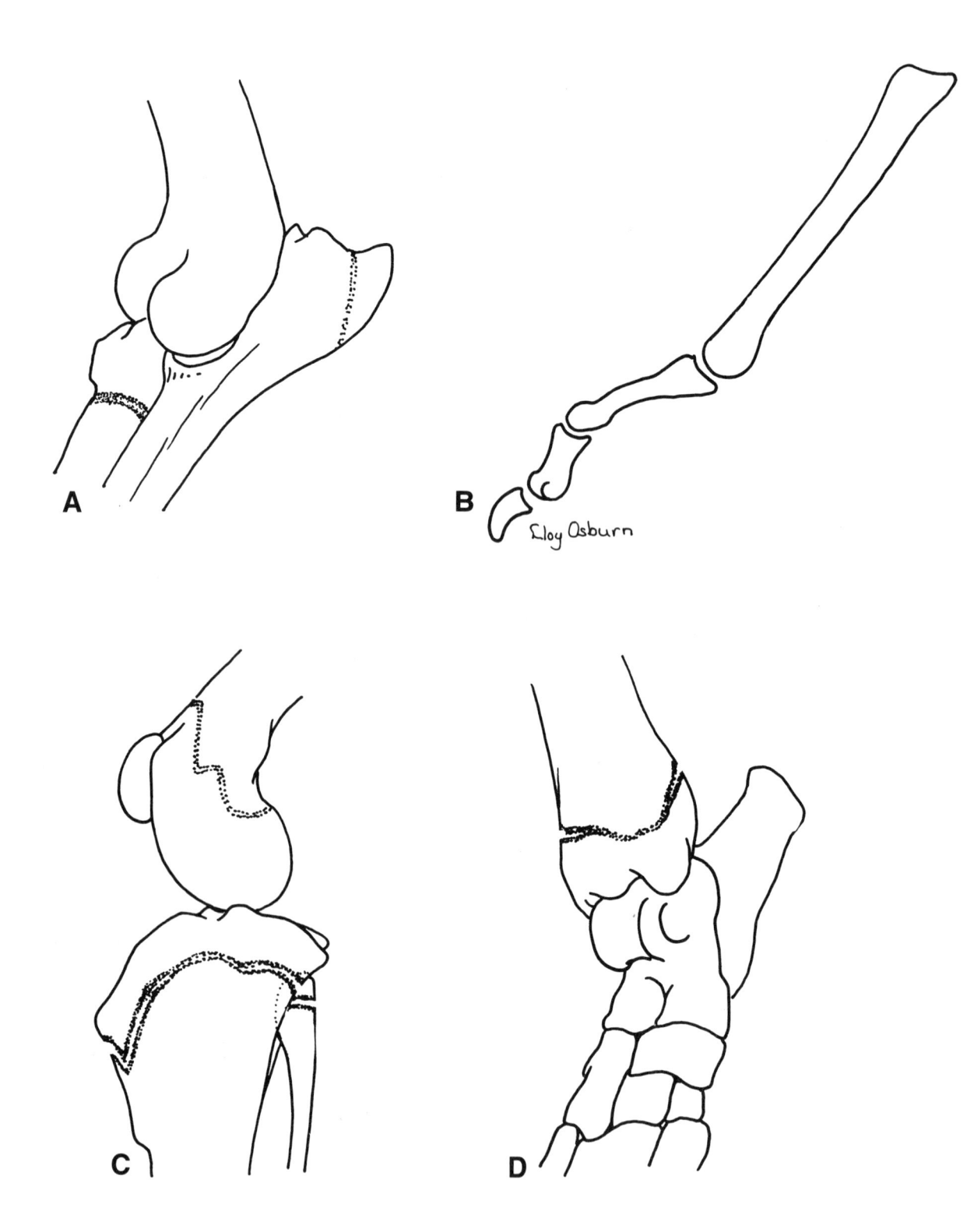

Figure 5 TRACINGS OF LATERAL RADIOGRAPHS AT 8 MONTHS: A, elbow; B, forepaw; C, stifle; and D, hock.

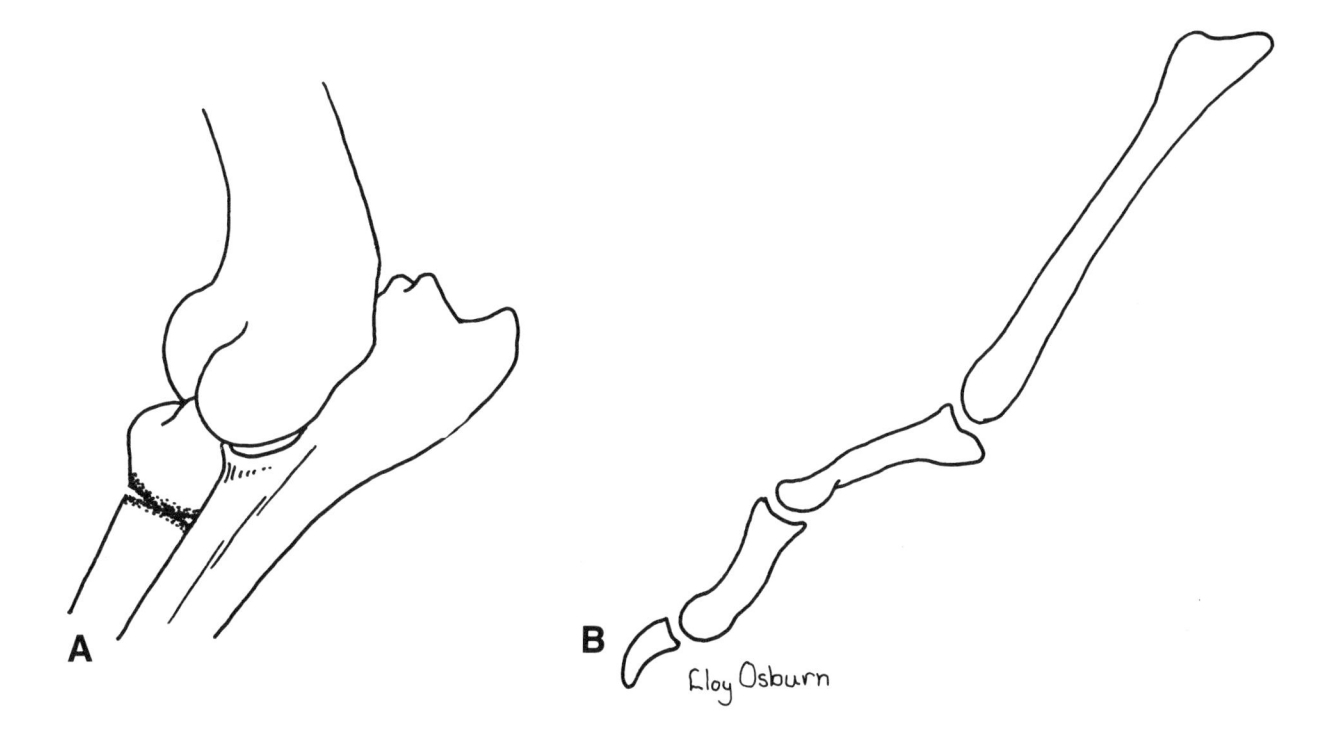

Figure 6 TRACINGS OF LATERAL RADIOGRAPHS AT 9 MONTHS: *A*, elbow; and *B*, hind paw.

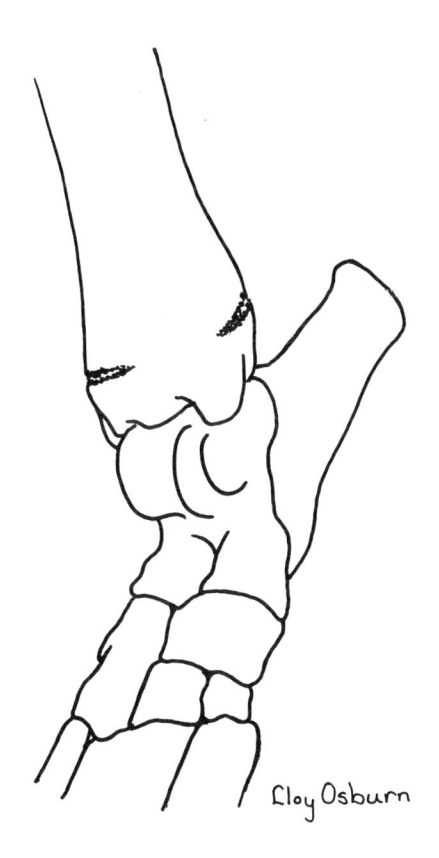

Figure 7 TRACING OF LATERAL RADIOGRAPH OF HOCK AT 10 MONTHS.

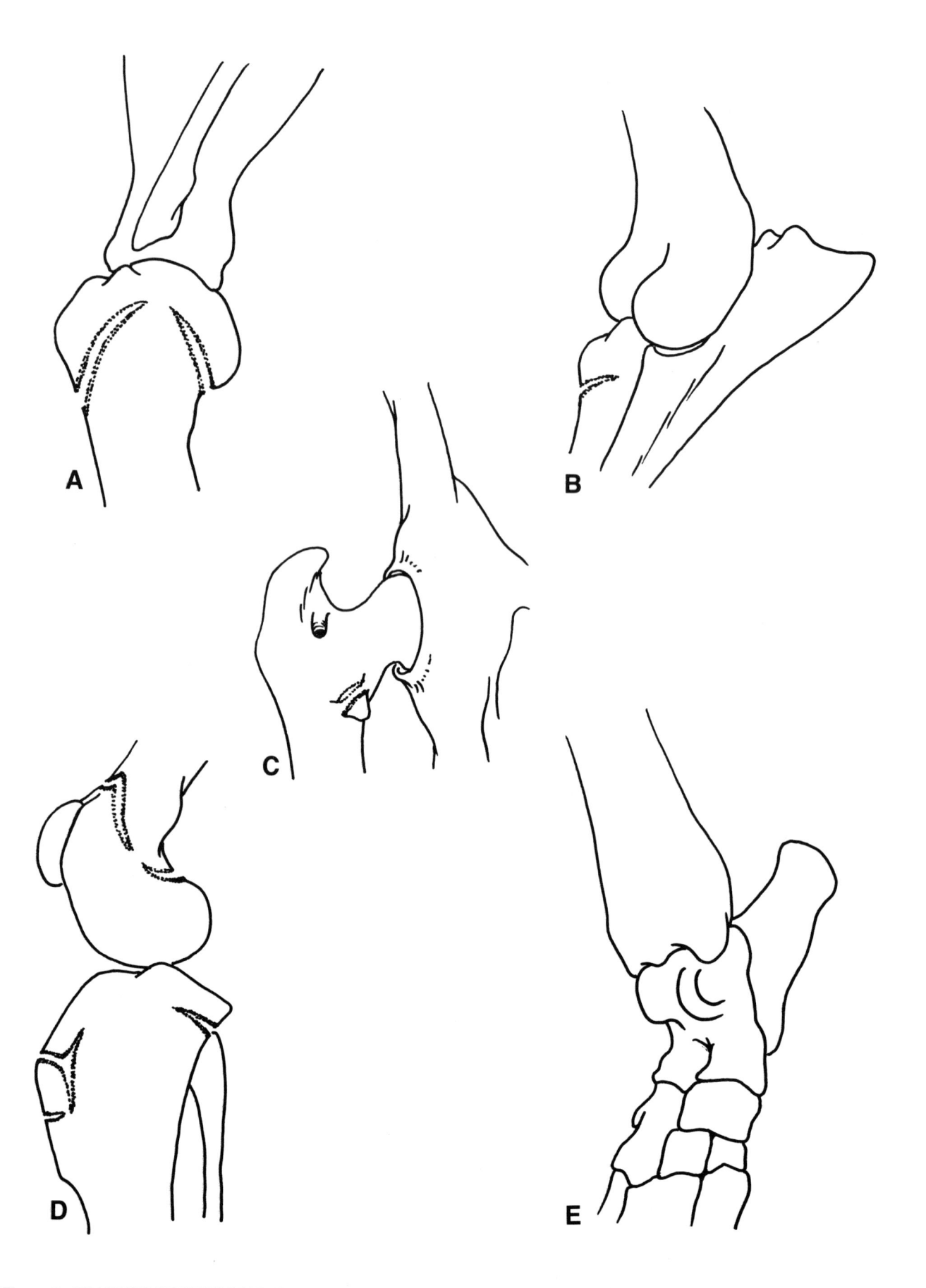

Figure 8 TRACINGS OF RADIOGRAPHS AT 11 MONTHS: *A*, lateral view of shoulder; *B*, lateral view of elbow; *C*, dorsal view of hip; *D*, lateral view of stifle; and *E*, lateral view of hock.

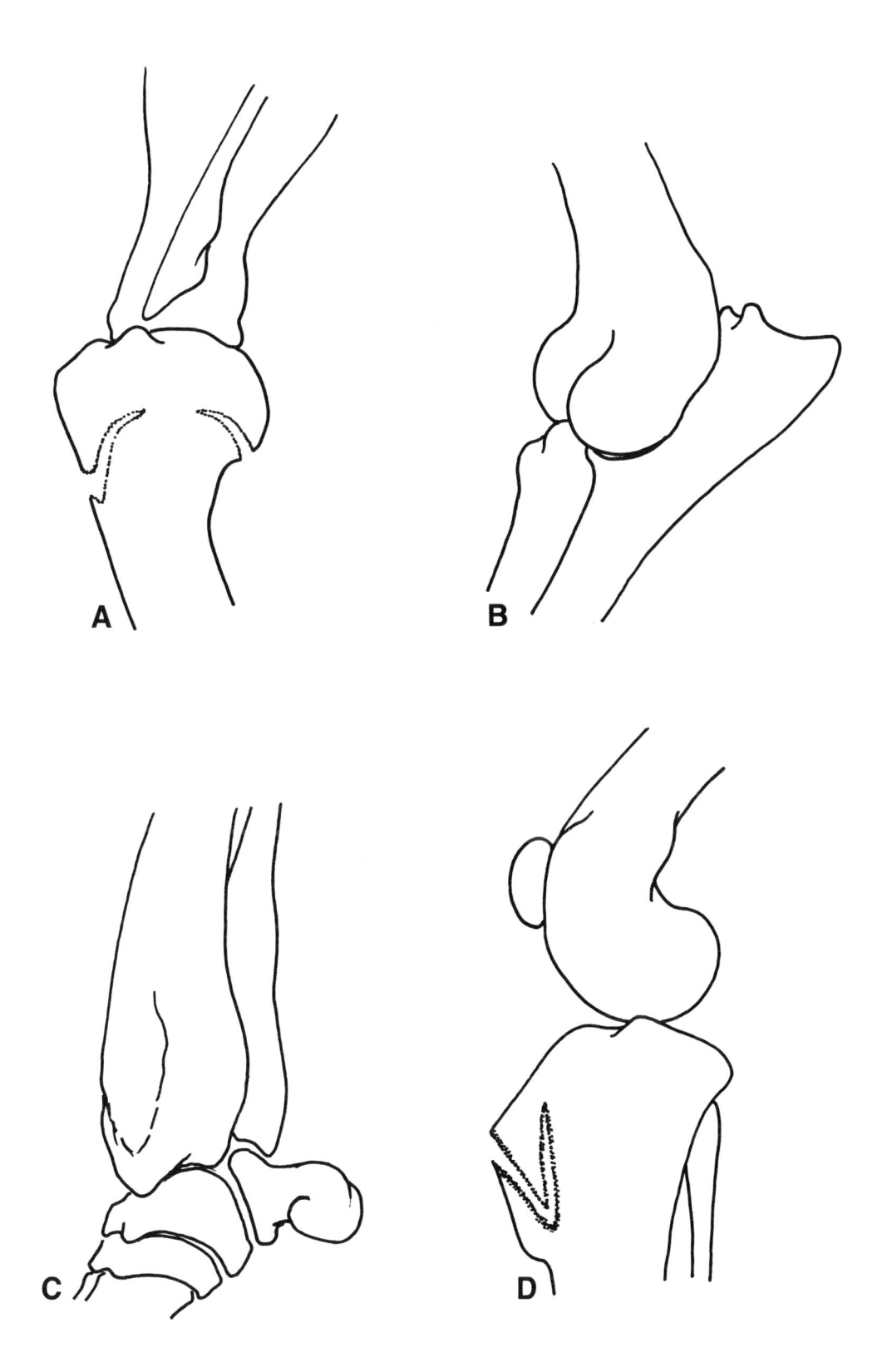

Figure 9 TRACINGS OF LATERAL RADIOGRAPHS AT 12 MONTHS: *A*, shoulder; *B*, elbow; *C*, carpus; and *D*, stifle.

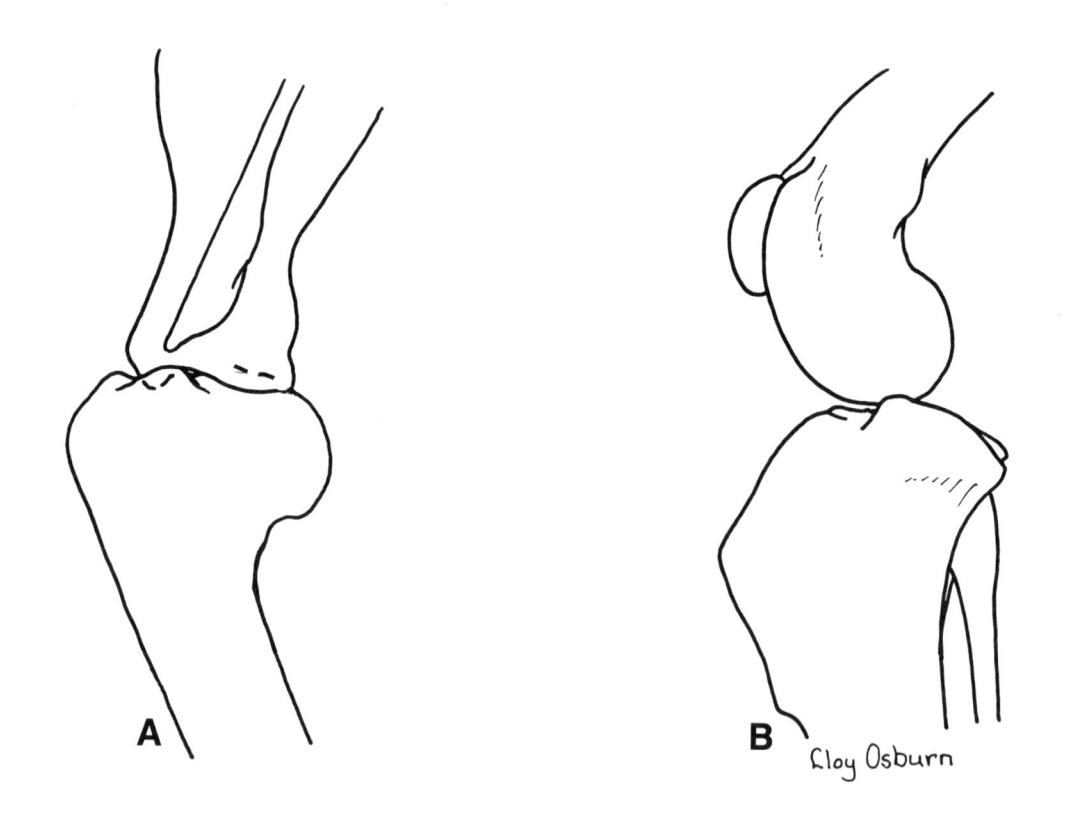

Figure 10 TRACINGS OF LATERAL RADIOGRAPHS AT 14 MONTHS: *A*, shoulder; and *B*, stifle.

INDEX

A

Acetabulum fracture, 82–83, 84–85
 conservative management, 82–83
 late complications, 82–83
 medical treatment, 83
 radiography, 82–83
 surgical management, 82–83
Airway obstruction, 196–197
Ameloblastoma, 182
Amputation
 in distal humerus fracture, 49
 in metacarpal/metatarsal-phalangeal subluxation, 70–71
 for pathologic fracture, 35
 in phalangeal fracture, 74–75
 in phalangeal luxation, 72–73
Antebrachial fracture, 56–57
 grafting in, 57
 radiography in, 56–57
 surgical management, 56–57
Antebrachiocarpal luxation/subluxation, 58–59
 arthrodesis, 58–59
 fracture/dislocation with, 58–59
 ligament tear with, 58–59
 radiography, 58–59
Antibiotics
 in bite wounds, 190–191
 in chronic stifle joint swelling, 118–119
 in elbow arthritis, 52–53
 in hematogenous osteomyelitis, 36–37
 in septic arthritis, 20–21
 in traumatic osteomyelitis, 38–39
Antinuclear antibody, in immune-mediated arthritis, 22–23
Apicoectomy, 189
Arthritis, 18–19. *See also specific sites*
 elbow pain and, 50–51
 hip pain and, 77
 medical therapy, 18–19
 surgical therapy, 18–19
 synovial fluid in, 200
Arthritis (immune-mediated), 22–23
 antinuclear antibody in, 22–23
 erosive vs nonerosive, 22–23
 medical therapy, 22–23
 radiography in, 22–23
 serology in, 22–23
 surgery in, 22–23
 synovial biopsy in, 22–23
 synovial fluid analysis, 22–23
Arthritis (septic), 20–21, 36
 aspiration in, 20–21
 chronic fistula with, 20–21
 infection origin, 20–21
 surgical management, 20–21
 synovial fluid in, 20–21
Arthrodesis
 in antebrachiocarpal luxation/subluxation, 58–59
 in atlantoaxial fracture, 166–167
 in arthritis, 18–19
 in calcaneous fracture, 145, 147
 carpal, 66–67
 in distal humerus fracture, 49
 in elbow arthritis, 52–53
 in immune-mediated arthritis, 22–23
 in intertarsal subluxation, 148–151
 in malleolar shearing injury, 137
 in osteochondritis dissecans, 24–25
 in phalangeal luxation, 72–73
 in proximal humerus fracture, 45
 in proximal intertarsal subluxation, 140–141
 in septic arthritis, 20–21
 in shoulder pain, 40–41
 tarsocrural, 152–153
 in tarsometatarsal joint subluxation, 162–163
Arthroplasty
 in acetabulum fracture, 82–83
 in femoral head and neck fracture, 106–107
 in hip dysplasia, 94–95
 after pelvic fracture, 87
 for sepsis with total hip replacement, 104–105
Arthroscopy
 in chronic stifle joint swelling, 118–119
 in osteochondritis dissecans, 24–25
Arthrotomy
 in chronic stifle joint swelling, 118–119
 with flap excision, in osteochondritis dissecans, 24–25
 in meniscal injury, 122–123
 in shoulder pain, 41
Aspiration, in stifle joint swelling, 118–119
Atlantoaxial-complex congenital lesions, 164–165
 prophylactic fusion, 164–165
 radiography, 164–165
 surgical management, 164–165
Atlantoaxial dislocation, 167
Atlantoaxial fracture, 166–167
 arthrodesis, 166–167
 radiography, 166–167
 surgical management, 166–167
Autoimmune factor, in lameness, 8
Avascular necrosis, 15
Axial pinning, 115

B

Bacteremia, in septic arthritis, 20
Bacterial culture
 in hematogenous osteomyelitis, 36–37
 in traumatic osteomyelitis, 38–39
Biopsy
 in chronic stifle joint swelling, 118–119
 in immune-mediated arthritis, 22–23
 in lameness, 8–9
 in pathologic fracture, 34–35
 in shoulder pain, 41
 in temporomandibular joint pain, 180–181
Bite wounds, 190–191
Blood loss, 196–197
Blood (fluid) transfusion, 196–197, 199
Bone cement, 168, 170
Bone cyst, 12–13
Bone tumor
 in pathologic fracture, 34–35
 radiation therapy, 35
 surgery for, 34–35
Bunnell suture, 117
Buttress plate, 113, 128–129

C

Calcaneus fracture, 144–147
 arthrodesis in, 145
 avulsions with, 144, 145
 radiography, 144, 145
 surgical management, 144–147
Caries, 189
Carpal arthrodesis, 66–67
 antebrachiocarpal, 66–67
 panarthrodesis, 66–67
 partial, 66–67
 radiography in, 66–67
Carpal bone (accessory) fracture, 62–63
 comminuted, 62–63
 radiography, 62–63
 surgical management, 62–63
 ventral vs dorsal avulsion, 62–63
Carpus
 in forelimb action, 4–5
 hyperextension, 12–13
 ligamentus laxity, 13
 retained carpus cores, 13
 valgus deformity, 13
Carpus lameness, in young animal, 13
Cement support, 35, 104–105
Cerclage, 65, 144–145
Cerebral edema, 174
Cervical spine fracture, 168–169
 radiography, 168–169
 surgical management, 168–169
Chlorhexidine, 184
Circulation failure, 196–197
Closed reduction
 in coxofemoral dislocation, 88–90
 in elbow arthritis, 52–53
 in elbow dislocation, 54–55
 in humerus shaft fracture, 46–47
 in metacarpal (metatarsal) fracture, 68–69
 in metacarpal/metatarsal-phalangeal subluxation/luxation, 70–71
 in proximal humeral fracture, 44–45
 in talus fracture, 142–143
 in tibial growth plate fracture, 131
 in tibial shaft fracture, 132–133
 in traumatic hip luxation, 92–93
Coccygeal fracture/luxation, 172–173
Compression plate, 47, 57
 in antebrachial fracture, 57
 in humerus shaft fracture, 46–47
Computed tomography

211

in atlantoaxial fracture, 167
in cervical spine fracture, 169
Condylectomy, in temporomandibular joint pain, 181
Congenital lesion, atlantoaxial-complex, 164–165
Contact Point, in forelimb action, 4
Contracture, in shoulder pain, 41
Corticosteroids
　in cranial fracture, 174
　in elbow arthritis, 52–53
　in immune-mediated arthritis, 22–23
Coxofemoral degenerative joint disease, 86–87
Coxofemoral dislocation, 88–91
　conservative management, 88–89
　degenerative joint disease with, 89, 91
　radiography, 88–89
　surgical management, 88–91
Crabbing, 3
Cranial fracture, 174–175
　comminuted, 174–175
　radiography, 175
　surgical management, 174–175
Craniomandibular osteopathy, 178–179
Cross pinning, 49, 67, 115, 130–131, 170
Curettage
　in foreleg lameness, 13
　in osteochondritis dissecans, 25
　in shoulder pain, 41
　in talus fracture, 143

D

Debridement
　in cranial fracture, 174–175
　in mandible fracture, 177
　in septic arthritis, 20–21
　in talus fracture, 143
　in tibial shaft fracture, 133
　in traumatic osteomyelitis, 38–39
Decompression
　in atlantoaxial-complex congenital lesion, 164–165
　in atlantoaxial fracture, 166–167
　in cervical spine fracture, 168–169
　in hematogenous bacterial osteomyelitis, 36–37
　in thoracolumbar spine fracture, 170–171
DeVita pin, 89
Dietary factor
　in forelimb lameness, 12–13
　in hind limb lameness, 15
Dislocation, 26–27. See also specific sites
Double hookplate, 111
Drainage
　in elbow arthritis, 53
　in septic arthritis, 21
　in traumatic osteomyelitis, 39
Drawer test, 120–121
Dynamic compression plate fixation, 148, 150

E

Ehmer sling, 89, 90
Elbow
　fragmented coronoid process, 13
　subluxation, 13
　ununited anconeal process, 13
Elbow arthritis, 52–53
　acute vs chronic, 52–53
　arthrodesis in, 52–53
　degenerative joint disease with, 53

fracture in, 53
inflammatory joint disease with, 52–53
joint luxation with, 52–53
medical therapy, 52–53
septic vs nonseptic, 52–53
surgical management, 52–53
Elbow dislocation, 54–55
　fracture with, 55
　neurovascular examination, 55
　radiography, 54–55
　surgical management, 54–55
Elbow joint, in forelimb action, 4–5
Elbow lameness, 10–11
　in young animal, 13
Elbow pain, 50–51
　arthritis and, 50–51
　fracture and, 50–51
　intrinsic vs extrinsic, 50–51
　joint disease and, 50–51
　musculotendinous, 50–51
　nerve injury and, 50–51
　osteochondritis dissecans, 50–51
　radiography, 50–51
　range of movement in, 50–51
Electrocardiography
　in distal humerus fracture, 49
　in proximal humerus fracture, 44–45
　in scapula fracture, 42–43
Emergency care, 196–199
　radiography, 197–199
Endodontic therapy, 189
Euthanasia
　in atlantoaxial-complex congenital lesions, 164–165
　in craniomandibular osteopathy, 178–179
　in hip dysplasia, 94–95
　in sacral injury, 172–173
　in septic arthritis, 20–21
Excision
　in arthritis, 18–19
　in carpal bone (accessory) fracture, 62–63
　in pathologic fracture, 35
　in radiocarpal bone fixation/luxation, 65

F

Femoral head and neck fracture, 106–107
　animal size factor, 106–107
　radiography, 106–107
　surgical management, 106–107
Femoral head and neck resection, in femoral neck fracture, 108–109
Femoral head excision arthroplasty, in canine hip dysplasia, 97
Femoral head necrosis, 84–85
Femoral head resection, 84–85
　in femoral head and neck fracture, 106–107
　in femoral neck fracture, 108–109
　in Legg-Calvé-Perthes disease, 102–103
　in slipped capital epiphysis, 100–101
Femoral neck fracture, 108–109
　animal size factor, 108–109
　surgical management, 108–109
Femoral osteotomy, 14–15
　in hip dysplasia, 94–95
Femoral shaft fracture, 112–113
　comminuted, 112–113
　conservative management, 112–113
　open vs closed, 112–113
　radiography, 112–113

surgical management, 112–113
Femoral thrombosis, 77
Femur, premature growth plate closure, 32–33
Femur (distal) fracture, 114–115
　growing vs adult animal, 114–115
　radiography, 114–115
　surgical management, 114–115
Femur (proximal) fracture, 84–85, 110–111
　radiography, 110–111
　surgical management, 110–111
Figure-of-eight wire, 59, 65, 69, 75, 138–139, 140–141, 144–147, 162–163
Fixation
　in acetabulum fracture, 82–83
　in antebrachial fracture, 57
　in antebrachiocarpal luxation/subluxation, 58–59
　in calcaneous fracture, 144–147
　in carpal arthrodesis, 66–67
　in carpal bone (accessory) fracture, 62–63
　in cranial fracture, 174–175
　in distal femoral fracture, 114–115
　in distal humerus fracture, 48–49
　in elbow arthritis, 53
　in elbow dislocation, 54–55
　in femoral head and neck fracture, 106–107
　in femoral neck fracture, 108–109
　in femoral shaft fracture, 112–113
　in fourth tarsal fracture, 160–161
　in fracture, 28–29, 31
　in fracture in immature animal, 28–29
　in growth plate fracture, 31
　in hip joint fracture, 84–85
　in humerus shaft fracture, 46–47
　in intertarsal subluxation, 148–151
　in malleolar fracture, 138–139
　in malleolar shearing injury, 136–137
　in mandible fracture, 177
　in metacarpal (metatarsal) fracture, 68–69
　in patella fracture, 116–117
　in pathologic fracture, 35
　in phalangeal fracture, 74–75
　in proximal femur fracture, 110–111
　in proximal humerus fracture, 44–45
　in proximal intertarsal subluxation, 140–141
　in radiocarpal bone fixation/luxation, 64–65
　in sacral injury, 172–173
　in scapula fracture, 42–43
　in second tarsal bone fracture, 156–157
　in slipped capital epiphysis, 100–101
　in styloid fracture, 60–61
　in talus fracture, 142–143
　in tarsal bone fracture, 154–155
　in tarsocrural joint instability, 152–153
　in traumatic hip luxation, 93
　in traumatic osteomyelitis, 38–39
　in tarsometatarsal joint subluxation, 162–163
　in third tarsal bone fracture, 158–159
　in thoracolumbar spine fracture, 170–171
　in tibial growth plate fracture, 130–131
　in tibial plateau fracture, 128–129
　in tibial shaft fracture, 132–133
Foot
　in fore limb action, 5

in hindlimb action, 6–7
Foot lameness, 10–11
Forage, in osteochondritis dissecans, 25
Forelimb
  anatomy, 4
  normal joint angles, 4
Forelimb action, 4–5
  goniometric angles, 4
Forelimb lameness
  curettage and grafting, 13
  dietary factor, 12–13
  fracture in, 12–13
  growth disorder in, 12
  radiography in, 12–13
  Stance Phase in, 10–11
  Swing Phase in, 11
  in young animal, 12–13
Fracture, 26–27. *See also specific sites*
  complete vs incomplete in immature animal, 28–29
  in degenerative joint disease, 16–17
  with elbow arthritis, 53
  elbow pain and, 50, 51
  external immobilization, 28–29
  in forelimb lameness, 12–13
  growth plate and, 28–29, 30–31
  in hind limb lameness, 15
  open vs closed procedures, 26–27
  radiography in, 26–27
  splinting in, 26–27
  stabilization in, 26–27
  surgical management, 28–29, 30–31
  suspected in immature animal, 28–29
  weight-bearing in, 28–29
Fracture (pathologic), 34–35
  biopsy in, 34–35
  blood examination, 35
  bone tumor in, 34–35
  radiography, 34–35
  surgery for, 34–35
  systemic disease and, 34–35
Fracture disease, 128
Freezing, 10, 11
Frenectomy, 185
Fusion
  in arthritis, 18–19
  in cervical spine fracture, 168–169
  for unfused odontoid process, 164–165

G

Gait, lameness examination, 3, 8–9
Gait patterns, 2
Genetic factor, in hip dysplasia, 94
Genu valgum, 14
Gingivectomy, 184–185
Gingivitis, 184–185
Gingivoplasty, 184–185
Gluteal area pain, 77
Grafting
  in atlantoaxial-complex congenital lesions, 164
  in antebrachial fracture, 57
  in central tarsal bone fracture, 155
  in distal humerus fracture, 48–49
  in femoral shaft fracture, 111
  in foreleg lameness, 13
  in humerus shaft fracture, 46–47
  in pathologic fracture, 35
  in premature growth plate closure, 32–33
  in proximal intertarsal subluxation, 141
  in tarsometatarsal joint subluxation, 162–163
  in tendon injury, 194–195
  in tibial plateau fracture, 128–129
  in traumatic osteomyelitis, 38–39
Groin pain, 77
Growth plate
  fracture and, 28–29, 30–31, 44–45
  fusion variation, 32–33
  injury with limb deviation, 32–33
  premature closure, 32–33
  surgical procedures, 32–33
Growth plate closure, 201–210
Growth plate fracture, proximal tibial in young animal, 130–131
Gunshot wound, 192–193

H

Hard palate fracture, 174–175
Head injury, emergency management, 198–199
Heart failure, 196–197
Hematoma, in cranial fracture, 174–175
Hemicerclage fixation, 144–145
Hemipelvectomy, partial, 86–87
Hind limb
  normal joint angles, 6
Hind limb action, 6–7
  goniometric angles, 6
Hind limb lameness, 10–11
  dietary factor, 15
  fracture in, 15
  radiography in, 15
  Stance Phase, 11
  surgical management, 15
  Swing Phase in, 10–11
  in young animal, 14–15
Hip, in hind limb action, 6–7
Hip arthroplasty
  in coxofemoral dislocation, 89, 91
  after pelvic fracture, 87
Hip dysplasia, 15, 93, 94–95
  euthanasia in, 94–95
  immature vs mature animal, 94–95
  medical management, 94–95
  radiography, 94–95
  surgical management, 94–95
Hip dysplasia (canine)
  breed factor, 96
  degenerative joint disease with, 96–97
  medical management, 97
  radiography, 96–97
  surgical management, 96–97
Hip joint fracture, 84–85
  conservative treatment, 84–85
  radiography, 84–85
  surgical management, 84–85
Hip lameness, 11
  in young animal, 15
Hip luxation (traumatic), 92–93
  complications, 92–93
  with fracture, 92–93
  radiography, 92–93
  surgical management, 92–93
Hip pain, 76–77
  breed factor, 76
  gait analysis, 77
  laboratory examination, 76–77
  medical management, 76–77
  radiography, 76–77
  surgical management, 76–77
Hip replacement
  in acetabulum fracture, 83
  in canine hip dysplasia, 97
  chemotherapy for sepsis, 104–105
  in hip joint fracture, 84–85
  in femoral head and neck fracture, 106–107
  in femoral neck fracture, 108–109
  in hip dysplasia, 94–95
  implantation revision with sepsis, 104–105
  sepsis with, 104–105
  in slipped capital epiphysis, 100–101
Hock, in hind limb action, 6–7
Hock lameness, 11
Humerus fracture (distal), 48–49
  amputation in, 49
  arthrodesis in, 49
  condylar, 48–49
  electrocardiography, 49
  grafting in, 48–49
  neurologic examination in, 48–49
  radiography, 48–49
  small vs large animal, 48–49
  supracondylar, 48–49
  surgical management, 48–49
Humerus fracture (proximal), 44–45
  electrocardiography in, 44–45
  greater tubercle, 44–45
  growth plate fracture, 44–45
  humeral head, 44–45
  humeral neck, 45
  neurologic examination, 45
  radiography in, 44–45
  surgical management, 44–45
Humerus shaft fracture, 46–47
  comminuted, 46–47
  configuration type, 46–47
  grafting in, 46–47
  long oblique, 46–47
  neurologic examination, 46–47
  short oblique, 47
  surgical management, 46–47
  transverse, 46–47
  young vs mature animal, 46–47
Hyperparathyroidism, 179
Hypertrophic osteopathy, 12–13

I

Immune factor, in arthritis, 22–23
Immunosuppressive agents, in immune-mediated arthritis, 22–23
Inguinal hernia, 77
Intertrochanteric osteotomy, in canine hip dysplasia, 97
Ischiatic nerve deficit, 86–87
Intertarsal subluxation, 148–151
  radiography, 148–149
  surgical management, 148–151
Intertarsal subluxation (proximal), 140–141, 146, 147
  radiography, 140–141
  surgical management, 140–141

J

Joint disease, elbow pain and, 50–51
Joint disease (degenerative), 16–17, 18–19
  Canadian classification, 96
  in elbow arthritis, 53
  fracture in, 16–17
  metabolic factor, 16–17
  shoulder pain and, 40–41
  synovial membrane in, 16–17
  traumatic factor, 16–17
Joint disease (inflammatory)
  in elbow arthritis, 52–53
Joint mice, 51
Joint replacement, in arthritis, 18–19

213

K

Kirschner-Ehmer apparatus, 112
Kirschner wire fixation, 49, 59, 65, 69, 114–115, 116, 128, 142, 168, 172
Küntscher nail, 112

L

Lag screw fixation, 45, 49, 59, 65, 69, 75, 111, 112–113, 114–115, 140–145, 148–149, 154–159, 172
Lameness, 8–9, 10–11
  autoimmune factor, 8
  biopsy in, 8–9
  gait examination, 3, 8–9
  metabolic factor, 8–9
  neurologic examination, 8–9
  organic disease in, 8–9
  palpation in, 8
  patient observation, 10–11
  radiography in, 8–9
  rate of onset, 8
  trauma in, 8
Lavage, in traumatic osteomyelitis, 39
Legg-Calvé-Perthes disease, 102–103
  conservative management, 102–103
  radiography, 102–103
  surgical management, 102–103
Limb gunshot wound, 192–193
Locomotion (normal), 2–3
Lumbosacral fracture/luxation, 172–173

M

Malleolar fracture, 138–139
  surgical management, 136–137
Malleolar shearing injury, 136–137
  arthrodesis in, 137
  radiography, 136–137
  surgical management, 136–137
Malocclusion, 186–187
  breed factor, 186
Mandible fistula, 178–179
Mandible fracture, 176–177
  radiography, 176–177
  surgical management, 176–177
Mandible pain, 178–179
  radiography, 178–179
Medullary nail, 113
Meniscal injury, 122–123
  surgical management, 122–123
  tibial compression test, 122–123
Meniscectomy, 122–123
Metabolic factor
  in degenerative joint disease, 16–17
  in lameness, 8–9
Metacarpal pad
  in forelimb action, 5
  in hind limb action, 7
Metacarpal (metatarsal) fracture, 68–69
  base avulsion, 68–69
  comminuted, 68–69
  of neck, 68–69
  nondisplaced vs displaced, 68–69
  radiography, 68–69
  of shaft, 68–69
  surgical management, 68–69
Metacarpal/metatarsal-phalangeal subluxation/luxation, 70–71
  amputation in, 70–71
  radiography, 71
  surgical management, 70–71
Metatarsal joint, in hind limb action, 6
Multiple pin fixation, 45, 47

N

Neoplasm, in shoulder pain, 41

Neurologic examination
  in distal humeral fracture, 48–49
  in humerus shaft fracture, 46–47
  in lameness, 8–9
  in proximal humerus fracture, 45
  in shoulder pain, 41
Neurovascular examination, in elbow dislocation, 55

O

Odontoid process defect, 164–165
Odontoma, 182
Odontoplasty, 185
Oligodontia, 182–183
Open reduction
  in acetabulum fracture, 82–83
  in antebrachial fracture, 57
  in cervical spine fracture, 168–169
  in coxofemoral dislocation, 89–90
  in cranial fracture, 174–175
  in elbow arthritis, 52–53
  in elbow dislocation, 55
  in fracture, 31
  in growth plate fracture, 31
  in humerus shaft fracture, 46–47
  in metacarpal/metatarsal-phalangeal subluxation/luxation, 70–71
  in patella fracture, 116–117
  in pelvic fracture, 80–81
  in proximal humerus fracture, 44–45
  in radiocarpal bone fracture/luxation, 65
  in sacral injury, 172–173
  in scapular fracture, 42–43
  in shoulder pain, 40–41
  in styloid fracture, 60–61
  in talus fracture, 142–143
  in temporomandibular joint pain, 181
  in thoracolumbar spine fracture, 170–171
  in tibial growth plate fracture, 131
  in tibial plateau fracture, 129
  in traumatic hip luxation, 92–93
Ostectomy, in premature growth plate closure, 32–33
Osteochondritis dissecans, 13, 15, 18–19, 24–25, 52–53, 142–143
  elbow pain and, 50–51
  medical management, 24–25
  radiography in, 24–25
  shoulder pain and, 40–41
  surgical management, 24–25
Osteochondrosis, 12–13, 15
Osteodystrophy (hypertrophic), 15
Osteoma, 34
Osteomalacia, 34
Osteomyelitis, 13, 15
  in shoulder pain, 41
Osteomyelitis (hematogenous), 36–37
  antibiotic therapy, 36–37
  culture in, 37
  radiography, 36–37
  surgical decompression in, 36–37
Osteomyelitis (traumatic), 38–39
  antibiotic therapy, 38–39
  culture in, 38–39
  drainage in, 38–39
  fixation revision in, 38–39
  grafting in, 38–39
  lavage in, 38–39
  radiography in, 38–39
  sequestrectomy in, 38–39
  surgical management, 38–39
Osteoporosis, 34
Osteosarcoma, 34
Osteotomy
  in hind limb lameness, 15
  in patella luxation, 127
  in premature growth plate closure, 32–33

P

Pace, 2–3
Panarthrodesis, 66–67
Panosteitis, 12–13, 15
Paradoxical breathing, 196–197
Patella fracture, 116–117
  articular surface intact vs disrupted, 117
  comminuted, 116–117
  patellectomy in, 116–117
  radiography, 116–117
  surgical management, 116–117
Patella ligament rupture, 116–117
  partial vs total, 116–117
  internal suturing plus wire support, 117
  surgical management, 116–117
Patella luxation, 14–15, 124–127
  breed factor, 124, 127
  congenital lateral, 124, 126, 127
  congenital medial, 124, 127
  surgical management, 124–127
  traumatic medial, 124, 126, 127
Patellectomy, 116–117
Pectinectomy, in hip dysplasia, 94–95
Pelvic collapse, 86–87
Pelvic dislocation, 78–79
Pelvic fracture, 78–79, 80–81
  complications management, 86–87
  conservative treatment, 80–81
  late complications, 80–81
  radiography, 80–81, 86–87
  surgical management, 80–81, 86–87
Pelvic osteotomy
  in canine hip dysplasia, 97
  in hip dysplasia, 94–95
Pelvic trauma, 78–79
  radiography, 78–79
  soft tissue complications, 78–79
  surgical management, 78–79
Peridontal tissue disease, 184–185
Phalangeal fracture, 74–75
  amputation, 74–75
  articular, 74–75
  radiography, 74–75
  of shaft, 74–75
  surgical management, 74–75
Phalangeal luxation, 72–73
  radiography, 73
  surgical management, 72–73
Pictineal tenotomy, in canine hip dysplasia, 96–97
Pin fixation, 47, 49, 59, 65, 67, 69, 130–133, 138–141, 144–147, 162–163, 175
Plaque, 184–185
Plate fixation, 33, 47, 57, 59, 67, 69, 74–75, 110–115, 132–133, 152–153, 170
Polyodontia, 182–183
Proximal intertarsal subluxation, 140–141
Pubic bone graft, 86–87
Pulpotomy, 189

R

Rabies, 190–191
Radial head excision, in elbow arthritis, 53
Radial nerves in antebrachial fracture,

56–57
Radiation therapy, for bone tumor, 35
Radiocarpal bone fracture/luxation, 64–65
 radiography, 64–65
 surgical management, 64–65
Radiography. See specific diagnoses
Radius, premature growth plate closure, 32–33
Radius fracture, 57
 styloid, 58–59
Reconstruction
 in antebranchiocarpal luxation/subluxation, 58–59
 in cranial fracture, 175
Renal osteodystrophy, 179
Replacement, in central tarsal bone fracture, 155
Rheumatoid arthritis, 18–19
 of elbow, 52–53
Rush pin (plate), 49

S

Sacral injury, 172–173
 conservative management, 172–173
 radiography, 172–173
 surgical management, 172–173
Sacral nerve injury, 172–173
Sacroiliac fracture/luxation, 172–173
Salter-Harris classification, 30–31, 44–45, 48–49, 114–115
Scapula displacement, 42–43
 luxation, 43
Scapula fracture, 42–43
 acromial, 42–43
 conservative management, 42–43
 electrocardiography in, 42–43
 glenoid, 42–43
 radiography in, 42–43
 scapular neck, 42–43
 with spine fracture, 42–43
 supraglenoid tubercle, 42–43
 surgical management, 42–43
Schröder-Thomas splint, 112
Screw fixation, 57, 63, 110–111, 128, 130–131, 136, 152–155, 160
Sepsis, with total hip replacement, 104–105
Sequestrectomy, in traumatic osteomyelitis, 38–39
Shoulder joint, in forelimb action, 4–5
Shoulder lameness
 "freezing" in, 10–11
 Swing Phase, 10
 in young animal, 13
Shoulder luxation/subluxation, 40–41
 congenital, 13
Shoulder pain, 40–41
 arthrodesis and, 41
 bicipetal tenosynovitis in, 41
 biopsy in, 41
 contracture in, 41
 degenerative joint disease and, 40–41
 luxation/subluxation and, 40–41
 medical management, 41
 musculotendinous causes, 41
 neoplasm and, 41
 neurologic factor, 41
 osteochondritis dissecans and, 40–41
 osteomyelitis and, 41
 radiography in, 41
 range of motion in, 40–41
 surgical management, 41
Singleton classification, 124–125
Slipped capital epiphysis, 100–101
 animal size factor, 100–101

 surgical management, 100–101
Soft tissue trauma, 78–79
Spinal disc disease, 77
Splinting
 in fracture, 26–27
 in metacarpal/metatarsal-phalangeal subluxation/luxation, 70–71
 in phalangeal luxation, 73
Stance Phase (retraction)
 forelimb action, 4, 5
 in forelimb lameness, 10–11
 hind limb action, 6–7
 in hind limb lameness, 11
Stapling, 33
Stay sutures, 130–131
Steinmann pin, 112
Sterilization
 in canine hip dysplasia, 97
 in hipdysplasia, 94–95
Stifle
 in hind limb action, 6–7
 in patella fracture, 116–117
Stifle area injury, 114–115
Stifle joint instability, 121
Stifle joint swelling (chronic), 118–119
 antibiotics in, 118–119
 arthroscopy, 118–119
 aspiration in, 118–119
 hot vs cold, 118–119
 radiography, 118–119
 surgical management, 118–119
 synovial biopsy, 118–119
Stifle lameness, 11
 in young animal, 15
Stifle ligament injury, 120–121
 cranial/caudal, 121
 drawer test, 120–121
 medial/lateral, 121
 stress radiography, 121
 surgical repair, 120–121
Stride, 2–3
 Contact Point, 2–3
 Lift Point, 2–3
 Stance Phase (retraction), 2–3
 Swing Phase (protraction), 2–3
Styloid fracture, 58–59, 60–61
 radiography, 61
 surgical management, 60–61
Suturing
 in metacarpal/metatarsal-phalangeal subluxation/luxation, 70–71
 in phalangeal luxation, 72–73
Swing Phase (protraction)
 in forelimb action, 4–5
 in forelimb lameness, 11
 in hind limb action, 6–7
 in hind limb lameness, 10–11
 in shoulder lameness, 10
Synovectomy
 in chronic stifle joint swelling, 118–119
 in elbow arthritis, 53
Synovial fluid
 in arthritis, 200
 in immune-mediated arthritis, 22–23
 in septic arthritis, 20–21
Synovial membrane, in degenerative joint disease, 16–17
Synovitis (proliferative), 18
Synsarcosis, 4, 5
Systemic lupus erythematosus, 22–23, 52

T

T-plate, 67
Tail amputation, in sacral injury,

142–143
Talus fracture, 142–143
 neck/head/body, 142–143
 with osteochondritis dissecans, 142–143
 peritalar, 142–143
 radiography, 143
 surgical management, 142–143
Tarsal bone fracture (central), 154–155
 radiography, 154–155
 surgical management, 154–155
 types, 154
Tarsal bone fracture (second), 156–157
 radiography, 156–157
 surgical management, 156–157
Tarsal bone fracture (third), 158–159
 radiography, 158–159
 surgical mangement, 158–159
Tarsal fracture (fourth), 160–161
 radiography, 160–161
 surgical management, 160–161
Tarsal joint nomenclature, 134–135
Tarsal lameness, 15
Tarsocrural arthrodesis, 152–153
Tarsocrural joint instability, 152–153
 surgical management, 152–153
Tarsometatarsal joint subluxation, 162–163
 arthrodesis, 162–163
 radiography, 162–163
 surgical management, 162–163
Tartar (tooth), 184–185
Temporomandibular joint fracture, 180–181
Temporomandibular joint luxation, 176–177, 180–181
Temporomandibular joint pain, 180–181
 surgical management, 180–181
Tendon injury, 194–195
Tenosynovitis (bicipetal), in shoulder pain, 41
Tenotomy, in shoulder pain, 41
Tension band wiring, 45, 47, 111, 116–117
Tension pneumothorax, 197
Tetanus, 180–181
Thoracentesis, 197
Thoracolumbar spine dislocation, 170–171
Thoracolumbar spine fracture, 170–171
 conservative management, 170–171
 radiography, 170–171
 stable vs unstable, 170–171
 surgical management, 170–171
Thoracotomy, 197
Tibia, premature growth plate closure, 32–33
Tibial compression test, 122–123
Tibial growth plate fracture (proximal) 130–131
 with epiphysis involvement, 131
 radiography, 130–131
 surgical management, 130–131
Tibial plateau fracture, 128–129
 comminuted, 129
 nondisplaced vs displaced, 128–129
 radiography, 128–129
 surgical management, 128–129
Tibial shaft fracture, 132–133
 closed vs open, 132–133
 radiography, 132–133
 surgical management, 132–133
Tibial tuberosity transposition, 15
 in hind limb lameness, 15
Tooth development, 182–183
Tooth disease, 188–189. See also

215

specific conditions
  radiography, 189
Tooth enamel hypoplasia, 182–183
Tooth extraction, 182–183, 184–185, 186–187, 189
Tooth fracture, 186–187, 189
Tooth impaction, 182–183
Tooth neoplasia, 182–183
Tracheotomy, 197
Trauma
  in degenerative joint disease, 16–17
  in lameness, 8
  in osteomyelitis, 38–39
Trochanter fracture, 110–111
Trochanteric pain, 77
Trochleoplasty, in patella luxation, 127
Trot, 2–3

U

Ulna, premature growth plate closure, 32–33
Ulna fracture, 57
Ulnar nerve, in antebrachial fracture, 56–57

V

Velpeau sling, 41, 42, 43
Ventilation support, 197

W

Walk, 2–3
Wedge recession, 15

in hind limb lameness, 15
Weight-bearing, in fracture, 28–29
Wounds, septic arthritis and, 20–21

Y

Young animal
  forelimb lameness, 12–13
  hind limb lameness, 14–15
  proximal tibial growth plate fracture, 130–131

Z

Zygomatic arch fracture, 174–175
Zygomatic arch resection, in temporomandibular joint pain, 180–181